Men's Fitness Magazine's Complete Guide to Health and Well-Being

Men's Fitness Magazine's

Complete Guide to Health and Well-Being

MEN'S FITNESS MAGAZINE
with Kevin Cobb

Produced by The Philip Lief Group, Inc.

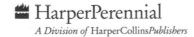

HarperPerennial
A Division of HarperCollinsPublishers

HarperCollins books may be purchased for educational, business, or sales promotional use. For information, please write to: Special Markets Department, HarperCollins Publishers, Inc., 10 East 53rd Street, New York, New York 10022.

First Edition

Library of Congress Cataloging-in-Publication Data

Men's fitness magazine's complete guide to health and well-being : the ultimate source-book for men's physical and emotional needs. — 1st ed.

p. cm.
ISBN 0-06-273354-0
1. Men—Health. 2. Physical fitness. I. Joe Weider's men's fitness.
RA777.8.M37 1996
613'.0423 dc20
95-39472
CIP

96 97 98 99 00 ❖/HC 10 9 8 7 6 5 4 3 2 1

CONTENTS

Advisory Board   viii

Contributors   xi

Foreword   xiv

1   To Be a Man: Our Total Well-Being   1

2   Men's Bodies—A Crash Course in Physiology   8
Men's Bodies: The Basics 9

3   The Healthy Man   27
The Physical Examination 27
The Results of Your Exam 31
Symptoms You Should Never Ignore 35
Men's Special Health Problems and Concerns 47
Alternative Health 70

4   Wellness and the Mind   83
Stress 84
Toxic Emotions 91
Other Common Behavioral and Emotional Problems 96
Therapeutic Approaches 105
Fitness and Mental Well-Being 111
Self-Healing Strategies 113

5   Body Image   131
The "New" Male Vanity 131
The High Price of a Perfect Body 134
What Makes a Good-Looking Man? 136
Grooming: The Basics 140

Your Skin and the Sun 145
Common Skin Problems 149
Caring for Your Hair 156
What to Do About Unwanted Weight 162
Fighting Body Fat 167
Eating Disorders: Not for Women Only 171
Posture 175

6 Healthy Living 178

Healthy Eating 178
Vitamins and Minerals for Men 201
Coffee, Tea and Thee 210
Environmental Health 216
A Healthy Lifestyle 225

7 Sexuality 235

A Layman's Guide to a Woman's Orgasm 236
Multiple Orgasms—for Men 240
Cerebral Sex 244
Beyond Condoms 246
Sexually Transmitted Diseases 248
Potency Problems 255
Are Your Sperm Healthy? 258
Performance Anxiety 262
Penis Size 264

8 Relationships 270

Making a Commitment 271
Monogomy 274
In the Heat of the Fight 279
Who Batters, and Why 282
Bitter Betrayals 286
Friends and Lovers 289
Of Human Bonding 291
Gay Relationships 294
Family Relationships 297

9 The Middle Years and Beyond 300

The Aging Process 301
Body Image Through the Ages 310
The Aging Athlete 314
Sexuality Through the Ages 317
Male Menopause 320
Does Heredity Equal Longevity? 322
Growing Through Grief 328

10 Fitness 331

Is the Fitness Boom Bust? 331
Stretching 334
The Weight-Room Lexicon 337
Basic Training: Starting a Weight Program 340
The 20-Minute Workout 348
Maximizing Aerobic Power 350
Exercise Addiction and Overtraining 356
Mind Fitness: Cross-Train Your Brain 359
Physically Challenged Athletes 362

11 Eight Myths about Men 367

Myth 1: Penis Size Doesn't Matter 367
Myth 2: Women Are Fatter than Men 368
Myth 3: Muscle Can Turn to Fat 369
Myth 4: Men Can't Have Sex with One or No Testicles 370
Myth 5: If Your Mother's Father Was Bald,
*   You'll Be Bald, Too 370*
Myth 6: Men Can't Do Aerobics 371
Myth 7: Men Are More Violent than Women 372
Myth 8: Flat Feet Pose a Health Risk 372

Index 375

ADVISORY BOARD

Behavioral Health

Morton H. Shaevitz, Ph.D.

> Director, Institute for Family and Work Relationships, La Jolla, CA; associate clinical professor of psychiatry, UC San Diego School of Medicine; author, *Lean & Mean: The No Hassle, Life-Extending Weight Loss Program for Men.*

Maria Simonson, Ph.D.

> Professor emeritus, Johns Hopkins Medical Institutions, Baltimore; founder and director, the Health, Weight and Stress Clinic.

Cardiology

John Cantwell, M.D.

> Director of preventive medicine and cardiac rehabilitation, Georgia Baptist Medical Center, Atlanta; team physician, Atlanta Braves.

Chiropractic

Paige Morgenthal, D.C.

> Associate Professor, Division of Clinical Sciences, Los Angeles College of Chiropractic, Whittier, CA.

Dentistry

Irwin D. Mandel, D.D.S.

> Professor emeritus, Columbia University School of Dental and Oral Surgery, New York City.

Dermatology

Arnold W. Klein, M.D.

> Associate professor of dermatology, UCLA Medical Center; in private practice, Beverly Hills, CA; co-author, *The Skin Book.*

Exercise Physiology

Bryant Stamford, Ph.D.

> Professor of allied health, School of Medicine, University of Louisville; director, Health Promotion Center, University of Louisville, Louisville, KY; author, *Fitness Without Exercise.*

James E. Wright, Ph.D.

Health and Science Editor, *Muscle & Fitness* magazine; former chief of strength research and exercise science, U.S. Army.

Nutrition

Susan Kleiner, Ph.D., R.D.

High-performance nutrition specialist; consultant to athletes and sports teams; in private practice in Seattle.

Jerzy Meduski, M.D.

Specialist in nutritional biochemistry; president, Nutritional Consultants Group, Inc., Los Angeles.

Podiatry

Douglas Richie Jr., D.P.M.

Specialist in podiatric sports medicine; in private practice, Seal Beach, CA.

Psychiatry

Mark Goulston, M.D.

Assistant clinical professor of psychiatry, UCLA Neuropsychiatric Institute, Los Angeles; diplomate, American Board of Psychiatry and Neurology; author, *Get Out of Your Own Way: Overcoming Self-Defeating Behavior.*

Andrew Slaby, M.D., Ph.D.

Clinical professor of psychiatry, New York University and New York Medical College; specialist in stress management and depression in private practice in New York City; author, *60 Ways to Make Stress Work for You* and *No One Saw My Pain.*

Psychotherapy

Sylvia Cary, M.F.C.C.

Specialist in addictive behavior; author, *Jolted Sober* and *The Alcoholic Man*; in private practice, Woodland Hills, CA.

Sexuality

Bernie Zilbergeld, Ph.D.

Specialist in marital and sexual issues; in private practice, Oakland, CA; author, *The New Male Sexuality.*

Sports Medicine

Nicholas A. DiNubile, M.D.

Special advisor to the President's Council on Physical Fitness and Sports; author, *The Exercise Prescription*; clinical assistant professor,

Department of Orthopedic Surgery, Hospital of the University of Pennsylvania.

Mauro DiPasquale, M.D.
Physician and author, *Drug Use and Detection in Amateur Sports.*

Sports Psychology
Charles Garfield, Ph.D.
Expert on the psychology of peak performance; associate clinical professor, University of California Medical School, San Francisco.

Training
A. Eugene Coleman, Ed.D.
Director, Human Performance Institute, University of Houston, Clear Lake; director of conditioning, Houston Astros.

Urology
Cappy Rothman, M.D.
Chief of urology and director, In Vitro Fertilization and Embryo Recovery Program, Century City Hospital, Los Angeles.

Weight Control
Howard Flaks, M.D.
Member, American Society of Bariatric Physicians (specialists in obesity treatment); in private practice, Beverly Hills, CA.

CONTRIBUTORS

We'd like to gratefully acknowledge and thank all those writers whose articles, which first appeared in *Men's Fitness* magazine, are now used in this book:

Randall Alford, "ADD Subtracts," July 1993; "Grief Relief," August 1993.

Gloria Auerbach, "Quality Time," December 1993.

Neil Ayers, "Staying Healthy in the Nineties," June 1993; "Walking Tall," June 1993; "Up-Sizing," February 1993.

Bob Barnett, "Do Diets Really Work?," April 1995.

Ron Bielicki, "You Can't Keep a Good Man Down," February 1993.

Jeffery Bland, "Well Groomed, Well Fed," March 1993.

Mark Caldwell, "A Shiver Runs Through It," February 1994; "Getting to Commit," March 1995; "In the Heat of the Fight," September 1994; "Bitter Betrayal," February 1995; "Friends and Lovers," May 1995; "Hot Flash," July 1994; "Forever Sorta Young," December 1995.

Sylvia Cary, "Guy Therapy," June 1994; "Is Someone You Know a Batterer?," October 1994.

Michael Castleman, "Caffeine Nation," March 1995; "A Man's Guide to Vitamins & Minerals," June 1994.

Victoria Clayton, "Meditation as Medicine," August 1992.

Sharon Cohen, "Toxic Avengers," July 1995.

Charlene Crabb, "Power Plants," February 1995.

Mubarak Dahir, "Too Vein," July 1993; "Tempest in a Teapot," April 1993.

Susan Davis, "Sunblock Surprise," June 1994; "Alcohol on Trial," June 1995; "Sleepless in America," August 1994.

Nicholas DiNubile, "Back Attack Risk-Profile Quiz," April 1993.

Kathleen Doheny, "Symptoms You Should Never Ignore," August 1993; Unconventional Healers," February 1994 "Toxic Emotions," January 1993; "Therapy for the Undisturbed," April 1993; "Crowning Achievements," November 1992.

Julie Sinclair Eakin, "Urban Renewal," September 1993.

Jeff Everson, "Terms of Enlargement," June 1995.

Bruce Feirstein; "You Gotta Have Friends," September 1993.

Kathleen Flinn, "It Takes All Types," March 1994.

Peter Gambaccini, "The Aging Athlete," July 1993.

Bill Geiger, "Circuit City," November 1995.

Tony Gervino, "Let's Get a Physical," July 1994.

Richard Gillett, "Change Your Mind," February 1993.

B. C. Gironda, "Worried to Death," September 1994.

Timothy Gower, "Eating Disorders," December 1994; "Sperm *und Drang*," November 1994.

Fred Hayward, "Gender Genocide," February 1993.

Laura Hilgers, "Lipid in the Gut," August 1994.

Therese Iknoian, "Mood Foods," August 1993.

Leah Ingram, "Shaving Grace," August 1994; "How Fit Are Your Torpedoes?," October 1993.

Ann Kearney-Cooke, "The High Price of a Perfect Body," January 1993.

David Levine, "Laughing Matters," November 1994.

David Lewis, "The Prostate: An Owner's Manual," July 1994.

Joan Lippert, "The Best Diet on Earth," October 1995; "Protein Power," December 1994; "All in the Family," November 1993.

John Little, "Basic Training," August 1993.

Jim Macak, "Two Who Survived," May 1992; "The Aging Process," August 1992; "You Can't Keep a Good Man Down," February 1993.

Ted Mason, "The New Male Vanity," June 1993.

Seth Matarasso, "Hold Back the Years," July 1995.

Steven Mirsky, "Thought Control," March 1995.

James Morelli, "Blood-Red Morning," January 1994.

Curtis Pesman, "Stage Fright," March 1994.

T. G. Rand, "Monogamy Chic," June 1994.

Ellen Rapp, "Clitoral Translations," February 1995.

David Reed, "What Makes a Good-Looking Man?," November 1991.

Jim Rosenthal, "Yoga Is No Laughing Matter," February 1991.

Jim Schmaltz, "The 20-Minute Working Man's Workout," March 1994.

Claire Schoen, "Ten Myths About Men," August 1992.

Lou Schuler, "CAT in the Sack," November 1992; "Too Much of a Good Thing," July 1995.

Steve Schwade, "Lab Readouts: Blood Simple," February 1993.

Arnold Schwarzenneger, "Advice for Aging Weight Trainers," July 1993.

Eric Sherman, "Down Time," December 1994.

Joel Silverman, "Of Human Bonding," August 1994; "The Fitness Evolution," May 1994.

R. D. Silverman, "The Question of Size," August 1991.

Todd H. Smith, "Strung Out on Workouts?," May 1992.

Bill Starr, "You're Getting Warm," September 1995.

Gayle Sato Stodder, "Home, Hazardous Home," October 1993; "Beyond Condoms," March 1993.

Mary Ellen Strote, "The Power of Prayer," October 1992; "Of Jowls and Jawlines," November 1993.

Beth Tomkiw, "The Skin Game," September 1995; "Tan, Gents," June 1995.

Evelyn Tribole, "Nutritional Cross Training," October 1992.

Chris Weygandt, "Deadly Skin," August 1991; "Monogamy," February 1991.

Larry Wichman, "The PSA: To Test or Not to Test," August 1993; "Come Again," April 1992; "Sexuality Through the Ages," July 1992.

FOREWORD

I'm convinced that the future belongs to the flexible. No, not those of us who can place our elbows on the ground from a standing position, but those who can successfully deal with constant change, from dating to office technology to . . . you name it. Once you had a doctor of your own choosing—today, your health plan won't allow you to make that choice. You used to work out to the point of injury—today, you know that will do you more harm than good. You used to eat and *enjoy* high fat foods—today, you have to be concerned with protecting your heart and watching your waistline. You used to play baseball—today, you're likely to be involved in a sport or activity that didn't exist a few years ago. You used to know about dating etiquette—today, you haven't a clue. Get used to it—things aren't going to get easier.

At *Men's Fitness*, we monitor these changes, and your attitudes toward them, very carefully. The idea of a true service magazine for men (women have known about service magazines for more than a hundred years) is thriving. We used to be the gender that refused to ask for directions. Now it's okay to seek advice on exercise, fitness, sports performance, nutrition, health, our emotions and sexuality. We want doable fitness and health, an approach that is logical, accepts us for what we are (lazy, sometimes), isn't too painful and even—is it possible?—*enjoyable*. Basically, I think we all want to live better lives as easily as possible.

That's where this book comes in. As we've done in *Men's Fitness* magazine and our brother electronic publication *Men's Fitness Online*, *Men's Fitness Magazine's Complete Guide to Health and Well-Being* provides essential information on living fit, healthy and smart with style and substance. From fitness and health to sports, behavior, sex and, as we say in the biz, "a whole lot more," this book tells you what you need to know.

Consider our new book a set of directions to your complete well-being. And you didn't even have to ask.

Peter Sikowitz
Editor-in-Chief, *Men's Fitness*

TO BE A MAN: OUR TOTAL WELL-BEING

What does it mean to be a man? If the man in question lives in America at a point in time near the end of the twentieth century, then that query has never been harder to answer. The purpose of *The Complete Guide to Health and Well-Being* is to provide the most thorough and current information on every aspect of a man's health, from diet and exercise to emotional health. But looming behind the detailed information found here is a simple yet elusive question: What does it mean to be a man?

The answer to this deceptively simple question has never been more evasive than it is today. Men's roles have changed enormously in the last few decades, and will no doubt continue to evolve in ways that are impossible to predict. Forecasting and evaluating the state of American manhood has in fact become something of a growth industry; a scholarly journal called the *Chronicle of Higher Education* reports that there are some thirty books about men and masculinity either on the shelves or on their way there. Whether these titles are the result of market research or a more heartfelt effort on the part of the authors to understand the changeable state of American men is unclear, but they do indicate that men are today reexamining their lives as never before.

While everyone's life has changed radically in the last fifty years, the alterations to the fabric of men's lives in this country hasn't been fully examined—especially by men themselves. We know that there has been enormous upheaval in nearly every aspect of our lives, yet we don't understand how it has affected our emotions and the way in which we view our place in the world. We need only think back to the lives our fathers led in the forties, fifties and early sixties—and then contrast them to the lives of our friends, our families, and ourselves today—to see the epochal shifts that have occurred in the roles men play in our society.

The most fundamental change has been to the structure of the family. "Family" in those prior decades almost always meant a father and a mother, most often with Dad as the primary breadwinner and Mom acting as homemaker and principle child-rearer. Men and women were thought to inhabit "separate spheres" in which males looked outward to face the challenges of the world while women turned inward, toward the family. That trend began in the nineteenth century and still exists today, though it's far from the norm for most families.

A family today might have a mom that goes off to work every morning and a dad who stays home with the kids. That dad might also be telecommuting via fax and modem to an office, or he may run some sort of business out of the home. Aside from the movies, there are very few "Mr. Moms" whose sole responsibility is running the household while their wives bring home the bacon; in the nineties—unlike the fifties—it generally takes *two* incomes to provide for all of the needs of a family.

The most typical arrangement today is one in which both parents work either full or part time, and share many more of the responsibilities of raising the kids and making a home. Permanent changes in the American economy—and more importantly, fundamental changes in the role of women in our society—ensure that the world of "Father Knows Best" and "Leave it to Beaver" will be forever relegated to "Nick at Night."

Some perceive this sea-change as bad, but a more positive view points to the new freedoms that men now enjoy. Most of today's fathers, for example, take a much more active role in the early life of their children, to the great benefit of all involved. Being a dad today requires more than changing the odd diaper or playing catch, and there's no greater example of that than childbirth itself. Where once men were exiled to the hospital waiting room to pace and smoke, fathers now participate in their partner's pregnancy in a way that would have been unimaginable thirty years ago. And the bond that comes from a father being present at the birth of a child sets the stage for a much more intimate, loving and honest relationship between parent and child right from the start. Fathers have moved beyond the merely titular "head of the family," and can now share fully in a far more important role—being an involved parent.

While men's role in the family has changed, families themselves have also been redefined. A family today can be a single parent of either sex—again, something uncommon just a few years ago, and nearly unheard of a few decades ago barring the death of a spouse. Men have demonstrated that they can create a home and provide for their children just as well as women can, and in child custody cases it's no longer automatically assumed that sons and daughters "belong with their mother." Fathers have earned the right under the law to be seen as equal to women when it comes to raising children, and courts can now make custody decisions based on what's best for a child—and not simply gender. (Regrettably, the workplace hasn't kept pace with the law; there's no such thing as a "Daddy track" in corporate America for fathers who want to spend time with their newborn children.) Then again, a family today might consist of two partners of the same sex.

While all of these changes to American society can seem overwhelming—and might make you nostalgic for the "good old days" that are better in hindsight than they ever were in the present—they really represent great opportunities for men. A man today can be straight, gay or bisexual; he can be single, married, divorced or widowed; he can choose to be a father, and have the freedom to assign the same priority in his life to that role as mothers traditionally have; and he can combine these aspects of himself in whatever way he sees fit—and with a level of acceptance from society that's never been witnessed before.

Despite the changes of the last fifty years to the circumstances of men, there is one area in which men haven't made great strides: our emotional life. What do men think and feel about the new options and responsibilities facing them? Who knows?—most men won't say. It's certainly not that men don't feel things as deeply as women, but rather that we haven't developed our own vocabulary for this aspect of ourselves. Moreover, the whole concept of expressing—or even experiencing—emotions is often seen as "unmasculine," and is tacitly discouraged by our society.

Much of this harkens back to the turn of the century, when raising a family really became "women's work." Men spent increasing amounts of time outside the home, concentrating more on career than the role of head-of-household. As women ran the home and assumed nearly all the responsibility for raising the children, men's familial role narrowed greatly. It suddenly became almost suspect to concentrate too much on duties that were now seen as "womanly." (It is interesting to note that this is the period in which the word "sissy" first came into the vocabulary). The nurturing role of fathers, and indeed anything that smacked of the softer side of being a man, became somehow unmanly.

Today, there is a large part of the male psyche that still views our emotional life as suspect, as if feelings by their very nature make us somehow less masculine. And we get conflicting information from society about what is expected of us. The media dish up the most extreme examples from either end of our expectations. The ultimate example of the emotionless, hard-driving male is the Terminator, a being that appears to be a man but is simply a machine wrapped in flesh. (It is significant that in the sequel to the film, the Terminator evolves his own set of emotions, and even admits to one character, "I know now why you cry.") At the other end of the spectrum is poor Alan Alda, who somehow became the piñata for those hoping to bash "the sensitive male." It is rare to see a man depicted anywhere who can be both strong and emotional.

It was precisely this male archetype that Robert Bly wrote about in his much-maligned book *Iron John*. Bly was attempting to provide a new mythology for a man, a "warrior ideal" for whom toughness and sensitivity were two sides of the same coin. One might argue with his approach, but there is clearly a need for a new model of masculinity—especially for our sons. As the social critic Christopher Lasch has written, "When adult manhood labors under such a heavy cloud of suspicion, young men have to choose between equally unsatisfactory alternatives: to become more like women or to embrace a masculine style that leaves no room for love and friendship with members of either sex."

With such unsatisfactory role models, it isn't surprising that so many men report feelings of isolation and dissatisfaction. The archetypes of our society don't point the way, and there's certainly no "men's movement" akin to the one that forever changed our notions of women's roles twenty-five years ago. There is a greater variety of accepted masculine roles today, yet men are still struggling to connect with each other and with themselves. Yale University psychiatrist Kyle Pruett observes that "men aren't any happier in the nineties than they were in the fifties, but their inner lives tend to be more complex. They are interested in feeling less isolated. They are stunned to find out how rich human relationships are." If we're not there yet, then at least the seeds of change seem to be sprouting and taking root within us.

If there aren't new archetypes to help guide us, is there something we can take from the old ones? Americans have always worshipped the pioneering spirit and the self-sufficiency that helped create our country. In an era when the old models have failed us, perhaps it's time to once again look to the concept of "being your own man." At first this might sound like the worldview that originally pushed men away from their families at the turn of the century and again during the careerist fifties, but it doesn't necessarily have to be that way.

The "pioneer spirit" or "rugged individualism" of today doesn't mean leaving the softer side of manhood behind, but rather integrating it into the whole. It doesn't mean forsaking family and friends for a quest; it means seeking out the ways that will best help you reconnect with them. It means assuming the responsibility for whatever course you've chosen in life. There probably won't ever be a large-scale social movement to aid you with this; it's something you have to discover and achieve for yourself. The process can start with simply being more open to other people's emotions, and more willing to share your own with friends and with family. Some might use therapy as a way to further uncover the self, while others could benefit from the shared experience of a men's group. Others still might find that becoming a father opens them up to a much wider range of experiences and emotions, and they use that opening to improve the other aspects of their inner life.

The world today is perfectly set up for this kind of approach to life—and not just on the emotional level. Individuals can now take much more control of their health and welfare than ever before. We know much more now about the effects of diet and exercise on quality of life and longevity. We know how the mind and the body can work in unison to the great benefit of both.

Heart disease is a prime example. It is the number one killer of men in America, claiming one out of every six men in the country. Yet it is a *lifestyle disease*, and one that is almost entirely avoidable—and even reversible—by those who can employ the knowledge and summon up the inner strength to make the changes that are really going to affect their lives: modifying diet, getting aerobic exercise and giving up cigarettes. The propaganda of the tobacco lobby notwithstanding, smoking kills 415,000 Americans annually—more than twice the number of those who die from AIDS, alcohol, cocaine, heroin, morphine, suicide, homicide, car accidents and fires *combined*.

And some fifteen years after the "fitness revolution" first swept America, the hard statistics on the number of people who have made regular, vigorous exercise an ongoing part of their lives isn't encouraging. In 1983, the National Health and Nutrition Exam Survey found that 26 percent of Americans were obese (or more than 20 percent above their normal body weight); in 1993, the same survey found that that number had *risen* to 34 percent. *Time* magazine was moved to write that same year that "the fitness movement has run out of recruits."

What is the message behind all of this grim news? It is simply that each individual has a tremendous say in the state of his own health. Most of us have our lives cut short by diseases that are largely within our own control, but we have to have the knowledge of which changes to make and the strength to see them through. The "new frontier" at the end of the twentieth century isn't exterior, it's interior. There are still plenty of worlds to conquer, but the first one we should address is within ourselves.

To that end, *The Complete Guide to Health and Well-Being* will serve as a resource for men who want the latest information about mind, body and spirit. We believe we have created the kind of sourcebook for men that's really never existed before. While women's health and issues related to it often occupy multiple shelves at the bookstore or library, books about men's health and well-being have been few and far between.

With this book, we give American men something they have long needed, and what no other men's book has delivered: a common-sense guide to their health, happiness and well-being. In the second chapter, we'll have a crash course in the male physiology and how best to look after it. The body is an incredibly complex mechanism, so a brief examination of its basic workings is a logical place to start. Chapter Three offers a guide to "wellness"—strategies for optimizing your health. It describes how to get the most from an exam by your doctor, and discusses the roles of both conventional and alternative therapies. We'll also look at some of the specific ills to which the male body is prone.

Chapter Four looks at wellness and the mind, with particular attention to the role of stress in our lives. Stress is probably the single greatest source of physical and emotional trauma in men's lives, and we'll offer specific ways to combat it. We'll examine the other aspects of our emotional lives, and point out sources for additional help. Chapter Five takes on the concept of body image, and how we perceive ourselves. Vanity is not just a women's issue; men are concerned with appearance as never before. We'll talk about a new male vanity—and the high price you might pay for it.

Chapter Six looks at healthy living, including guidelines for optimal nutrition, a 30-Day High Performance Menu, a look at the most important supplements for men and a guide to some potentially hazardous environmental conditions. Sexuality in all of its myriad forms is the topic of Chapter Seven. We'll suggest new techniques that can greatly improve your sex life, including something you might have considered impossible: multiple orgasms for men. Fertility and safe sex are also highlighted.

Relationships and how to improve them fall within Chapter Eight. We'll look at love relationships and friendships—and the sometimes slippery path between the two. We'll concentrate on the wonderful things that relationships bring to our lives, but we won't shy away from their dark side—abusive and violent behavior. Chapter Nine brings us to men and aging, with emphasis on the pleasures and potentials of growing older. We'll also tell you how to use your family history to determine what hazards might face you as you age.

Chapter Ten concentrates on fitness and training, including recommendations for getting the most physical and mental benefits from your workouts. We'll pay close attention to that mysterious place, the weight room, and define its arcane terminology. Finally, the book will conclude with eight myths about men—a section that will give both serious and tongue-in-cheek perceptions on men today.

Throughout the book, we'll use charts, sidebar articles, boxes, self-tests and other elements to help make this vast amount of material as easily accessible as possible. And beyond that, we will present this information as free of jargon as we can—and with as much humor and good spirit as the subject will allow. After all, our sense of humor is an important part of who we are. (And as you'll see in Chapter Four, a sense of humor can also be a determining factor in how healthy we are.)

The Complete Guide to Health and Well-Being offers innumerable ways to improve all aspects of your life, but it never really answers the most fundamental question of all: What does it mean to be a man? Perhaps the best thing it can do is pose that maddeningly simple question, point you to some of the options available, and give you the chance to answer it in whatever way best suits your life and your goals.

What does it mean to be a man? The answer to that question is pretty much up to you.

2

MEN'S BODIES—A CRASH COURSE IN PHYSIOLOGY

Inhabiting a male body is much like having a bank account: as long as it's healthy, you don't think much about it. Compared with the female body, it is a low-maintenence proposition: a shower now and then, trim the fingernails every ten days, a haircut once a month . . . A man and his body are like a boy and the buddy who has a driver's license and the use of his father's car for the evening; one goes along, gratefully, for the ride.

—JOHN UPDIKE

If you think of your body as being like a car (and if you're a man, that's the kind of analogy that probably appeals to you), then you are in possession of a remarkably low-maintenance vehicle. Men's bodies are for the most part stronger and less complex than the comparatively exotic variety piloted by the opposite sex. Our bodies are much more straightforward, from our heavier skeletons and denser muscle mass to our external genitalia. We can't bear children, of course, but we also aren't subject to the enormous hormonal changes that affect women from the beginning of menstruation to the onset of menopause. Our life expectancy is shorter by about seven years, yet we are less often sick; according to a study on sex differences published in *U.S. News & World Report*, women spend 40 percent more days sick in bed than do men. Our bodies are, simply, *simpler*. If women's bodies seem like complex and sophisticated European cars—with beautifully sculpted lines, graceful curves and mysterious, finelytuned inner workings—then men are more akin to a '57 Chevy: gas it up and go.

We may be simpler in design, but men's bodies come with their own unique set of problems. The same hormonal tides that control women's reproductive physiology also protects them from heart disease; men are much more likely to die of heart attacks than are women—at least until menopause, when the numbers begin to even out. Women are sick more often than men and are more likely to be afflicted with chronic diseases, but men stubbornly avoid visits to the doctor; by the time a disease is discovered in a man it's much more likely to be fatal. Men also suffer higher death rates from certain cancers, from accidents, from AIDS and from suicide. The unfortunate bottom line is that the overall risk of death is higher for males at all ages, and for every leading cause of death.

On the positive side, it's somewhat easier for men to mitigate some of these risk factors. Heart disease and diabetes, for example, are often related to poor nutrition and obesity—that is, being more than 20 percent above ideal weight for your height, age and body type. But men seem to have an easier time losing and maintaining weight than do women, whose bodies naturally carry a higher percentage of fat. Our heavier muscle mass makes it easier for us to add muscle, which in turn can help control weight and protect the strength of our bones. Those bones are also less subject to osteoporosis, or the diminishing of bone density, that can be a problem as we age. The good news in all of this is that many of the risk factors men face are lifestyle-related, and so are well within our control.

MEN'S BODIES: THE BASICS

The following is a head-to-toe examination of the male physiology. We are, of course, more similar to women than we are different; we are all human animals. But men's bodies exhibit fundamental differences from those of the opposite sex, and understanding those areas of divergence can help us better appreciate what it means to be a man on the physical level, and how best to maintain and improve our bodies.

The Brain and Nervous System

From the vagaries of thought and creativity to the nuts-and-bolts business of regulating the body's functions, the duties of the brain and nervous system are phenomenally complex. The brain tells the lungs to breathe, the heart to beat, the eyes to see, the legs to run, the intestines to digest. As if those tasks weren't enough, the brain also creates our emotions; love may feel as though it resides in the heart, but it occupies the penthouse. And of course, the brain is home to all of our conscious and unconscious thoughts, hopes and dreams. Exactly how the brain does all this is still one of life's great mysteries.

While much of the brain's business remains a riddle, its structures and composition are well understood. The brain weighs in at about three pounds, and is comprised of three different areas: the *cerebrum*, the *cere-*

bellum and the *brain stem*. The cerebrum is the largest part of the brain; it's the dome-shaped structure that resembles a shelled walnut, and consists of four lobes—the frontal, temporal, parietal and occipital. Most of the brain's information is stored on the surface of the cerebrum, which is called the cerebral cortex. Beneath the cerebrum is the plum-sized cerebellum, whose primary function is to coordinate muscle movement. The brain stem connects to the cerebrum just forward of the cerebellum, and attaches the brain to the spinal cord and the rest of the nervous system.

Communication within the brain is the result of an amazing electrochemical process that passes messages from one nerve cell to another. Neural messages travel at a speed of less than 1/1000 of a second (slightly faster if you've just had some caffeine), and must "jump" from cell to cell over a small void called a *synaptic cleft*. Individual brain cells are not directly linked to each other—yet a single cell may be connected to over 10,000 other cells. The brain's astoundingly complex communications system is controlled by thirty different chemicals called *neurotransmitters* that govern which messages are passed and which aren't. Diseases like chronic depression and schizophrenia are the result of imbalances in minute amounts of neurotransmitters, which alter how information is sent and received within the brain—and drastically revise the way that person sees the world.

The brain and spinal cord make up the *central nervous system*, while the rest of the body's nerves comprise the *peripheral nervous system*. The spinal cord, protected by the bony column of vertebrae that surrounds it, is the place where the central nervous system communicates with the peripheral nervous system and the rest of the body. The foot soldiers of the peripheral nervous system are the nerves that radiate out from the spinal cord to every inch of the body, carrying out the instructions of the brain and in return relaying information about the status of different body parts and stimuli from the outside world.

Although structurally identical, the brains of men and women function quite differently. Testosterone, the primary male sex hormone, seems to play a direct role in how the male brain develops—and may explain why it is so different from the female brain. Bruce McEwen, a neuroendocrinologist at Rockefeller University in New York City, has discovered profound changes between male and female animal brains at the cellular level. "Brain cells respond to testosterone by becoming larger and developing different kinds of connections," he notes. The brain, it seems, is "sexed" early in life by the sex hormones, beginning as soon as six months after conception.

The early sexing of the brain may well determine the kind of skills you have. Some studies suggest that men exhibit greater development in the region of the brain governing visual stimuli, while women show more complex neural pathways in the areas related to speech and language. Women also seem to house language ability in both hemispheres of the brain, while in men that trait is localized in the left hemisphere. The *corpus callosum*—the thick mass of nerves that sits between the two hemispheres and connects them—seems to be thicker in women, and might allow for more communication between the brain's two halves. This may explain why a stroke to the left side of the brain is three times as likely to affect a man's speech as a woman's.

The developmental emphasis on the visual within men's brains would seem to explain the undisputed male edge in terms of visual-spacial ability—or the ability to see, understand and manipulate objects in a three-dimensional environment—an advantage that first shows up at about age eight and continues throughout life. Infant girls have an edge when it comes to visualizing *faces*, however, as opposed to objects. Many studies show that female infants as young as five or six months can detect differences in photographs of human faces, but boys of that age can't. The girls will smile and vocalize only to faces, whereas the boys will also react to inanimate objects and blinking lights. Researchers theorize that there may be a biological predisposition in females to react to other humans more strongly because they will need those bonding skills when they become mothers.

Men's greater visual-spacial acumen might account for another characteristic: a shorter attention span. Teachers have long made this observation, and studies with preschool-age children bear it out. One researcher found that in a twenty-minute interval, the young boys would engage in an average of 4.5 activities, while girls from the same age group concentrated on just 2.5 tasks. The girls, however, started and completed more projects than the boys, who were much more distractible. In fact, the boys interrupted their play to look at something about four times as often as the girls, and spent more time simply looking at the other children. One possible explanation might be that boys are simply more visually oriented, and spend more time scanning their environment for information.

It isn't at all clear that these cognitive differences result in a meaningful division in the mental skills of men and women. Men might have better visual acuity while women might be slightly more advanced in language or conceptualization, but individual differences in intelligence and acumen are much more important than any generalized traits in the gross anatomy of men's and women's brains.

On the other hand, the way in which the brain processes impressions into emotional responses does seem to be significantly different for the two sexes. The research into how our emotions are created within the physical anatomy of the brain indicates that men and women actually use different parts of their brains to create similar feelings.

Scientists used to believe that the brain had a single, central "emotional center" that was responsible for the creation of our feelings from the input reaching us through our senses. Using the newest generation of imaging systems such as PET (positron-emission tomography) scans, researchers can now take a "snapshot" of different parts of the brain while a person is experiencing an emotion, and measure the different activity levels.

For generations scientists believed that our emotional life was tied to the *limbic system*, the structures surrounding the brain stem that are thought to be the oldest region of the brain. But the new scanning techniques show that several different regions of the brain can create an emotional response—and that different areas can respond with contradictory emotions at the same time. This might explain the seemingly conflicted emotions we sometimes feel, as when an event makes us both happy and sad. The limbic system does seem to be primarily responsible for sadness, while the outer layer of the brain—the cerebral cortex—seems to house more of the areas associated with happiness.

When they are sad, women seem to activate the limbic section of the brain more strongly than men do. They are capable of greater electrical activity in this region when they are in the grips of sadness—and apparently, are capable of a deeper experience of that emotion. Mark George, M.D., a psychiatrist and neurologist with the National Institute of Mental Health whose research first noted these differences, reports that, "Women seem to experience a more profound sadness than do men. It makes me wonder if this might be related to why women have twice the risk of depression as do men." While the limbic system provides an intriguing clue, science has yet to explain why men and women can feel sadness so differently.

If men have a biological advantage when it comes to feeling the most profound levels of sadness, we might not do as well in some other areas— most notably, anger. Both blind rage and anger can effect either sex, but strike men disproportionally to women. (Houston psychiatrist Kenneth Wetcher, M.D, speculates that male anger may be part of our innate make-up because it once had a positive societal purpose: enraged men were more inclined to do battle in order to protect their families and communities.) With the help of PET scans and other imaging systems, we should have in the near future a much better understanding of the physical mechanisms behind our emotional states. With luck, that knowledge will translate into new therapies and techniques to keep us on a more even emotional keel.

The early sexing of the brain not only affects our skills and emotions, but our behavior as well. Indeed, testosterone is the primary reason for one of the greatest behavioral differences between males and females: aggression. Men are more aggressive than women; and this difference begins to show itself as early as age two and continues through adulthood. It's also seen across cultures from every corner of the world. Males whose brain cells are abnormally insensitive to testosterone tend, like women, to have higher scores than average men in verbal ability while demonstrating less mechanical ability—as well as being less aggressive.

The developmental differences between male and female brains are found throughout life, from infancy to old age. For example, recent research has confirmed an unfortunate notion that neurologists have long suspected: the brain diminishes in size as we get older. Worse still, this diminishment appears more often and in greater variety in males than in females. A study at the University of Pennsylvania used MRI (magnetic-resonance imaging) to analyze the brains of healthy adults from ages 18–80, and found that most of the shrinkage in male brains took place in the left hemisphere—the area controlling speech and analytical abilities. Women show shrinkage on both sides of the brain but at a slower rate, and with less apparent functional damage. There's not much you can do about a withering brain, except apply the same rule you should to your muscles: use it or lose it. People who stay mentally active into old age keep their facilities intact the longest.

The Cardiopulmonary System

The term *cardiopulmonary system* refers to the way the heart and lungs function together as a unit. When we breathe in, the lungs bring fresh oxygen into the body and the heart pumps blood into the capillaries of the lungs where it can be it can be recharged with oxygen. The heart then circulates this oxygen-rich blood throughout the body via the arteries, and returns the oxygen-depleted blood to the heart via the veins. The heart pumps the depleted blood into the lungs where carbon dioxide collected from the body is exchanged for oxygen. We exhale the carbon dioxide, breathe in fresh air, and the whole remarkable process begins again.

The Lungs

The lungs are roughly cone shaped and are divided into lobes. The lung on your right side has three lobes, while the one on your left has only two; the left lung sacrifices a lobe in order to make room for its cardiopulmonary partner, the heart. The lungs might be the most well-protected organs in the body; they're surrounded by the spinal column, ribs, the breastbone and the respiratory muscles. The bottom of this enclosure is a vaulted sheet of muscle called the *diaphragm*, which supports the lungs and allows them to fully expand during deep breaths.

When you breathe in, the air is drawn into each lung by a tube called the *primary bronchus*. As the air moves deeper into the lung the bronchus branches out into ever-smaller passages called *bronchioles*. The most minute pathways dead-end into tiny sacs called *alveoli*, which is where the actual interface between breath and blood takes place. Each person has about 300 million alveoli in each lung; if the alveoli within just one lung were spread out in an even layer they would cover half of a tennis court. The lungs are real workhorses, processing about 3,500 gallons of air every day.

The Heart

Your heart is roughly the size of your fist with your opposite hand wrapped around it—5 inches long, 3.5 inches wide and 2.5 inches thick. A man's heart is larger than a woman's by about 2 ounces, yet *still* weighs in at a mere 10.5 ounces. By the time you reach the age of sixty-five, it's your heart that should feel like retiring; it will have pumped blood through your circulatory system over 2.5 billion times.

But those numbers are just the tip of the iceberg. All of the blood vessels in your body if placed end-to-end would circle the earth's equator three times, for a total of about 60,000 miles—yet it takes just 23 seconds for your heart to circulate blood through your entire body. (If you happen to be 25 pounds overweight, your ticker has to pump through an extra 5,000 miles of vessels.) The heart squeezes out roughly 2.5 ounces of blood with every beat, which adds up to 2,500 gallons of blood a day. But in all of these statistics perhaps the most arresting notion is the simplest: your heart has been working *continually*, without rest, since the day you were born, and baring catastrophe will continue to do so into your ripe old age. The heart is the proverbial "Little Engine That Could."

Men have larger hearts (and greater lung capacity) than women in proportion to their generally larger bodies; and larger lungs and hearts translate into increased aerobic capacity—the ability of the heart to circulate oxygen-rich blood to the muscles. Indeed, the heart actually craves aerobic exercise. Regular, moderate and sustained aerobic exercise helps condition the heart muscle *itself* so that in time it becomes more efficient, pumping more blood with each beat and using fewer beats to circulate blood throughout the body. And these benefits are the return on a surprisingly small investment of time and energy on your part.

While regular aerobic exercise is the most important ingredient in the recipe for a more healthy heart, diet and stress-reduction are both key elements. Reducing fat intake to less than 20 percent of your total diet and lowering the blood-cholesterol level to below 200 milligrams should be goals for anyone, especially those with a family history of heart disease; this will also help keep your weight near your desired level for your age and build, which also greatly benefits your heart. (But it isn't just your cardiovascular system that reaps the benefits of diet and exercise: research from the Netherlands indicates that plaque build-up within the arterial walls of the brain might be at the root of the mental decline that so often accompanies old age, and that those with cleaner arteries performed better on mental tests regardless of age.) Diet will be discussed in more detail in Chapter Six, while stress and the best methods for dealing with it will be examined in Chapter Four. Strategies for optimizing your cardiovascular health will be examined in the next chapter.

Bones, Muscles and Joints

A man's frame—his skeletal system and the muscles that strengthen and support it—is a wonderful argument both for and against evolution. *Homo sapiens* is unique among his primate brothers: we are the only member of the clan who is fully erect and bipedal. Though the apes might spend considerable time on two feet, they occasionally revert to four; only man moves around fully upright—and we can even walk backwards, something our ape relatives can't manage. Unfortunately, our reach might have exceeded our grasp. It's not clear that our bones and muscles are up to the task of being fully erect, as is evidenced by the amount of backache and joint problems we have. When was the last time you heard King Kong moaning about his lumbar region?

Ailments of the frame—most notably back pain—rank first among disease groups that affect the quality of life, according to research from the Yale School of Medicine. It's the most common musculoskeletal ailment for which both men and women seek medical attention. About 80 percent of the population will, at some point, be sidelined with significant back pain at a national cost of over $16 billion dollars. Next to the common cold, it's the biggest reason most people will miss a day of work. Backache also strikes men disproportionally; jobs in the trucking, lumber, mining and construction fields—which are still predominantly male—lead all other careers in incidence of back problems.

BACK ATTACK RISK-PROFILE QUIZ

As you answer the following questions, add the designated points for every "yes" response.

1. My job involves sitting 50 percent or more of the time, or for several consecutive hours, on a regular basis. **3 points**
2. I am more than 10 percent above my ideal body weight. **2 points**
3. I have had at least one "back attack." **4 points**
4. I do not exercise regularly (three times a week) with specific attention to aerobic conditioning, abdominal-muscle and lower-back strengthening, and hamstring stretching. **4 points**
5. I am a smoker. **2 points**
6. My job requires frequent bending and lifting. **3 points**
7. I am not happy with my job, or even hate it. **2 points**

Zero to 2 points: Mild risk
3 to 6 points: Moderate risk
Over 6 points: High risk
If you scored higher than 2, you should be doing preventive lower-back exercises and making the necessary lifestyle adjustments (significant enough to change your answers to the above questions) to lower your risk for serious back trouble down the road

The Skeletal System

The vagaries of evolution aside, the skeletal system is a remarkable feat of architecture. We are born with 350 bones, most comprised of soft, watery material called *cartilage*. Even the skull of a newborn baby is surprisingly malleable, an indication of just how soft our new bones really are. As the infant grows, cartilage begins to stiffen as it absorbs calcium ingested by the body. The calcified cartilage is then replaced by "true bone," which is mostly calcium at the outer layer. In the process many of the original 350 separate pieces of bone begin to knit together, eventually forming the total of 206 that most of us end up with (some have two additional ribs and/or an extra one in the tailbone, or coccyx).

Bones not only form the framework of our skeletal system, they play another key role: creating red blood cells that form the most important element of our blood, as well as the white blood cells that help us fight disease. These blood components are created in the *marrow*, the gelatinous center of a bone. There are about five million red blood cells per cubic millimeter of blood, and they are continually reproduced and released by the marrow.

Though the hardest, outer layer of bone might seem to be dead, it is actually the newest part of a bone. Bone grows from the outside in, with the newest layer forming on top of the previous one, while the older layer is gradually absorbed into the interior of the bone. Under a microscope, the interior of bone looks like coral: lacey and full of holes. The more holes there are in the interior, the less dense the bone is. At the center of the bone is the softest layer, the marrow.

Bone stops increasing in length at about age twenty in males, but this process of reabsorption and reformation never ends. Through adolescence, reformation is greater than reabsorption; after age forty, reabsorption gradually outpaces reformation and we begin to lose bone mass. Later in life, bones can give way to the slow leeching of calcium known as osteoporosis. Although the condition is most often associated with post-menopausal women, men can also be at risk as they age—though to a lesser extent than women. Good nutrition, with adequate levels of vitamin D (the Reference Daily Intake, or RDI, is 400 international units per day for adults) and calcium, can help maintain strong bones. Calcium is the fifth most abundant element in the human body, and the majority of it is found in our bones. (In addition to strengthening bones and teeth, it also aids nerve-impulse transmission, muscle contraction, heart function, blood-pressure regulation, and helps protect against colon cancer.) Current government guidelines call for 800 milligrams of calcium a day for men, and many experts feel that should be raised to 1,000. Most men, unfortunately, consume only about 75 percent of their RDI of calcium. Green, leafy vegetables and lowfat dairy products are the best sources.

Exercise is another great way to build and maintain your skeletal system; bones grow stronger with use and atrophy with neglect. Weight-bearing exercise, like running or walking, and weight lifting are the best ways to improve bone density. Bone strengthens when it has to support your body against the force of gravity. Even just standing will build bone; by one estimate, men should be standing or moving around on their feet a minimum of three hours a day to maintain bone strength. Mood can also apparently alter bone density. A study in the *American Journal of Psychiatry* reported that severe depression has been found to reduce bone density in some patients, possibly because of hormonal changes.

The Muscular System

Bones supply the body's architecture, but it is the muscles that allow that superstructure to move from place to place, and with an impressive measure of speed and grace. We associate muscles with movement, but they perform many other less obvious functions in the body. They circulate the blood, move air and food through the body and provide the mechanical power behind the organs. They are the body's furnace, converting the chemical energy of food into mechanical energy and in the process making our lives possible.

Of the roughly six hundred muscles found throughout the body, there are three distinct varieties. *Skeletal muscle* is the kind we are most familiar with; it's the type that weight-lifters develop in order to display their arms, backs and legs to maximum effect. Less obvious but in some ways more important are the *smooth muscles*; they perform the maintenance for our bodies that we are nearly unaware of—helping blood through the vessels and food and waste products through the digestive system. They also control functions like the expansion and contraction of the pupil, the stiffening of hair follicles and motion of the tongue through the complex act of swallowing. The *heart muscle* is unique; no other muscular tissue could do the heart's job without quickly becoming exhausted.

For our purposes, it's most important to learn about the skeletal muscles because these are largely *voluntary*—they can be controlled by conscious command from the brain. Most smooth muscles (and the heart muscle) are called *involuntary* because they do their job automatically. Many muscles—like the tongue—can respond in both ways, and a number of involuntary muscles can learn to act voluntarily with the right training. Students of some Eastern religions, as well as those who study biofeedback techniques, can learn to control even such fundamental processes as heart rate or blood pressure.

The skeletal muscles come in pairs of opposed groups. All muscles work by contraction—they pull, not push. So it takes groups of opposed muscles to lift your arm, for example: one to raise it, another to lower it. Even the simplest task requires a carefully coordinated symphony of movement, often involving the use of several different muscle groups simultaneously. The complexity of this symphony is apparent in illnesses like Parkinson's disease or stroke that effect muscle control and coordination; those afflicted have great difficulty with simple movement, and often must relearn how to perform basic tasks. When you turn your mind to more complex motions—like running the high hurdles, performing gymnastics or throwing a curve ball—the feats performed by the muscular system take on their proper magnitude.

Each muscle is made up of minute strands of fiber, ranging from a half-inch long to as much as a foot, gathered into bundles. There are some six trillion muscle fibers in the body, each capable of supporting 1,000 times its own weight. When activated, each fiber pulls at full capacity, but the brain can determine how many fibers are fired and thus control and coordinate the action of the muscle. It is this remarkable communication between brain and muscle that allows for the graceful movement and precise use of strength of which the body is so capable.

As mentioned, just as the heart muscle strengthens and becomes more efficient through aerobic exercise, all muscles become stronger with use. The more a muscle is utilized, the more it builds itself with nutrients and blood vessels, expanding its capacity for future demands. Stronger muscles also help reinforce and protect the bones they surround, making the body's frame a better structural unit. And as with the heart, the muscular system responds very positively to exercise by pumping blood more efficiently and expanding its ability to use oxygen, its primary fuel.

Even those who have no interest in bodybuilding or weightlifting will discover that a couple of weight-training sessions every week will pay off tremendously, especially if combined with aerobic workouts. More importantly, weight training increases bone density, lowers cholesterol and blood pressure and even speeds the "transit time" of food through your digestive system—which can help protect you from colon cancer.

The Joints

The muscles and bones are linked together by a variety of mechanical devices called joints. Joints are the unsung heroes of the musculoskeletal system: they permit a vast range of motion for bones that must meet and function together—but not touch. They must fasten two or more bones to each other firmly, yet cushion them from one another while providing lubrication for movement. They range from simple hinges like the ones found in the finger to the sophisticated ball-and-socket arrangement of the shoulder, and they must be strong enough to bear the pressures of running and jumping. The wrist alone contains thirty-four joints linking eight bones; perhaps this is what Walt Whitman had in mind when he said, "The narrowest hinge on my hand puts to scorn all machinery."

From the simplest to the most complex, all joints are made of the same materials. The joint is enclosed by a membrane of tough connective tissue, and surrounded by a lubricant called *synovial fluid*. Ligaments surround this package and link the two bones together while limiting the joint's range of motion. In larger joints, where muscle tissue is attached by nearby tendons, small lubricating sacks called bursas separate the tissue from the joint.

WHEN GOOD JOINTS GO BAD

With the yeoman's job that joints perform, it's not surprising that they are a frequent source of complaint. Some joints simply wear out over the course of a lifetime; after all, they're called upon to service a body that now lasts twice as long as those of our prehistoric ancestors. Others fail because of disease or infection. Fortunately, joint replacement—especially for the hip—has become a routine antidote for this worst form of joint injury. Much more common are complaints focusing on the dreaded "itis"—inflammations of the various components that make up a joint. Tendinitis and bursitis affect the tendons and bursas; arthritis—which can appear in over one hundred different forms—attacks the joint itself, often causing debilitating pain and severe loss of motion. The most serious form of arthritis is the rheumatoid variety; more than simply pain in the joints, it's actually a disease affecting the entire immune system of the body and can involve organs as well as joints.

Men have an advantage when it comes to most forms of arthritis: it's often much more acute when it strikes women. Degenerative arthritis of the hip, however, seems to strike white males about three to six times as often as Native Americans or those from Pacific Rim countries, and no one knows why. All forms of arthritis respond best to early treatment, so any persistent pain in any joint is reason enough to see your doctor. Osteoarthritis, the degenerative form of the disease, also has a definite link to body weight. If you're twenty or more pounds overweight in your twenties, you have nearly twice as great a chance of developing osteoarthritis of the knee or hip later in life, according to researchers from the Johns Hopkins Medical School.

The Digestive System

The digestive system is one of the lowest maintenance body systems there is. For most men, the process is a no-brainer: food goes in one end, nutrients are extracted, waste comes out the other end.

The digestive system really begins in your mouth, where you chew your food and combine it with saliva. Eating breaks down foods into a manageable size, while each subsequent step in the process breaks the food down further until it disassembles into its basic chemical components.

Saliva is just the first of the digestive juices your lunch will face in its thirty-foot journey through the digestive tract. The physical act of chewing also raises or lowers the temperature of your food to the proper temperature for digestion.

The food travels from your mouth to the *esophagus*, the muscular tube that leads to the stomach. The food is actually squeezed downward in a complex muscular motion to the top of the stomach, where a circular muscle opens to admit it. As each bite of food enters the stomach it's stored in an area called the *fundus* until the stomach moves it to the *antrium*, where the pool of gastric juice awaits. The stomach then churns and mixes the food and gastric juice, and the food is converted into a semi-liquid pulp called *chyme* over the course of the next three to six hours.

The chyme then passes through the duodenum to the small intestine, where most of its nutrient value is absorbed by the body. The complex folds of the intestinal wall contain billions of *villi* and *microvilli*—cells that secrete digestive juices and absorb nutrients. The villi pass the nutrients on to the blood, which distribute them throughout the body. The leftover waste products—which may represent only 5 percent of your original meal—are passed to the large intestine, or bowel. The remaining water from the chyme is reabsorbed, and the colon forms the remaining waste matter into feces. These are then expelled by the body, perhaps twenty-four hours after you sat down to lunch (depending on what you ate and the speed of your system).

Although both regular exercise and weight training will help your overall digestive functioning, the digestive system requires little but good food and adequate fiber and water to eliminate waste products.

Skin, Nails and Hair

The Skin

Although many men assume that skin is simply an enormous wrapper that holds everything else in place, it's actually an organ in its own right. It's responsibilities include regulating body temperature and respiration. Your skin breathes, which is why Goldfinger's victims died of asphyxiation after being painted gold from head to foot in the old James Bond film.

That said, your skin *is* like an enormous wrapper. It's the place where your body meets the outside world, and it helps protect the most delicate internal structures from the environment. The top two layers of the skin, the *epidermis*, offers the most protection; it's meant to be quickly and easily replaced by the layers beneath, ridding the body of any minor damage inflicted by day-to-day living. At its thickest, on the palms and soles of the feet, the epidermis is a mere 1.5 millimeters thick; on the thin-skinned eyelids, that depth shrinks to .10 millimeters.

The epidermal-layer cells are composed largely of keratin, the same protein that forms hair and nails. And like hair and nails, these cells are dead. They are pushed up from the *dermis*—the thick, living layer of skin beneath the epidermis—where they form the body's protective layer. After four to six weeks of guard duty, they flake off and are replaced by a new layer. This is why minor scrapes, burns and blemishes will disappear over time.

When men are accused of being "thick-skinned," the charge is true—at least as far as the epidermis is concerned. We do seem to have tougher hides than do females, and that difference can show up in unexpected ways. Women's skin is thought to be more sensitive, probably because of the difference in thickness. One sex researcher named Rebecca Chalker theorizes that this extra sensitivity might explain why women may enjoy foreplay more than men: they may appreciate the subtle sensations more. Their softer, thinner skin might make them somewhat more prone to wrinkles, however, and here men enjoy a distinct cultural advantage. After all, no one expects men to have smooth, perfect complexions.

Men do have their own skin worries, of course, and shaving is right at the top of the list. Shaving, sun protection, acne care and other issues relating to men and their skin will be addressed in Chapter Five. Aside from these worries, the skin is virtually maintenance-free. Like hair and nails, skin is built and nurtured from the inside so good nutrition and overall health are the most important aspects.

REAL MEN USE MOISTURIZER

Dryness and the sun are the skin's worst enemies. Soap commercials aside, it isn't necessary—or desirable—to lather yourself until you look like a snowman; soap dries out the skin and diminishes the elasticity we naturally lose as we age. Use soap more sparingly, focusing more on the armpits and genitals. High-detergent soaps may leave you with a "manly" smell, but can also irritate and dry out your skin; instead choose a mild soap with a minimum of ingredients. Also, avoid vigorous scrubbing of the skin—especially the thinner, more delicate skin of the face. If you live in a dry area or are subject to arid winter air, using a moisturizing lotion after your shower will help the skin retain its own moisture. (Don't worry: they make unscented varieties so you won't smell like Aunt Ruth.)

The Nails

Men have fewer complaints about their nails than women, primarily because we tend not to think about them. The exposed part of the nail, called the nail plate, is composed of keratin—just like the hair and skin. And like hair, the nail plates are lifeless. The living section of a nail lies under the skin, and is called the *matrix* or root. Most of the problems of the nail and nailbed (the area under the nail plate) experienced by women are the result of growing their nails long and applying polishes and varnishes to them. For most men, this obviously isn't a problem.

The Hair

Hair, like nails and the outer layer of skin, consists primarily of dead keratin. But never has a mass of dead cells been the focus of so much poetry and pathos as is the case with hair. And men are just as guilty as women on this score—probably because hair loss affects so many more males than females. Trying to tell yourself that hair is just a collection of dead cells isn't much consolation when an increasing amount of yours turns up in the shower drain and in your brush. Hair loss and the strategies for dealing with it are discussed in full in Chapter Five.

The Teeth

A tooth consists of a *crown* and a *root*, embedded—permanently, one hopes—in a socket in the gum. The outer layer of enamel encases a layer of dentin, which surrounds the tooth's pulpy center and the nerves and blood vessels found there. The long "legs" of the tooth that anchor it in the jawbone are called the *centiums*. Adults have twenty-eight teeth (excluding wisdom teeth) that perform four different jobs—biting, tearing, crushing and mashing—with amazing precision and efficiency. Given a small amount of care, they last a lifetime.

Women pay more attention to their oral hygiene than men; by one estimate, about 60 percent of males between 20 and 24 already have bleeding gums—a sure sign that their teeth are well along the road to ruin. Healthy teeth and gums require minimal amounts of maintenance, but they need it every day. Those who can find the ten minutes or so daily that it takes to care for the teeth can probably enjoy them for the rest of their lives. Those who can't can expect to visit a brave new world filled with new acquaintances with names like *implant, bridge, extraction, caps* and *root canal*. This is not a place you ever want to visit. For more information on maintaining healthy teeth and gums, see Chapter Five.

CRACKED TOOTH SYNDROME?

Thought your mouth didn't give you enough problems? The men of the Nineties seem to have invented a new one: Cracked Tooth Syndrome.

CTS is defined by pain in a seemingly normal tooth that has a fine-line crack in it, one so small it might not show up on X-rays. Air can enter the fissure, irritating the nerve below. The causes of CTS are the byproduct of our stress-filled lives: the gnashing of teeth while sleeping, working or under tension (clenched jaw muscles are a clue). Even the popular antidote for stress—the gym—can cause problems; CTS is common among weight-lifters who clench their teeth while lifting. They can avoid the problem by using mouthguards (like those worn by football players), and everyone else can minimize it by fighting stress and being aware of that clench-jawed feeling. Caps on the affected teeth will eliminate the symptoms.

The Urinary Tract and the Reproductive System

As similar as are the male and female bodies, here is the one area where they are indisputably different. In the broadest terms, the difference comes down to an external genital and urinary system verses an internal one. Because so much of our reproductive system is out in the open, men are exposed to more traumas to their sexual organs than are women (as anyone who plays contact sports will quickly remind you). In fact, nearly 17 percent of men who suffered an episode of "significant testicular trauma" in childhood were found to have abnormalities in the quantity or quality of their sperm as adults, according to a study by the University of Wisconsin.

The primary external structures of the male reproductive system are the penis and testicles. The penis allows for the easy passage of urine and semen; the testicles—housed in the scrotum—produce sperm and testosterone, the male sex hormone. Inside the body, the structures are a bit less straightforward. The *urethra* is the tube that carries urine from the bladder to the opening at the end of the penis; it also does double duty as the conduit for semen during sex. Sperm is stored and matured in the *epididymis*, a thin, coiled tube that resides beside each testicle.

When the sperm is mature enough to do its job, it travels from the outside of the abdomen to the inside, up a canal called the *vas deferens* that stores the sperm and leads it to the urethra. The vas deferens terminates at the *prostate*, which links it to the urethra and adds (along with the *seminal vesicles* and the *bulbourethral glands*) the other components to the sperm that make up semen. As for the urinary system, the kidneys are linked to the bladder by the *ureters*. The bladder sits just above the prostate; urine must pass through a tube in that gland in order to reach the urethra.

Men's external genitalia are much easier to examine, and are generally less problematic than their female equivalents; a man is spared the seemingly innumerable trips to the gynecologist that are a part of a woman's routine. Our external sexual organs should make it much easier for men to stay apprised of their own sexual health. Unfortunately, most men never learn how to self-examine for testicular or prostate problems. If men were as diligent about examining their testicles as women are about checking the health of their breasts, then testicular cancer—the number-one cancer among men 20–35, despite a 95 percent cure rate—wouldn't be nearly the threat it is today. (The self-exam for testicular irregularities is described in Chapter Three.)

While the male body is a low-maintenence vehicle, it's certainly not a no-maintenance one. And there are a number of problem areas that affect men more than women, or that are entirely unique to us. But attending to the maintenance—in the form of a good diet, regular exercise and fighting stress—can go a long way toward steering you clear of the problems to which the male body is prone. In the coming chapters, you'll discover the best ways to perform the minimal maintenance work your body requires. Who knows? You might even be inspired to do an overhaul.

MEN'S BODIES THROUGH THE AGES

Since men's bodies are so much simpler than women's, you might suppose that they represent the basic blueprint for the human form. Wrong. We all started out as females, but somewhere along the second month of existence in the womb you fought the odds and became a male. Here are some of the crucial male/female developmental differences at various stages of life.

The Fetus:

At first, the embryo has all the equipment to become either sex. The only clue to its destiny is buried deep in the genetic code, in the twenty-third chromosome pair. In the sixth week of development, if the embryo has inherited a Y chromosome from its father, a gene signals the start of male development. In both sexes, hormones begin to prepare the brain for the changes of puberty a dozen years away.

At about eight weeks into the pregnancy, male and female fetuses are still virtually identical. Both have begun to create the ovaries or testicles that will determine gender. But it is not until the testicles begin to secrete male hormones that sexual differentiation begins to take shape. (If they don't secrete, the baby is born a genetic—but sterile—female.) At that point, the penis, scrotum, prostate and spermatic duct begin to form, and the die is cast.

Infant:

The skeletons of boys are slightly less mature than those of girls at birth. Some studies have suggested that newborn girls are slightly more responsive to touch and that infant boys spend more time awake. There is also evidence that boy infants respond somewhat earlier to visual stimuli, girls to sounds and smells.

Toddler:

Boys gain and pass girls in skeletal maturity by the end of the first year. At the age of 2, boys begin to show signs of greater aggressiveness. At 3, a slight, early female edge in verbal ability disappears—but by 10 or 11, it is back. Boys begin to show superiority in spatial skills at the age of 8 or so, and at 10 or 11, they start outperforming girls in math.

Adolescent:

Girls begin to fall behind in body strength. In both male and female, reproductive organs develop rapidly. Both spurt in height; when it is over, the average male will be 10 percent taller than the female. Meanwhile, the female superiority in verbal skills increases, as does the male edge in spatial skills and math.

Adult:

The mature woman carries twice as much body fat as a man. And the man carries 1.5 times as much muscle and bone. Because of the female hormone estrogen, which works to keep women's bodies in peak childbearing condition, women have some built-in health advantages—including more pliable blood vessels and the ability to process fat more efficiently and safely than men.

Old Age:

The male can continue sperm production into his late eighties and even early nineties. After menopause, the female's estrogen production drops off, and they lose some of the protection the hormone formerly provided. But the advantages of her fertile decades persist: blood vessels become more rigid more slowly, though eventually women's risk of cardiovascular disease will match that of men.

3 THE HEALTHY MAN

There are innumerable ways to improve nearly every aspect of your physical well being, but the first step is to get a concrete idea of how your various body systems are currently functioning and which ones need the most attention. The best way to accomplish this is to make an appointment with your doctor for a complete physical examination. There will be other tests later in the book that you can take at the gym, and others still you can address while you read this book, but the foundation for all that follows is the basic information on your overall state of health—and to determine that you need your doctor's help. And of course, he'll need your help, too.

THE PHYSICAL EXAMINATION

A physical exam should be an interactive experience. No, that doesn't mean that you get to perform an exam on your physician ("Cough please, Doctor"); it means that you have to be frank with him about your aches and pains, your diet, your lifestyle and many other aspects of yourself that you might not really want to dwell on. Good doctors are good listeners; the blood tests and proddings are important too, but the best doctors will pay attention to what you say—and don't say—about the way you live in your body. That means your job is to be as honest and as thorough as possible. You're not dropping off your VCR for service, you're here to work with your doctor to determine the state of your health and to improve it. That commitment goes both ways: If your doctor doesn't answer your questions completely, or is too rushed to spend adequate time with you, then it's time to look for a new physician.

Shopping around for the best doctor might be a lot to expect from men, especially since we have such a hard time dragging ourselves to any doctor, for any reason. Every year, women in this country account for 150 million more visits to the doctor than men; OB/GYN appointments make up some of this difference, but women are clearly more willing to seek medical attention than we are. A recent survey of 1,500 doctors conducted by a nonprofit group called the Men's Health Network confirms this: 94 percent of physicians believe men are less likely to seek medical attention than women, and 92 percent say that men are more likely to delay getting help—often until a problem becomes severe or even life-threatening. Waiting until an illness or disease has progressed before getting treatment means a higher death rate, and as we noted earlier men have a higher death rate at all ages throughout their lives. The reluctance to see a doctor may help explain why men die younger than women; as with smoking or exercise, getting regular exams is a "risk factor" that's entirely within your control.

So you've made an appointment for a physical. What can you do to get the most out of the time (and money) you'll spend in the doctor's office, and what should you expect him to do? The best thing you can do is make a list of any symptoms, pains or changes to your health that you've noticed since your last checkup. If you have a copy of your last medical evaluation, read it and see if you notice any differences between the state of your health then and now. Also, write down any questions you have, either specific ones about a complaint or more general ones ("What should I do about ear wax?"). Most people show up at the doctor's with a mental list of queries, and immediately forget their questions once the exam starts. Write it down, and take it with you.

What can you expect from the visit? Unless you live in a small town or pay out-of-pocket for your health care, you can probably expect to see an unfamiliar doctor. Ideally patients should have a long-term relationship with their physicians; they should know you, your habits, your problems and your health goals. As more health care is administered by health maintenance organizations (HMOs), that's less likely to happen. Since you may well be seeing an unknown doc, communication is that much more important. (To be fair, doctors are under more "cost-containment" pressure than ever before, and are encouraged to speed through routine exams. One study found that a doctor today spends an average of just *seventeen seconds* before interrupting a patient during an exam—so much for being a good listener.)

The physical usually starts with your medical history, and how your doctor handles this is often an indication of whether or not you're in capable hands. These are some must-ask questions: Have you ever been hospitalized? Any reactions to medications? Any allergies or extended illnesses? Does anyone in your family have cancer, and which kind? Does your father have a heart condition? Did any relatives die young? Do any close relatives have unusually high cholesterol? As the history continues, expect the questions to become more personal. Do you ever use drugs or alcohol? Smoke? Are you sexually active, and what is your orientation? Have you had an AIDS test? The final question your doctor asks is often the hardest to answer: In general, how are you feeling? You should give that one some thought long before reaching the exam room.

CHECKUP CHECKLIST

Some doctors will talk to you for a half-hour during an exam and run you through a full battery of tests; others might just check your blood pressure and call it *bueno*. How do you know if you're getting a good exam? The number of tests isn't a good yardstick, as some might not be indicated for your age or lifestyle. But don't leave the consulting room until you've at least discussed these with your doctor:

1. **Medical history.** The most crucial part of the exam.
2. **Head-to-toe physical.** Provides baseline for future exams, and should include an inch-by-inch skin exam.
3. **Testicular exam.** Screens out problems from cancer to varicoceles to hernias.
4. **Rectal exam.** Patients over 40 should have one, including a digital prostate exam.
5. **Urinalysis.** Measures sugar and protein levels in the urine and tests kidney function.
6. **Complete blood count (CBC).** Measures red blood cell count for anemia.
7. **SMAC blood test.** Tests liver, heart and kidney function; measures blood sugar, cholesterol, blood gases and electrolytes.
8. **Electrocardiogram (EKG).** Tests the heart's electrical impulses, which in turn gives a measure of how well it's moving blood through the chambers.
9. **HIV test.** If you haven't always used a condom, you should take it.

To screen for cancer, men between 20 and 39 should be examined every three years with particular attention to the mouth, testicles, skin, thyroid gland and lymph nodes. From age 40 to 49, those checkups should become annual events and add a digital rectal exam to the above tests. Above age 50, the annual tests should also include an exam for precancerous polyps in the colon with a special flexible viewer called a sigmoidoscope, a stool test to determine the presence of blood (a sign of colon cancer) and perhaps a prostate-specific antigen (PSA) test (See "The Prostate" later in this chapter).

The next phase is the physical exam and the collection of samples for testing. After urinating into the specimen cup provided, you'll be weighed and measured for height. Blood pressure will be assessed. The doctor will want blood for cholesterol and blood sugar tests, carbon-dioxide levels (a measure of cardiovascular health) and routine screenings of liver and kidney function. You might be asked if you want an AIDS test; if you've ever had unprotected sex or shared a needle with someone, the answer to this should definitely be "yes." From there, the doctor will examine your ears for a ruptured eardrum or impacted wax, shine a light in your eyes to observe your body's only visible blood vessels (high blood pressure can reveal itself as burst vessels within the eye), check your tonsils, thyroid gland and lymph nodes for swelling that might indicate infection and listen to your heart and lungs with a stethoscope.

Next the doctor will check your skin for any moles or lesions to make sure there are no signs of skin cancer. He'll check your reflexes with a small rubber hammer; your "kick response" gives a clue about the functioning of your peripheral nervous system. Then comes the unpleasant stuff: he'll ask you to drop your shorts so that he can examine your testicles for swelling (which might indicate cancer). He'll then ask you to "turn your head and cough"—this is to check for the presence of hernias, which most often appear as a bulge in the scrotum. Coughing causes the opening from the scrotum to the abdomen to close, and by placing his finger at that juncture the doctor can easily check for the presence of a hernia. Many doctors at this point will also slip on the dreaded rubber glove and ask you to bend over so that they can examine the prostate gland digitally. This is unpleasant but very necessary; it's the best way to check for swelling of the gland that can indicate cancerous or benign prostate enlargement, and if there is a problem an early diagnosis is key to successful treatment.

THE RESULTS OF YOUR EXAM

Ideally, you should have another appointment with your doctor to discuss the findings of the lab tests he ordered. More typically, you'll only be scheduled if a test reveals that there is a problem or the strong potential for one. Most men receive the result of blood work and other tests in the mail, perhaps accompanied by a short note from the doctor clarifying some of the scores and indicating areas that might present problems down the road. If you have further questions or are confused about the readouts, it's up to you to contact the doctor and ask for more explanation—in person, if necessary.

In the absence of an unusual test result indicating a serious underlying health condition, the areas where most men will find room for improvement is in their resting heart rates, blood pressure and cholesterol tests. Regular exercise and an improved diet can bring all of the results back into the normal range; if you're already in pretty good shape, these lifestyle improvements can pump you into the "optimal" category. If you're already under a doctor's care for high blood pressure or seriously high cholesterol, a conscientious diet and exercise program can allow you to reduce or even eliminate the medications you're taking to address these problems. Your doctor can help plan such a program—and only your doctor can decide when medication should be altered or reduced. Don't try to do that yourself.

Here are the ranges for the tests that reflect the state of your circulatory system:

RESTING HEART RATE	BLOOD PRESSURE	CHOLESTEROL
Optimal: 60 beats per minute	110/70 millimeters	180 ml/dec
Average: 72 to 80	120/80	220
Poor: 90 and above	140/90	240 and up

Your resting heart rate is a terrific indicator of how well your heart is working. As you train aerobically and the heart strengthens, your resting rate will drop to reflect your improved conditioning. (It's not unusual for elite athletes and marathoners to have resting rates below 50; Tour de France champion Miguel Indurain's is 28.) If you want to check your rate for improvement, take it at your wrist pulse-point first thing in the morning, before you get out of bed. Simply count the number of heartbeats that occur during a ten-second interval (use a clock with a second hand to measure this) and then multiply that number by six. The result will tell you the number of heartbeats over the course of a minute.

A NEW HEART TEST

A new technology allows doctors to get a much clearer picture of how your heart is working—and without expensive and invasive tests. The new device is called an ultra-fast CT (or computerized tomography) scanner, and it gives the clearest picture ever of how much buildup there is inside the arteries of your heart, which is the best way to determine whether you're at risk for a heart attack.

The ultrafast CT test, also marketed as "Heartscan," uses high-speed video imaging to take a snapshot of your heart and the surrounding arteries (and the buildup within). Best of all, the test is totally noninvasive and costs less than $400. Many feel that this is the heart test of the future, and will soon become a standard diagnostic tool. If you have risk factors for cardiac disease, ask your doctor whether ultrafast CT is the right diagnostic test for you.

A lowered blood pressure puts less stress on vital organs like the heart and kidneys. High blood pressure is also associated with stroke, and may indicate that there is already some hardening of the arteries present. The blood cholesterol level is harder to interpret. Everyone agrees that lower numbers are desirable, but higher readings don't necessarily make you a candidate for heart disease. A better indicator is the amount of high-density lipoprotein (HDL) in your blood; this is the protective substance that carries fat away from the walls of your arteries. The ratio of HDL to total cholesterol, according to some studies, is at least 15 percent more accurate than a simple cholesterol level in predicting heart disease. Any abnormal readings mean that you need to be retested two or three more times for a confirmed diagnosis.

There are two other test results to which you should pay particular attention. Inconspicuous among the laundry list of numbers on your lab readout is *creatinine,* a by-product of muscle-protein breakdown. Elevated levels can indicate undetected kidney disease; more importantly, a study of 11,000 high-blood-pressure patients conducted by Emory University confirms that high creatinine level *plus* high blood pressure can be a warning sign that a patient is at risk for early death from heart disease or stroke. The Emory researchers think that this warning sign is much more valuable than cholesterol as a predictor of disease. The normal range on a lab readout is 0.7 to 1.5; patients with levels above 1.7 had a mortality rate from stroke and heart disease that was more than *triple* that of patients in the normal range. If you fall into that category, talk to your doctor. High creatinine levels can result from weight training since they reflect the breakdown of muscle protein, so lay off the iron for a couple of days before your exam so that you don't skew the results.

Another important test result is the one for *blood glucose.* This is critical because it is the major predictor for adult-onset diabetes—and as many as half the people with this problem are unaware that they have it. Diabetes, a condition in which the insulin balance within the body becomes disrupted, is the U.S.'s fourth-largest killer. Complications from the disease are horrible: blindness, kidney failure, amputation from poor circulation, heart disease and impotence—which strikes 60 percent of men with diabetes. The disease is treatable (and responds well to diet and exercise) but early diagnosis and intervention are the keys. Be sure to ask your doctor about your blood glucose level, especially if you have a family history of diabetes.

AVOIDING MALPRACTICE

Every year, hundreds of thousands of Americans are seriously injured through medical negligence in hospitals; about 80,000 of them die. That death toll is worse than that from AIDS and traffic fatalities combined. Your odds of becoming a malpractice victim are directly proportional to how much medical care you receive. If you're young and healthy, you're probably not susceptible to the things that most often put people in hospitals—strokes, heart attacks and cancer. But you do face one big threat: accidents. A spill on a motorcycle or a fall from a ladder could suddenly land you on a gurney.

Nobody is suggesting that you avoid doctors or hospitals when you need them. But there are ways to cut your odds of feeling like a clay pigeon on a shooting range when you seek help. To be savvy about your medical care, follow these rules:

- Stick with research hospitals. As a general rule, the chances of getting excellent treatment are better at a university or research hospital, where physicians and staff are more likely to keep up with cutting-edge advances and to have the latest medical equipment on hand. The doctors are also more likely to be leaders in their fields. A Harvard malpractice study revealed less negligence in teaching hospitals than in other institutions.
- Select physicians carefully. "Don't select a doctor based on factors such as ethnicity, location or religion," Wachsman says. "Pick a physician based on his or her merits." That means speaking with patients who have direct experience with that doctor.
- Find out where your doctor did his medical training and whether he's certified in his field. After graduating from medical school, a doctor can practice any kind of medicine, even surgery, without advanced training. Make sure your doctor is certified by one of two dozen specialty boards recognized by the American Medical Association. You can find out his

or her status by calling the American Board of Medical Specialties at 800-776-CERT.
- Play detective. Determine whether anyone has filed suit against your doctor (a "defendants' index" at the local courthouse will tell you if he or she has ever been sued there). Also contact your state's medical board, which is empowered to discipline physicians. Keep in mind, however, that a lot of watchdog licensing boards are toothless pussycats. Consumer advocate Ralph Nader's group, Public Citizen, regularly ranks states by how well they keep lousy practitioners out of circulation. (For $15, Public Citizen will send you a list of doctors in your state who have been disciplined. Write to its Publications Department, 2000 P St. N.W., Suite 600, Washington, DC 20036.) According to the group, some of the more conscientious states are West Virginia, Oklahoma, North Dakota, Georgia and Iowa. Among the clunkers are Massachusetts, New Hampshire, Pennsylvania and the District of Columbia, which in 1993 had the distinction of not disciplining a single one of its 4,100 doctors.
- Be inquisitive and assertive. "You absolutely have to do research, ask questions and never sign a consent form unless you're 100 percent sure of what's going on," advises Sandra Gainer, associate director of the National Center for Patients' Rights in New York City. "Stop your doctor and say, 'Explain this to me.' You just have to speak up." Never fear getting a second opinion: In fact, when it comes to major procedures, many insurance companies now require doing so.

• Know what malpractice is. Only one of the following two scenarios constitutes true malpractice. Can you figure out which one? (1) Your doctor gives you penicillin, a drug you've never taken before, for strep throat. You have a severe allergic reaction, end up in the hospital for two weeks and miss months of work.

(2) A year later, a doctor fails to read in your chart that you're allergic to penicillin. You end up in the hospital again.

Only in the second case is your doctor negligent. Why? Because he or she had the means to learn of your allergy and failed to do so.

SYMPTOMS YOU SHOULD NEVER IGNORE

By simply going to the doctor for a checkup, you've put yourself in a rare group among men. Far too many men wait until they are seriously ill before darkening a doctor's doorstep. This accounts for the 150 million fewer doctor visits by men than women every year—and quite possibly, for our shorter lifespans. For many men, acknowledging a symptom—and the possibility of a trip to the doctor, or worse—is a sign of weakness, and a fate worse than death. For men ignoring symptoms is the rule, not the exception.

The good news is that many symptoms deserve to be ignored. The problem is deciding which ones warrant a professional opinion. Generally, any symptom that persists over time should be addressed; even a stuffy nose should be looked at if it's been that way for weeks. Here are the most important common symptoms and their implications.

Headaches

You don't have to be as hypochondrical as a Woody Allen character to think that your headache is a brain tumor—it's a common reaction, but an uncommon cause. For a tumor to be the problem, the headache would have to be relatively constant and focused on one area of the head. More likely culprits are stress, fatigue, sinus infection or a hangover. But if headaches strike with daily or even weekly frequency, it's time to see a doctor.

The most important recent advances in headache research have significance for the more than 45 million Americans who get headaches regularly, and for virtually all of us who get them at least occasionally. Hardest hit, of course, is the 10 percent of the population who suffer from the most debilitating types of headaches: migraines and cluster headaches. These are now believed to be associated with a drop in levels of serotonin, the brain chemical that's popularly linked with relaxation and plays a role in the constriction of blood vessels. When serotonin levels decrease, blood vessels become inflamed, exerting pain along the scalp and forehead. Why that pain assumes so many forms and degrees of severity remains a mystery.

But the serotonin/headache connection has led to the development of the first remedy specifically designed to combat the notoriously difficult-to-treat migraine headache, and one that's somewhat effective against the more demonic pain of cluster headaches as well. Sometimes it's even used to ward off the mere possibility of a headache—among susceptible athletes who are about to engage in competition, for example. Formerly available only in an injectable form, an oral preparation is also now available.

When should a headache steer you toward the doctor's office? "If someone has a severe headache for the first time in his life, that's one indication to investigate," says Ninan T. Mathew, M.D., director of the Houston Headache Clinic. A headache that comes on very suddenly, steadily worsens or is accompanied by other problems such as weakness, fever, seizures or mental confusion should prompt a trip to a physician as well. And any headache that regularly interferes with your exercise routine or other aspects of daily life is worth special attention.

Tension headaches

Cause: stress, fatigue. The most common headache type. Symptoms: dull, constant throbbing; tightness in the facial muscles and around the scalp. Pain can be on one or both sides of the head; it can feel like a tight band around your head. Duration: anywhere from an hour to several days, though more than half a day is unusual. Relief: heat or ice pack; a soothing bath or shower; aspirin, ibuprofen or acetaminophen; stress-reduction techniques like controlled breathing or meditation. Anti-depressant medicines may be effective against some chronic tension headaches.

Migraine headaches

Cause: possibly a genetic deficiency in the way mood-enhancing serotonin is released in the brain. Can be precipitated by stress, sleep deprivation and certain foods. About 17 percent of women and 5 percent of men get them.

Symptoms: debilitating throbbing, usually on one side of the head, often accompanied by nausea, vomiting and sensitivity to light or noise. Some people get a warning "aura" before the attack, from visual disturbances to a curious sense of well-being. Duration: two hours to two days. May strike as often as several times a week or only once every few years. Relief: sumatriptan. An herbal remedy known as feverfew has been shown to reduce the frequency, duration and severity of migraines, but it must be taken consistently.

Cluster headaches

Cause: unknown. Though they're rare, afflicting only about 1 percent of the population, 90 percent of those affected are men. Potential triggers include alcohol and naps. Symptoms: severe, searing, drill-like pain centered around one eye. Duration: a few minutes to several hours. Clusters are actually waves of headaches that can go on for weeks or even months, hitting one to eight times a day and usually at exactly the same time each day and the same seasons each year (usually spring or fall). May go away for years, only to return. Relief: anything that works. Some patients find breathing pure oxygen helps; others have found relief with sumatriptan or Indocin, a prescription painkiller that actually causes headaches more often than it cures them; in some people, however, it's effective. Physicians may try other prescription medications, including antidepressants, as well.

Exertional headaches

Cause: anything from exercise to sex. Afflicts about 10 percent of headache sufferers but is more common in men. Can be frightening. Symptoms: pain that runs the spectrum from mild, tension-like discomfort to severe migraine. Duration: anywhere from a few seconds to several hours. Relief: Some people get exertional headaches when they begin a new exercise regimen or return to one after a break. Exercising for shorter periods of time may solve the problem. However, getting regular headaches as a result of exercise is a different situation. Many people who experience such headaches can banish or control them using Indocin.

Sinus headaches

"Sinus headaches are misdiagnosed by family doctors, and over-diagnosed," says Dr. Seymour Diamond. "Even people with severe sinusitis—infection of the sinuses—rarely get headaches from it." More likely, you have a migraine, cluster or tension headache. True sinus headaches are caused by pressure on swollen sinus linings, and tend to get worse through the day. They are cured by eliminating the underlying sinus infection.

HOW TO MAKE YOUR HEADACHES HISTORY

As many as 90 percent of headaches are avoidable. If you suffer from chronic headaches, keep a journal tracking their onset, severity and duration. Doing so may help you identify and eliminate one or more of the following common triggers:

- Inertia. Exercise is most effective against tension headaches but has also been shown to reduce migraines. However, exercising during a migraine episode can exacerbate the pain.
- Alcohol. In some people, the trigger is a specific type of alcoholic beverage, most commonly wine.
- Hunger. Hunger headaches result from overzealous dieting, skipping meals or fasting.
- Sleep. Poor or inconsistent sleep patterns can be a trigger. Some people experience these headaches on weekends without realizing why.
- Caffeine. If you're hooked, at least avoid caffeine when you feel a headache coming on.
- Stress. For chronic tension headache sufferers, employing a stress-management technique, such as meditation, the "relaxation response" or biofeedback, can be helpful.
- Medicines. Frequent use of aspirin or similar painkilling drugs can cause "rebound" headaches.
- Tobacco. Many migraine sufferers find that cigarette smoke is a headache trigger, and cluster headaches are more common among smokers.
- Eyestrain. If you find that reading, going to the movies or driving gives you a headache, you may simply need corrective lenses. Also, bright light can trigger some migraines.
- Altitude. If you live in the lowlands but go to higher altitudes to ski, climb or hike, take it easy during your first day or two out.

For more information, contact the National Headache Foundation at 800–843–2256.

Chest pain

Chances are that at some time or another you're going to have to decide what to do about pain or discomfort in your chest. That decision may have to be made in a hurry, under stress and without benefit of a second opinion. The farther the pain is from the center of the chest, the *less* likely it is to be a heart attack. If the pain inches into the arm or jaw or is accompanied by nausea or sweating, call 911. If you're unsure what to do, have someone take you to the emergency room—or at the very least, call your doctor. According to Isadore Rosenfeld, M.D., author of the book *Symptoms*, "Any adult who suddenly experiences discomfort in the chest must assume that it has something to do with the heart. If it turns out to be a false alarm, you've lost nothing. But if it indeed was the heart, you may have saved your life." You're much better off safe than sorry with this symptom. For young, healthy men the most likely explanation is that you've pulled a muscle in the chest wall, from exercise or even coughing.

Now, if your heart is not the source of the trouble, what else can it be? The chest is a very busy place, with several different organs and nerves, all of which can produce symptoms simulating those of a heart attack. Among the possible perpetrators are the lungs; the esophagus; a hiatal hernia; nerve irritation; and the muscles of the chest wall.

The True Heart Attack

Many people think that cardiac pain is sharp and stabbing or that it arises in the left side of the chest. In fact, the typical pain of a heart attack is pressurelike. It is located mainly in the center of the chest, behind the breastbone, whence it can radiate to either shoulder, through to the back, the arms or the hands (it's usually but not always the left arm, the left shoulder and the left hand), the jaw or the ears.

If closure of the artery is complete, the symptoms do not disappear when you stop whatever it is you're doing. A nitroglycerin tablet under the tongue may give relief for a few minutes, but then the pain recurs. The patient is pale, weak and short of breath, breaks out into a cold sweat and is usually very apprehensive. There may be a cough, palpitations (an awareness of the heartbeat), dizziness and lightheadedness. Things may improve somewhat in the sitting position.

That's the description of a classic heart attack, but the picture may vary considerably, depending on your particular threshold for pain, as well as on the severity and the location of the damage within the heart. Indeed, a heart attack may be "silent" and unrecognized by the victim, who may either live through it despite a lack of treatment—or die.

Angina pectoris is another cardiac condition that produces chest pain similar in nature to a heart attack: pressing or squeezing, often beginning in the middle of the chest and radiating to the left arm, shoulder or hand. Angina is less severe, is not usually associated with weakness, sweating or other symptoms and, most important, is of short duration. An anginal attack is frequently precipitated by some unusual stress—physical (like walking too fast up a hill, especially in cold or windy weather) or mental (like a heated argument or an exciting football game) and disappears quickly when the exertion or stress is over. Angina usually reflects a partial blockage of the coronary arteries by arteriosclerosis rather than the complete obstruction that causes most heart attacks. Repeated or increasing frequency of angina, especially when it comes on at rest or during the night, is a warning that a heart attack is imminent. See your doctor immediately!

The heart can generate another kind of pain, due to an entirely different disorder, one that affects the wrapper that envelops it—the pericardium. When the pericardium becomes inflamed or infected by a virus, the result is pericarditis. Its symptoms mimic those of a heart attack, except that the pain worsens when you take a deep breath.

The only sure way to tell these two very different conditions apart is by a good physical exam and an electrocardiogram. Never make that diagnosis yourself. Simple viral pericarditis usually runs a benign course, requiring only rest and aspirin for treatment. However, the condition may also stem from more serious causes—everything from a heart attack to a cancer that's spread to the pericardium. Medical treatment will depend on the underlying cause.

Chest Pain from the Lungs

There will be times when you think your chest pain is coming from the heart, but it's actually originating in the lungs. That can happen in two common conditions of which you should be aware. One is dangerous and requires immediate attention; the other can make you really sick but is not usually a threat to life. Let's look at the less serious situation first. It's fairly easy to recognize in its typical form.

Pleurisy

The lungs are covered by a two-layered envelope called the pleura, which can become inflamed, irritated or infected, a condition called pleurisy. If you have pleurisy, the two layers of this lung wrapper rub together so that you feel a sharp pain near the end of each deep breath. The pleura are a particularly attractive target for viruses. Viral pleurisy is often accompanied by fever and a cough. Pneumonia also frequently begins as pleurisy.

In either case, because it hurts so much to breathe deeply, you find yourself taking only shallow breaths. Moving about doesn't usually aggravate matters, but coughing really hurts. Viral pleurisy usually lasts for a few days, then clears up on its own. The pain goes away because the pleura produce a lubricating fluid between the two layers, so that now when you breathe they glide smoothly over each other without friction. The outlook for and treatment of the pain of pleurisy, however, depend on what's causing it. There's usually nothing to worry about in simple viral pleurisy. However, pleurisy can result from a number of serious underlying illnesses. One such disorder, a blood clot to the lungs, is often heralded by pleurisy.

Embolism

A clot originating somewhere in the body (usually in the legs or the pelvis) travels along a network of veins into the lung, where it becomes lodged. In so doing, it cuts off the circulation to a portion of the lung, damaging it. The pleura are irritated in the process, causing the pain. The severity of the attack depends on the size of the blood clot and how much pulmonary tissue is injured.

So the spectrum of symptoms in a pulmonary embolism can range from sudden pain anywhere in the chest, which worsens when you breathe, to spitting blood, a sharp fall in blood pressure (shock) and even death. If you suspect an embolism because of any of these symptoms, you've got to move just as fast as if it were a heart attack. The consequences are potentially as serious.

Just as there are factors which predispose you to a heart attack, so are there circumstances which should lead you to think of a lung embolism. They include:

- Recent phlebitis, an inflammation of the veins in the legs. A clot forms within the vein, and a piece breaks off and travels to the lung. This is most likely to happen if you have been confined to bed for some reason or have been sitting for hours in a car or on an airplane.
- Injury to the legs can damage the veins too, causing clot formation. If the affected vessel is situated deep in the leg, you may not be aware of this injury-induced phlebitis until the embolism actually occurs.
- Prolonged bed rest results in sludging of the blood flow and so predisposes to clot formation. As a rule of thumb: No matter what it is that has put you to bed, get up and get moving as soon as you possibly can.
- Almost any operation, especially one in the pelvis, leaves you more vulnerable to traveling blood clots.

As a general rule, chest pain which has the characteristics of pleurisy (it hurts when you breathe deeply and especially when you cough), while not always a medical emergency, is something that should be evaluated by your doctor quickly.

There is one rather dramatic condition which can cause sudden chest pain and shortness of breath together. That's what happens when a portion of one lung suddenly collapses. This condition, called *spontaneous pneumothorax* is usually the result of the rupture of a small blister on the lung, which allows air to escape into the chest cavity, where the resulting pressure can lead to the collapse of part or all of the lung. Before that rupture occurs, there are no symptoms. Pneumothorax can also result if an injection is given in the chest wall and the needle is inserted too deeply. If you ever receive such an injection and suddenly become short of breath, you'll know why! Under whatever circumstances it occurs, you must see your doctor as soon as possible to prevent more of the lung from collapsing.

Heartburn

You've been moderate in your eating and drinking, yet when you lie down, swallow, eat a large meal or bend over, you feel a burning sensation in your lower chest and upper abdomen. Instinctively, you stand up or drink some liquids and you feel better. Diagnosis: heartburn. Heartburn results from the acid in your stomach backing up into your food pipe (esophagus). The muscle designed to prevent this from happening sometimes goes lax, causing reflux of the acid and the characteristic burning sensation. This is most likely to happen when a portion of the stomach slips up through the diaphragm and into the chest (you then have a hiatus hernia).

If you have "heartburn" and are in a high-risk group for heart disease by virtue of your sex (male), your age (over 40) and other risk factors (high blood pressure, high cholesterol, bad family history, diabetes, cigarette smoking), you should have an electrocardiogram and a stress test to make sure that what you're suffering from is indeed a reflux of acid into the food pipe and not cardiac pain.

Fatigue

"Healthy" fatigue is the wasted feeling you might have at the end of a workout in which you've really pushed yourself. Persistent fatigue that hits you even when you're well rested is a warning sign. You could simply be working out too hard and not giving your body time to recover (see

"Overtraining" in Chapter Ten). Disrupted sleep patterns can also give you that leaden feeling. Any significant physical or emotional ill—from a cold to a depression—can leave you fatigued, either from lack of sleep or from the stress that the illness inflicts on your body. Fatigue can also be the result of lifestyle: staying up too late, eating poorly, not exercising, drinking to excess, smoking, being overweight or burning the candle at both ends. In addition, a variety of prescription and over-the-counter medications—including those for blood pressure, allergy, motion sickness, sleeping disorders, heart problems and psychological ills—can leave you dragging. If it occurs during the winter, fatigue might be the result of seasonal affective disorder (SAD), the metabolic slow-down that some people experience as a response to lack of sunlight during that time of year.

Among the more serious physiological causes of fatigue are mononucleosis, chronic fatigue syndrome, a low-grade infection, diabetes or a low blood-sugar level. Hepatitis or a malfunctioning thyroid can also be the cause. Fatigue might also signal cardiopulmonary problems like plaque buildup in the coronary arteries, pleurisy or embolism—or even a minor heart attack that's gone unnoticed. If your unexplained fatigue lasts for more than two weeks, it's time to see the doctor.

Bleeding

Dark blood in the stool (resulting in a tarlike appearance) can signal bleeding somewhere in the intestinal tract, perhaps from polyps in the colon. Bright-colored blood, on the other hand, probably comes from hemorrhoids. Occasional nosebleeds are no sweat, but freeflowing ones two or three times a week may signal high blood pressure or chronic allergies. The tendency to bleed easily or profusely can be a sign of leukemia, especially if accompanied by fatigue. A little bleeding in the gums is okay if you're new to flossing or haven't been brushing regularly; more than that indicates a periodontal problem. In smokers, persistent bleeding in the mouth might indicate oral cancer.

Bruises

If you bruise easily, that should be evaluated; it may mean that your blood is low in platelets, the component that helps your blood clot. Bruising may indicate a bad reaction to over-the-counter or prescribed drugs, especially anticoagulants, aspirin, antihistamines, anesthetics, penicillin, antidepressants, cortisone or anticonvulsants. It may also be a sign of a deficiency in vitamin C, riboflavin or folic acid if the symptom is accompanied by bleeding gums. Bruising can even be a sign of HIV infection. A tendency to bruise or bleed easily might indicate leukemia, especially if fatigue is also present; it's also a symptom of aplastic anemia, allergies, infections and a blood disorder called thrombocytopenic purpura.

Heavy sweating

An overactive thyroid or being overweight can cause heavy sweating, as can a simple fever. Sweating with chest pain may signal angina or a heart attack; if it accompanies faintness, nausea, panting, a rapid pulse or clammyness it could indicate shock. Sweating combined with hand tremors are a sign of hyperthyroidism. Drenching sweats (not related to weather or exercise) or night sweats that soak the sheets indicate that an infection is present, and may also indicate leukemia.

Coughing

Coughing can signal a cold, pneumonia, influenza, gastrointestinal reflux (stomach acids splashing back into the esophagus) or even lung cancer; a blood clot or tumor in the lungs might also be suspected. Coughing can also point to an environmental irritant, from smoking to fumes to molds. "Productive" coughs (those that bring forth mucus or any other substance) means the body is trying to rid itself of something, but if it persists past one week seek help—and do so immediately if you cough up blood. Persistent unproductive coughs might mean an underlying heart or lung problem, especially if accompanied by chest pain or shortness of breath. With any cough that lasts past a week (unrelated to a cold), see the doctor.

Hoarseness

Unless you have a cold or have been screaming at a ballgame, this bears investigation. The more benign possibilities are smoking, postnasal drainage, infection, stress or a chronic irritation of the vocal cords. More serious causes include growths on the vocal cords; these strike men more often than women, and may be benign, precancerous or cancerous. Smokers may suspect cancer of the voicebox. Hoarseness from yelling or talking too much will disappear within three days. If it persists beyond that, or is accompanied by difficulty with swallowing or chest pain, see your doctor immediately.

Abdominal pain

Usually this is the price of an overactive appetite, but it can indicate appendicitis if the pain begins in the middle of the abdomen and moves to your lower-right abdomen (near the front point of your hip bone). Persistent or spasmodic pain centered on one side of the lower abdomen—especially if accompanied by gas, bloating, nausea, constipation or diarrhea—may point to irritable bowel syndrome. Other suspected illnesses are ulcers, colitis, pancreatitis, gallbladder disease, diverticulitis, or cancers of the stomach, large intestine or pancreas. All-over pain in the abdomen probably means a bowel problem; try a diet of clear liquids for two days. If that's no help, see the doctor. It could be a bowel obstruction or a hernia.

Weight loss

Sudden, unexplained weight loss always warrants a trip to the doctor. Unless you've radically upped your aerobic work while dieting severely (which is the wrong method for long-term weight loss), this is always a very serious symptom. Illnesses that can bring on sudden weight loss include hyperthyroidism, pernicious anemia, Addison's disease, anorexia, diabetes, tuberculosis and several forms of cancer. If accompanied by skin lesions, fatigue or difficulty in breathing, this symptom could indicate AIDS

Mysterious lumps

Lumps can mean anything from a small benign growth to cancer. Lumps may come from sources as diverse as insect bites, cysts, swollen sweat glands and a host of skin diseases. Lumps on the neck, armpits or groin can mean that the body's lymph system is fighting off a disease, or could indicate Hodgkin's disease—a form of cancer that's highly curable if it's caught early. Painless lumps on the joints of the arms or legs are a sign of rheumatic fever. Lumps under the earlobes and accompanied by pain and difficulty in swallowing indicate mumps. Other lumps can indicate migrating internal organs, abscesses, hernias or obstructed veins. Go to the doctor for a lump that doesn't disappear on its own after 10 days or so to rule out the more serious possibilities.

Erection problems

Many men think of erectile trouble—difficulty in obtaining or maintaining an erection—as an indication of a psychological or relationship problem, not a physical symptom. This certainly can be the case: stress, fatigue, depression or unresolved marital issues like infidelity can all play themselves out in the bedroom. (Even witnessing natural childbirth has been known to cause impotence in husbands.) But 75 percent of the time the problem has a physical cause. Impotence can be a sign of vascular problems, diabetes or high blood pressure. Drugs prescribed for ulcers, epilepsy, high blood pressure, hormonal imbalances or chronic pain can have potency problems as a side effect. Prostate surgery can damage nerves to the penis, as can drugs designed to reduce the size of the prostate. An occasional problem with erections is perfectly normal; it happens to most men from time to time. But if erection problems have been ongoing for months then it's time to see your doctor.

Urinary problems

Loss of bladder control is *not* a normal part of aging for men, and any ongoing problems in this area really need to be addressed by an M.D. Other urinary symptoms that warrant a trip to the doctor include a weak or interrupted urinary stream; difficulty starting urination; frequent need to urinate, especially at night; dribbling after you think you've completely emptied your bladder; painful urination; or persistent pain in the lower back, pelvis or lower abdomen. Difficulty in urinating combined with lethargy might indicate kidney failure; constant desire to urinate combined with abdominal pain, fever, and cloudy or light red urine points to a bacterial infection of the kidneys. Pain that starts in the back and moves into the urinary tract probably indicates a kidney stone.

Aches, pains and anomalies are your body's early-warning system. As such, they shouldn't be ignored; if they persist, see your doctor. They also shouldn't be ignored *by* your doctor. If symptoms persist and your doctor can't explain them, get another opinion and have any tests you've undergone repeated. Doctors do make mistakes. Keep listening to your body and keep looking until you find someone who can help you discover what it's trying to tell you.

CAN ILLNESS MAKE YOU WELL?

One of the basic principles of healing is: interpret the symptom and find the cure. But a new philosophy of addressing ills, called "Darwinian medicine," says just the opposite. For the Darwinians, sickness may actually be good for you.

The logic is that fighting off certain symptoms of an illness may be counterproductive, even harmful. People with colds take anti-fever medications, for example, yet studies at the Johns Hopkins School of Hygiene and Public Health show those who don't fight their fevers get well sooner. The fever helps the body fight and kill the cold virus. Some diseases like malaria live on the body's supply of iron, so the body "hides" iron in the liver as a defense mechanism. But a doctor may find that the patient has "iron-poor blood" and order additional iron supplements—which is just what the invading organism wants.

Our bodies and the diseases that prey on them have evolved over eons by natural selection: survival of the fittest. Sometimes modern medicine can outsmart the body's own defenses. The medical Darwinians have recognized this, and are trying to adapt treatments to reflect this new thinking. The body has a remarkable ability to cure itself. That's the reason why so many symptoms clear up on their own, and why it's sometimes best to leave them alone.

MEN'S SPECIAL HEALTH PROBLEMS AND CONCERNS

The Heart and Circulatory System

You'll encounter a great deal of information in this book about the heart, and especially about the way the entire circulatory system responds to exercise and a proper diet. There's a good reason for this: heart disease is men's worst enemy. If you take nothing else from this book, at least remember this: Heart disease is the greatest killer of American males, and in almost all cases it's totally preventable.

Perhaps the most feared aspect of heart disease is the catastrophic event known as a *heart attack*. What is a heart attack? Simply, it is the cutting off of the supply of blood to a part of the heart, resulting in the severe damage or death of the tissue at that site. (The medical term for heart attack, *myocardial infarction*, literally means "death of heart muscle.") A heart attack is the final stage of the gradual narrowing of the arteries, called *atherosclerosis*, that nourish the heart itself. (When this narrowing occurs in the arteries leading to the brain, brain tissue can die, resulting in a *stroke*.) When one artery becomes so clogged from atherosclerosis or a blood clot that blood can no longer reach that part of the heart, the rhythm of the heartbeat is interrupted—the heart either stops pumping partially or altogther. If surgery isn't quickly performed to clear or bypass the clogged artery, death is the inevitable result. All too often, the heart attack *itself* is the first and only symptom that a person has of coronary-artery disease; roughly 1.5 million Americans will experience a heart attack this year, and one-third of them will die from it.

For those who already have some form of heart disease there are a number of drug therapies and surgical options that didn't exist even ten years ago—from alpha- and beta-blockers to balloon angioplasty—that are literal life-savers, and coronary-artery bypass surgery is now practically a routine operation. For healthy men who want to steer clear of cardiac problems, the news is even better: regular aerobic exercise along with relatively minor lifestyle changes can go a long way towards insuring that the most lethal killer of American men doesn't pay you a visit.

Later chapters will deal with additional specifics concerning nutrition, stress reduction and exercise, but here is a quick checklist of the changes you can make to improve your heart today—and to avoid the deadly consequences of heart disease tomorrow.

Quit Smoking. You'll be doing both your heart and your lungs an enormous favor. By now you probably know about the damage smoking does to your lungs, but that burning tobacco leaf also hurts your heart. The average smoker is more than twice as likely as a nonsmoker to have a heart attack, and dies from them twice as often. Researchers at Oxford University recently discovered that smokers in their thirties and forties suffer five times as many heart attacks as their nonsmoking counterparts. Smoking contributes to atherosclerosis—a leading cause of heart disease and stroke—by causing an imbalance in nerve impulses in blood vessels, causing them to constrict. That constriction, in turn raises blood pressure. Nicotine also causes the heart rate to speed up. The Mayo Clinic of Rochester, Minnesota, reports that smoking permanently damages the carotid arteries (the ones that carry blood to your brain). This may explain why the risk for stroke is also 50 percent higher for smokers. And the University of California at San Francisco recently found that even secondhand smoke causes blood platelets to become sticky, forming clots that can disrupt the flow of blood to the heart or brain.

Start Exercising. A sensible exercise program can greatly reduce your risk of heart disease. Stanford University researchers found that men and women who run on a regular basis have significantly lower cholesterol levels than do nonexercisers. Even moderate fitness levels are associated with strikingly reduced risk of death. According to David Goldstein, M.D., medical director of the Fitness Institute in Ontario, Canada, writing in *The Physician and Sportsmedicine*: "Research has shown that moderate regular exercise [stationary bicycling for forty minutes a day, three days a week, for example] reduces mild hypertension in sedentary, middle-aged subjects who are not taking blood pressure medication." And the benefits of exercise certainly don't stop with your heart: better circulation, better breathing, greater strength, less fat, a clearer head and better self-image. According to Dr. Frans Wacker of Yale University, "Exercise may work synergistically to help control a host of independent risk factors for coronary heart disease, including obesity, stress, high blood pressure and high levels of blood lipids; in addition, it helps stimulate or reinforce other positive lifestyle changes such as better nutrition or smoking cessation." What are you waiting for?

Men may have a disproportionate level of heart disease when compared to women, but we also have a built-in advantage when it comes to building aerobic strength—the ability of the heart to use and transport oxygen. "Aerobic" exercise takes its name from the Greek word for "air," because during this type of exercise blood is continually pumped to the large muscles of the body, forcing the heart and lungs to replenish the blood with oxygen. The heart becomes more efficient the more it is used, pumping more blood with less effort. The heart muscle itself expands in size and builds larger vessels to supply itself with more blood to meet the extra work it's called upon to do (just the opposite of what happens in the case of atherosclerosis).

This increase in heart-muscle mass and lung capacity is the engine behind all of the direct and secondary benefits we get from aerobic exercise—especially a reduced risk of heart disease. In addition to the improved capacity of the heart muscle, aerobic exercise also causes changes in blood chemistry and composition. Overall cholesterol drops, the ratio of "good" to "bad" lipoproteins improves, and the level of circulating blood lipids called triglycerides falls; the net effect is that blood is less likely to stick to artery walls and cause obstructions—in fact, the build-up in your arteries can reverse itself by regular aerobic exercise (especially when combined with a low-fat diet). Aerobic exercise also causes a rise in the body's metabolic rate, so you burn more calories even when you're not exercising. This helps you lose fat, which also helps the heart.

"Anaerobic" exercise, on the other hand, is defined by short bursts of strenuous exertion—as with weight lifting or sprinting—as opposed to long periods of sustained effort. To fuel this exertion during exercise, the body uses its small stores of a carbohydrate called glycogen; oxygen isn't called for as a fuel, so the heart and lungs don't get a workout. Anaerobic exercise has its own benefits; the more muscle you have, the greater the percentage of lean-muscle mass your body contains, and muscle needs more fuel than fat to sustain itself. So adding muscle mass can help you burn fat even when you're not exercising.

Both aerobic and anaerobic exercise will be explored in much more detail in Chapter Ten, but for now the important thing to remember is this: aside from the cessation of smoking and good nutrition (which will be discussed in Chapter Six) regular aerobic workouts are the single best way to strengthen the heart and improve the functioning of your entire circulatory system. If stressed in a *positive* way by the demands of a regular aerobic schedule, your heart and lungs will grow stronger and better able to meet the rigors of life; if stressed in a *negative* way—by smoking, a sedentary existence and a bad diet—then their capacity to function will be greatly diminished, as will the overall quality of your life. And besides, it's enjoyable. As Dr. Frans Wacker notes, "Unlike many health-enhancing measures, exercise adds something pleasant to one's existence rather than taking something away. "

Cut Out the Fat. Eating less fat means eating less of the stuff that clogs arteries, and the less fat you eat the less body fat you'll have to lose down the road. Every extra pound of fat you carry has to be supported by an additional *15 to 25 miles* of blood vessels, putting an obvious and unnecessary strain on the entire circulatory system. The USDA says a normal, healthy man should get no more than 30 percent of his calories from fat—and most nutrition experts recommend a maximum of 20 to 25 percent. (Dean Ornish, M.D., the San Francisco-based low-fat apostle, puts his cardiac patients on a 10 percent fat diet, and has had demonstrable success in reversing heart disease.) Eat lean meats like fish and chicken or lean cuts of beef or pork. Dry beans, soy products and peas are good alternate protein sources. When you do eat meat, trim off the fat; avoid meat sauces made with butter, cream, lard or shortening; and bake or broil instead of fry. And by all means avoid dairy products made with whole milk; skim or low-fat milk is the better way to go. If you always put premium in your tank, your engine will run better.

Cut Out the Cholesterol. The National Cholesterol Education Program recommends that you take in less than 300 milligrams of cholesterol a day. Unfortunately, according to the American Medical Association, the average American eats an extra 350 to 450 milligrams daily. This can lead to a buildup of plaque on the walls of your blood vessels, one of the leading causes of heart attack and stroke. So clean out those pipes. Exercise is one way to reduce your cholesterol level; it can lower both total cholesterol and raise the "good" HDL cholesterol—possibly by helping to reduce body fat. Substituting low-fat foods for those high in saturated fat is another. Generally, avoid fatty cuts of meat, egg yolks, whole milk and whole-milk products—ice cream, butter- or cream-rich sauces and hydrogenated oils. The new labels on food packages make it easier than ever to see exactly what's contained in a product, so use those numbers to keep a diary of how much cholesterol and fat you're consuming during the day.

Watch Your Blood Pressure. Almost 60 million Americans have high blood pressure, or hypertension, which dramatically increases the risk of heart disease and stroke. Millions of them don't know they have it, so the first step is to get your blood pressure checked. A "normal" blood-pressure reading is 120/80; the upper or *systolic* number and the lower or *diastolic* number represent the range of pressure within your arteries as the heart expands and contracts. Have your pressure checked by your doctor or a qualified health professional who can properly interpret these numbers and tell you what they represent for you. If you have borderline hypertension and you're using diet and exercise to combat it, you might want to invest in a home blood pressure kit so you can monitor your progress. But make sure that your *first* reading is done by someone qualified.

Larry W. Gibbons, M.D., medical director of the world-renowned Cooper Clinic in Dallas, says you can reduce your blood pressure by adopting some healthful habits. Changes in diet and exercise can bring great results. Avoid immoderate alcohol use as well as obesity and excessive stress. All these contribute to hypertension. Avoid sodium: according to the USDA, populations with low sodium consumption rarely suffer from high blood pressure, while high blood pressure is common in those with high sodium intakes. When you consider that your body needs only about 0.20 grams of sodium each day—but that most Americans get from 6 to 18 grams a day—you begin to realize how much you can cut from your diet. Leave that shaker alone; you can learn to enjoy less salty foods. Or try one of the many salt substitutes that are available at your supermarket. When cooking, don't add salt until the dish is done; you'll get more salt flavor from less salt this way. Also, while most foods naturally contain sodium, processed foods usually have lots of added salt. Try to eat food in as close to its natural state as possible.

Relax. Excessive stress has been linked to heart disease in numerous medical studies. Eliminating all stress from your life is impossible. After all, life is filled with challenges—we would all be pretty bored without them, and even joyful events cause some stress. The more practical solution is to learn to cope with stress in a healthy way. Dean Ornish, M.D., of the Preventive Medicine Research Institute in San Francisco, conducted a study that showed relaxation and meditation can actually help reverse atherosclerosis. He and many other doctors have begun to seriously study the tremendous potential of the mind in healing the body or in preventing disease in the first place. There are many simple things you can do to relieve tension: quietly relaxing alone, meditating, exercising, even laughing. Therapists, doctors, stress-reduction programs and relevant books can help you learn to relax using a variety of techniques. See Chapter Four for more information on the best ways to fight tension and promote relaxation.

Drink Moderately—If At All. People usually consider only the dangers of becoming addicted to alcohol when they swear to go on the wagon. Alcoholism is the best reason to quit drinking, but there are other evils lurking in the bottle. As a food source, alcoholic beverages are bad news. They have loads of calories and few nutrients. A long list of diseases is attributable to heavy drinking, including cirrhosis of the liver and cancers of the mouth, throat and liver. And aside from hindering general health, excessive alcohol promotes hypertension, thus increasing your risk of heart disease. There have been studies linking alcohol used in moderation with increased levels of high-density lipoproteins (HDL), the "good" cholesterol that helps prevent heart attacks, but some doctors think the increase is of a harmful subgroup of HDL, not the beneficial stuff. So because of this confusion, you shouldn't just start knocking back a few, saying, "It guards against heart attacks." No responsible doctor would tell a patient to begin ingesting a drug as powerful and dangerous as alcohol for such a dubious benefit. Either quit altogether, or limit yourself to no more than one drink a day (1.5 ounces of 100-proof liquor; 5 ounces of wine; 12 ounces of beer).

Volunteer. A recent study conducted by the New-York based Institute for the Advancement of Health showed overwhelmingly what many have always suspected: Volunteering to help others is beneficial to your health. The survey of 3,300 volunteers found that the more often people give their time, the better they feel. In fact, those who helped others at least once a week were ten times more likely to say they were healthy than those who volunteered only once a year. Pent-up hostility, frustration, loneliness—all these health wreckers slide right off your back when you stop to give someone a hand. Find a needy cause where you live; they'll be glad to have you.

Fall in Love. Although its symptoms—shortness of breath, palpitations, dizziness, insomnia—may resemble some signs of a heart attack, true love can be good for your health. In fact, new studies show that married men, smokers and nonsmokers alike, live longer. According to Gershon M. Lesser, M.D., loneliness is a killer, and connecting with others may spare you from all sorts of catastrophic physical ills. Start by getting involved in a dynamic group—environmental, political, arts-related, business, religious or personal-growth—whatever you'd like to explore. These groups are wonderful resources for forging relationships with people who share your interests. Who knows? You may even find that special someone there. But no matter where you find them, positive emotional connections are always good for your heart.

THE HEART'S RED HERRINGS—SYMPTOMS YOU SHOULDN'T WORRY ABOUT

As an adult, the information you get from your buddies about heart disease is about as accurate as the information you got from them about sex when you were a kid on the playground. Here are some problems you might think relate to heart attacks, but don't necessarily represent a problem:

Palpitations

"Everyone's heart goes bump in the night every once in a while," says Fredric Pashkow, M.D., director of the cardiac health improvement and rehabilitation program at the Cleveland Clinic. Healthy men who experience occasional, short-lived arrhythmia generally have nothing to worry about; skipping a beat is not a risk factor for heart disease. When you should be concerned: if the irregularity is sustained for more than 20 or 30 seconds or if it happens several times in a day.

Blood-pressure pills

Don't panic if you're one of the six million Americans who take blood pressure-lowering drugs known as *calcium channel blockers*. A recent study from the University of Washington seemed to indicate that these drugs can increase heart-attack risk, but the subtleties of this research went unreported in the subsequent media frenzy—so the conclusion is far from clear. A far greater risk would be to quit taking your medicine. Your best course of action is to talk to your doctor about your treatment options.

Heart murmur

It's something your doctor will pick up with a stethoscope: the sound of blood trickling back through a valve in the heart when it shouldn't. It has nothing to do with your risk of a heart attack. Many murmurs pose no problem, but some require treatment ranging from antibiotics to keep the valve from getting infected, to replacement of the valve to ensure it continues working properly.

Excess iron

Some researchers have suggested that excess iron in fortified foods or vitamins designed for women puts men at greater risk of heart disease. Other studies challenge this assertion. The bottom line is it's still open to debate. If you happen to get extra iron in your diet or from a food supplement, there's no cause for alarm.

Success

Remember the "type-A personality," whose hard-charging drive for success doomed his heart to premature problems? The broad idea that striving for—and achieving—success automatically raises risk of heart disease has fallen out of favor now that specific dangers such as hostility and depression have been shown to be the real issue. After all, many successful men *are* happy.

SILENT HEART ATTACKS?

Icelandic researchers who tracked nearly 10,000 men for almost 30 years discovered a disturbing phenomenon: a third of the men in their study who had heart attacks didn't even *know* it. They felt no pain and experienced no symptoms.

Silent heart attacks occur for the same reasons as the regular variety, and go unnoticed because they affect a less-critical part of the heart or because the victim has an abnormally high threshold for pain. The researchers discovered the heart attacks only because all of the men were receiving electrocardiograms (EKG) every few years. When they noticed a result in a patient that was radically different from his prior EKG exam, they discovered the "silent" heart attack.

This is one reason why many doctors recommend that men get a "baseline" EKG at age 40 or so; that way there's something to compare results to later in life. Those with strong cardiac risk factors—such as high blood pressure or diabetes—should have an EKG at least every few years so that problems (even silent ones) don't go unnoticed.

The Urinary Tract

Nature has given men a few advantages when it comes to the urinary tract. Because men urinate through the penis, our urethras—the tube that carries urine from the bladder—are long enough to isolate the bladder from germs. Women have much shorter urethras, and germs can more easily migrate "upstream" to the bladder. While bladder infections, or *cystitis*, is relatively common among women, it is not much of a problem for men. Later in life, if the prostate swells enough to obstruct the flow of urine, men can experience the same problem. (The prostate is discussed later in this chapter.)

Regardless of age, what are euphemistically referred to as *bladder control problems* indicate an underlying medical condition and should be addressed by your internist or urologist. Inability to control the bladder is often a sign of diabetes or a neurological problem, conditions that are much more serious than a simple loss of continence. Forcing yourself to "hold it in" can cause even more problems; it can cause the bladder to expand, and make it harder to completely empty it when you urinate—which in turn can lead to other forms of urinary tract dysfunction.

Athletes may experience a urinary problem even more disquieting than incontinence: peeing red. *Hematuria*, or blood in the urine, takes two basic forms, and both can occur as the result of strenuous activity. The first indicates that whole red blood cells have leaked into the urine. The second means that both whole and damaged red blood cells are present. Both conditions are most often the result of "microtraumas" to the bladder during exercise; the jarring experienced by the body causes capillaries inside the bladder to leak.

As upsetting as vermilion urine might be, it's most often not a reason for serious concern. Dehydration is thought to play a major role; an insufficiently watered athlete's dry bladder is more apt to bleed from cracks along its dried-out lining. For runners, the problem may lie further south. The constant pounding of feet against pavement can smash blood cells down at foot level as well as jar the bladder. Athletes who prefer impact sports are much more susceptible to hematuria, while it is uncommon among swimmers or cyclists—even if they become dehydrated. Regardless of your sport, make sure you drink enough water before, during and after your workout. If hematuria persists you need to be seen by a urologist, who can eliminate the other possible causes for the bleeding (such as kidney stones, cancer or tuberculosis) and prescribe the best course of treatment.

One urinary complication that favors men over women is *kidney stones*. Perhaps 10 percent of all males will experience these painful little demons at some point in their lives—over twice the rate for women. And they don't just afflict older men; the first attack typically happens in the late twenties. In about 80 percent of cases, the problem results from an overabundance of calcium in the system, often combined with a salt called oxalate; when they mix, stones can result. High levels of uric acid, or low levels of citrate—a chemical that keeps calcium dissolved—are also culprits. As with hematuria, dehydration is also a factor; the higher your water intake and subsequent urine output, the lower your chances are for kidney stones.

The problem usually presents itself when the body tries to expel the stone. As it moves from the kidney through the ureter and the passage of urine is partially blocked, the pain grows from mild itching to something approaching the sensation of childbirth. You may also experience nausea, chills, sweating, vomiting, hematuria or even shock. If the urine backs up into the kidneys enough to damage the organs, even death can result. Fortunately, the pain and other symptoms drive almost everyone to the doctor long before that happens.

Once you're diagnosed, treatment for small stones usually involves lots of water (and pain killers) as the stone works its way out over the course of the next several hours or days. Stones causing an obstruction to the ureter have to be dealt with by a cystoscope, a basketlike instrument that travels up the urethra to the ureter and snags the stone. Larger stones are pulverized with ultrasound waves, making them small enough to pass.

Luckily, 70 percent of kidney-stone cases are entirely preventable. The first step is a blood screening and a urine sample to determine levels of calcium, oxalate, uric acid, sodium and citrate. Your doctor may then recommend a diet lower in calcium or foods that are rich in uric acids: organ meats, sardines, mussels and mushrooms. Drug therapies including a diuretic called HCTZ may also be indicated. And again, water intake is essential: two or three quarts a day to minimize the chances of occurrence or recurrence. Concentrate on getting plenty of water before you exercise and early in the day, when you're more likely to be dry.

Hernia

Because of anatomical differences, *hernias* are practically a male-only condition: men get them at thirty times the rate of women. And unfortunately, they can strike us at any age—including infancy—and there's not much that can be done to prevent them.

A visible lump in the groin region is called an *inguinal hernia*, and is caused when the lining of the abdomen, a portion of the intestine, the spermatic cord or a combination of these parts pushes through the transverse fascia—the sheet of connective tissue that separates the organs from the abdominal muscles. Although they can occur as the result of heavy lifting or straining, hernias can also happen during a cough or sneeze. Often there's no pain involved, and you might not even be aware of the hernia until you notice a golf-ball size lump or protrusion in the groin. Athletes occasionally realize they have a hernia when they notice a steady reduction in their physical performance, such as when a runner notices he's clocking slower times.

A recent surgical innovation is a great leap forward in correcting hernias. In the past, surgeons simply pushed the protrusion back in and then stitched muscles together over the hole. Recovery time from this procedure was prolonged: three or four days in the hospital, and no real physical activity for up to two months. Worse still was the relatively high failure rate of about 10 percent; the tension in the stitched-up muscles often caused another tear along the suture line. The new method is called "tension-free hernioplasty," and places a polypropylene patch over the hole—and requires no muscle stitching. The failure rate is about one in a thousand, and patients are on their feet and active in less than a week. Men have often used the long downtime associated with the old operation as an excuse to avoid fixing the hernia; the new one requires only a local anesthetic and less than an hour to perform. With this new procedure, there's no excuse not to get your hernia fixed.

The Testicles

"A sack of worms" is how the word *varicocele* roughly translates from its French origins. It's a rather graphic description of a condition in the scrotum that can leave a man feeling as if he's carrying around exactly what the word's origin suggests. On the other hand, he might not even know he has it.

Varicoceles (varuh-koh-seals) have been medically recognized since at least A.D. 500, when the Greek physician Celcus described how one man's veins were "swollen and twisted over the testicle, which has become smaller than its fellow, inasmuch as its nutrition has become defective." Besides leading to atrophy of the testicle and being uncomfortable, a varicocele can cause infertility. The condition affects 16–18 percent of men, according to Cappy Rothman, M.D., clinical instructor of surgery at UCLA and director of the in-vitro fertilization center at Century City Hospital in

Los Angeles. Furthermore, he says, it's found in approximately 45 percent of infertile men.

Doctors agree that a varicocele should be treated if it causes pain or is the suspected source of a patient's infertility. But Michael Warren, M.D., chief of the division of urology at the University of Texas Medical Branch in Galveston, says most varicoceles are present at birth and many never pose a problem. "It's possible to have one and not have to worry about it," Warren says. "You could have been born with it, have no pain and father ten children. If that's the case, it's most likely nothing to worry about."

Varicoceles are formed when the veins that transport blood from the scrotum become stretched and dilated, preventing normal blood flow and causing "pooling" of blood in the vessels. Those veins start in the scrotum, move through the spermatic cord and pass into the abdomen, where they empty into the inferior vena cava, a major vein that takes blood back to the heart. On the right side of the body, the vein from the scrotum usually empties directly into the inferior vena cava. But on the left, the vein drains into the left renal vein, the one that carries blood from the left kidney, and then into the inferior vena cava. This makes the vein on the left longer and, consequently, more susceptible to damage by compression from other parts of the body. Its length also makes it more prone to backflow of blood. As a result, about 80 percent of varicoceles occur around the left testicle.

A varicocele may also result from anything that disrupts proper drainage of the left renal vein, such as a kidney tumor or pressure from severe exertion of the abdominal muscles. Activities such as training with weights and doing abdominal crunches may exacerbate varicocele damage, though they're unlikely to cause the problem. You shouldn't have to give up your workout routine as long as you closely monitor the varicocele and consult with your doctor. The sudden onset of a varicocele is more likely to signal something more serious, such as an obstruction in the kidneys or perhaps a local tumor, than is a longtime or congenital varicocele. If you're uncertain whether it's new or not, seek medical advice.

Troublesome varicoceles may cause mild pain or a heavy feeling in the scrotum, but most have no symptoms. Therefore, Warren and Rothman encourage men to do regular testicular self-examinations. "Every man under the age of fifty should check himself each time he showers," says Warren. "And if you notice anything different from the last self-exam, you should seek medical attention." As of now, Rothman points out, the vast majority of varicoceles are diagnosed when men go to a doctor for infertility problems. The theory is that the warm blood backlogged in a varicocele may prevent the scrotum from keeping the testicles at the optimum sperm-making temperature.

Although it's not clear exactly how, the abnormal blood flow caused by a varicocele can also interfere with testosterone concentration in the testes, which can inhibit sperm production. It may also decrease the availability of oxygen and nutrients necessary for sperm development. The sperm of men with varicoceles frequently exhibit decreased motility and are often "tapered," or deformed, as well.

Rothman says correcting a varicocele results in an 80 percent chance of improved sperm production and a 35 percent chance for pregnancy if other functions in both partners are normal. Historically, the veins were treated by such methods as cauterization, acupuncture, sometimes even castration. Today, "the testicles aren't even touched," Rothman says. He says the actual operation takes just fifteen minutes, though the patient should expect to spend three to four hours in the clinic before heading home. The goal of the surgery is to separate and tie off the dilated veins so that blood flows normally. The best place to achieve that is not in the scrotum, with its many small veins, but in the lower abdomen, where those smaller veins merge into larger ones. The operation, including the surgeon's, anesthesiologist's and doctor's fees, should cost about $2,500. Although it's a standard medical procedure, an increasing number of insurance companies classify it as elective infertility treatment. Several new, nonsurgical methods to correct varicoceles are being developed as well. One, laparoscopy, involves inserting a laser tube into the abdomen. Another involves injecting a drug, balloon or coil into an abdominal vein to block blood to the problem veins. A recently publicized study found that blood was effectively blocked in 95 percent of 523 cases observed. While these might one day be the preferred methods of treatment, they're still experimental right now.

There is good news and bad about *testicular cancer*. First, the good: the cure rate has risen dramatically—up from 78 percent in the mid–'70s to about 93 percent today, according to the National Cancer Institute. Now the bad news. Testicular cancer primarily strikes young men, focusing on those in the 20–34 age group. Whites are especially vulnerable; Native Americans, Hispanics and Asians experience it less often, and African Americans almost not at all.

Perhaps the worst news is that none of the thousands of cases of testicular cancer diagnosed every year ever needs to go undetected. Women understand the importance of checking their breasts for changes or abnormalities, but men have yet to follow this example by regularly examining their testicles. Identified and treated, this cancer is among the most curable;

ignored, it can quickly spread to the lymph nodes and other structures. If men simply checked themselves regularly, virtually all testicular cancer could be caught and cured.

If you discover a lump on a testicle, it may be a simple cyst. Your doctor should be able to determine the nature of the problem with a physical exam; if doubt remains, a sonogram is used to differentiate between a cyst and a tumor. If a tumor is discovered, doctors generally remove the testicle and *then* perform a biopsy—just the opposite of what happens with other cancers. The testicle is removed for biopsy because the risk of spreading cancer cells into the scrotum is too great. If the tumor is cancerous, then the patient may undergo more extensive testing, radiation therapy, chemotherapy, more surgery or a combination of these procedures.

Even with a single testicle, a man can still produce more than enough sperm and testosterone to father a child and provide adequate amounts of male hormones for the health of his body. Although there can be complications from chemotherapy and other related procedures, most men don't experience long-term problems with either fertility or sexual performance. Most importantly, the chance for a recurrence can be as low as 1 percent.

As with all cancers, early detection is the key. Take a minute *now* and learn how to examine your testicles—and then use that knowledge every time you shower.

TESTICULAR SELF-EXAMINATION

Perform your self-exam during or after a shower or warm bath, when the scrotal sac is relaxed. Check one testicle at a time. Put your index and middle fingers of both hands under the testicle, and rest your thumbs on top. Gently roll the testicle between the thumbs and fingers and feel for any small lumps. Also feel for swelling or hardening of the entire testicle. Though it's common for one testicle to be larger than the other, take note if one is larger than it normally is.

Other signs you should watch for: a dull ache in the lower abdomen or the groin, pain or discomfort in the testicle or scrotum or fluid in the scrotum. If any of these symptom last as long as two weeks, call your doctor.

For more information about testicular cancer, call the National Cancer Institute at (800) 422–6237 or the American Cancer Society at (800) 227–2345.

The Penis

The penis is, fortunately, a relatively trouble-free organ. Sexual problems like impotence originate in the mind, nervous system or the circulatory system—but not in the penis itself. The organs surrounding the penis, particularly the testicles and the prostate, are much more prone to disease than the penis.

Circumcision, or the surgical removal of the foreskin that envelops the tip of a nonerect penis, is a relatively routine procedure in America and some other parts of the world. It usually is performed shortly after birth. While the routine use of circumcision is somewhat controversial, it is thought to impart a number of health benefits. Penile cancer, though rare in the first place, is almost unknown among circumcised men; it accounts for 10 percent of the male cancers in parts of the world where circumcision is uncommon, while Israel has the lowest incidence of penile cancer in the world (all Jewish males are circumcised). Urinary tract infections and sexually transmitted diseases are also less prevalent among men without foreskins. Most American doctors still favor the routine circumcision of newborn boys, though not very many would recommend the procedure in adult men who weren't circumcised in childhood. If you are "intact," careful daily washing of the area under the foreskin should be a routine.

If circumcision is so great, then why is there a controversy? Uncircumcised penises are thought to be more sensitive; the uncovered tip of a circumcised penis develops more layers of skin to protect itself, and those extra layers theoretically diminish the sensation of sex. Others object to the practice because they think it's a cruel thing to do to an infant, and that simple washing can reduce any problems associated with having a foreskin. For some, their religion mandates that boys be circumcised. If you're not in that category and you're expecting a boy, circumcision is a decision that you and your wife should make together in consultation with your doctor.

Any red spot, bump or eruption appearing on the penis should be seen by your doctor. It's possibly some form of sexually transmitted disease, but could be an early sign of cancer. If you're having problems achieving or maintaining an erection, your doctor can evaluate the situation and tell you if the problem is physical or psychological, then recommend the best course of treatment.

The Skin

Men pay far less attention to their skin than women, which is both good and bad. The good part is that we don't inflict on ourselves the facial peels, heavy makeup and other regimens that can irritate the skin. The bad part is that since we ignore the skin almost entirely, we're less likely to notice any changes that might signal the start of skin cancer.

Skin cancer is the most common form of the disease in the US, and has increased rapidly in the past few years. The American Academy of Dermatology estimates that your lifetime probability of developing the disease in the 1930s was 1 in 1,500; today it's 1 in 120, and by the year 2000 it could be 1 in 75. Contrary to popular opinion, malignant *melanomas*, the most deadly skin cancers, can strike the young as well as the old. Of those who develop the disease, 25 percent are under the age of 40.

It's important to monitor changes in the size or shape of moles, and to keep an eye out for reddish patches, smooth growths, colored nodules (pink, blue or black) or any rapid growth on or under the skin— particularly if you have a fair complexion. The easiest way to do this is with a head-to-toe self-exam of the skin performed about once a month. To do this, shed your clothes and stand before a full-length mirror in a brightly-lit room. Use the mirror to examine the front, back and sides of your body, then check the arms and hands. Make a mental note of the size and location of moles. Using a hand mirror, give special attention to the scalp, shoulders and neck—prime areas for skin cancer. Finally, sit down and check the soles of your feet. You should now have a good sense of the state of your skin, and be in a better position to spot any changes.

While it is essential that you take an active part in early detection, you can't do it alone; you also need the help of a dermatologist. Ideally you should see the dermatologist once a year, and the easiest way to remember to do that is to schedule an appointment on or near your birthday (to get your "birthday suit" examined). With both of you working together—and with the regular use of sunscreen—skin cancer needn't be a worry.

THE ABCDs OF MELANOMA

Keep an eye out for these abnormalities as you examine your skin, particularly if you're blond or a redhead, have a family history of melanomas, were a sun worshipper or worked outdoors as a youngster, have significant freckling on the back, or have the precancerous condition called *actinic keratosis*.

A stands for asymmetry. One half of a mole doesn't match the other.

B stands for *border irregularity*. The edges are ragged, notched or blurred.

C stands for *color*. Pigmentation isn't uniform; shades of tan, brown, blue or black are present. Dashes of red, white or blue add to mottled appearance.

D stands for *diameter*. The size is greater than six millimeters (about the same as a pencil eraser). Any growth in the size of a mole should be a concern.

The Prostate

The prostate represents both everything that men most cherish and everything they most fear. While it fuels orgasms and makes fertility possible, it can also squeeze so tight you aren't even able to urinate.

Nestled beneath the bladder, the prostate has a hole in the center through which sections of the tubes from the bladder and the scrotum run. These tubes carry urine and semen through the gland on their way out of the urethra. In adolescence the prostate is about the size of a pea; in a healthy adult it is roughly the size of a walnut—but can grow to near grapefruit-like proportions when diseased.

As if it's growth characteristics weren't strange enough, the prostate is anomalous in other ways. It's both a gland—secreting fluids that contribute to the composition of semen—and a muscle, contracting in a way that contributes to the experience of an orgasm. The muscular part is outside; the glandular part is the pulpy tissue on the inside. Much of the prostate's function is still a mystery, including exactly what ingredients it adds to semen. What is known is that its crowded location within a delicate part of the male anatomy makes it capable of interfering with several essential functions.

For young men, *prostatitis* is the greatest worry—although prostate cancer can occur occasionally in males under 40. Prostatitis is the most common problem of the prostate, and accounts for 25 percent of all urological office visits. Its symptoms are chronic pain in the lower abdomen, difficult and painful urination, or a brownish discharge from the penis. Some 28 percent of all men will have a bout of it at some point in their lives, according to the National Prostate Cancer Education Council. Prostatitis is often caused by a bacterial infection, but can also flare-up for no apparent reason.

Antibiotics cure the bacterial form of the disease, but nonbacterial prostatitis can be as hard to cure as it can be to diagnose. It often clears up by itself, but the real problem is discovering what caused it in the first place. Both coffee and alcohol can inflame the prostates of some men, as can spicy foods; if you have to urinate five minutes after a beer or a cup of coffee, you have your culprit.

Stress is often a cause of prostatitis, and many men notice that their pain miraculously clears up after a vacation, a change of job, a massage, a session of yoga, etc. The prostate muscle reacts to stress by "clamping down," but meditation and other forms of relaxation can make it loosen up. Stop-and-go urination is also a suspect; starting and stopping your stream (like a Shower Massage on the "pulse" setting) can force urine back into the prostate. Just let it flow, and don't stop until you're done.

A surprisingly common cause of nonbacterial prostatitis is simple dehydration. This can make the urine very concentrated, which in turn can inflame the prostate. Those who live and work in hot climates need to be especially careful to drink lots of water all day long; eight glasses is a minimum. Working out can quickly cause dehydration: drink water before, during and after your exercise sessions. The color of your urine is a good barometer. If it's clear, then you're getting enough fluids through your system.

Sex can also play a role in prostatitis. A change in sexual habits, from celibate to active or vice versa, can cause the gland to become congested or irritated. This usually clears up as your prostate adjusts to the new situation. Unprotected vaginal sex can also introduce bacteria into your urethra if your partner has a urinary-tract infection; unprotected anal sex is another potential cause. And if you're looking for an excuse to have sex, take note: ejaculation seems to be good for the prostate. Urologists believe that ejaculating every two or three days keeps the prostate from becoming congested by its own secretions.

In men over forty, another common prostate affliction is *benign prostate hyperplasia* (BPH), a noncancerous but bothersome enlargement of the gland that can squeeze the urethral tubes so tightly that urination becomes difficult—and sometimes impossible. Though it rarely gets to that stage, the urinary difficulties caused by BPH affect about 80 percent of men above age sixty at one point or another.

The causes of BHP are mysterious. Since castrated men don't get it, it's thought that the disorder must be linked to testosterone production. High levels of cholesterol also seem to be implicated, as does high blood pressure. If you're overweight—and especially if you carry your extra pounds as a "spare tire" around the middle—you may be setting yourself up for BHP; men with waists larger than 43 inches are twice as likely to have enlarged prostates as those with a size 35 or smaller belt size. Doctors usually treat BPH with alpha-blocker drugs, which relieve pressure on the urethra, and a drug with the trade name Proscar. If those don't work, then surgery may be necessary to enlarge the passageways surrounding the ure-thral tubes. Often the best course is to do nothing; BPH disappears on its own about 75 percent of the time.

As with so many other aspects of this enigmatic organ, the statistics on the occurrence of *prostate cancer* are a bit inscrutable. The American Cancer Society estimates that by the time you're 70 you have a 10 percent chance of contracting prostate cancer; other experts point out that the dis-ease can progress so slowly and asymptomatically that the actual percent-age might be much higher. (Prostate cancer can also strike rapidly.) Around 80 percent of all prostate cancer strikes men above age 65.

What is especially worrisome is the fact that prostate cancer can hit without producing any noticeable symptoms at all. When symptoms do appear, they may mimic those of prostatitis or BHP. By the time pain becomes intense enough for men to seek treatment, the cancer may have already spread to the bones or other parts of the body. The test for the dis-ease, called the prostate-specific antigen (PSA) test, isn't very reliable; a new screening technique developed by the University of St. Louis called the "free PSA" test looks very promising—correctly diagnosing the cancer almost 90 percent of the time—but is still experimental. Those with a family history of prostate cancer should consider the PSA test. If you're not in that category, ask your doctor whether it makes more sense to wait for the new test to prove its worth.

Treating prostate cancer can also be a tricky affair. In older men, hor-mone and radiation therapies can effectively control the cancer—if caught in time—for the patient's remaining lifespan. In younger men when the condition has been detected early, a more aggressive surgical approach that removes all or part of the diseased organ is often used. A newer technique uses cryosurgery—the freezing of the tumor by insertion of a tubular device containing liquid oxygen. It's thought that cryosurgery greatly minimizes the impotence and urinary incontinence that can accompany conventional surgery.

To help avoid prostate cancer, there are three steps you can take. First, minimize high-fat foods, especially red meat: a Harvard study associates a diet with more than five servings of red meat a week with late-stage prostate cancer. Second, stay trim: men who are overweight face a greater risk for this cancer. Last, take vitamin E: this antioxidant can reduce the risk for prostate cancer by 34 percent. A good supplemental daily dose of the vitamin is 400 international units.

THE PSA—TO TEST OR NOT TO TEST?

There's nothing like a good controversy to get the blood flowing, and if the controversy is at all sexual in nature, so much the better. Experts have long regarded the dreaded digital rectal exam as the gold standard for prostate cancer detection. While most still believe it's adequate for younger men with no family history of the disease, many urologists and national health organizations now recommend that high-risk men undergo a two-tiered approach that includes the newly developed prostate-specific antigen (PSA) blood screening. The newest method of identifying the disease in its early stages is on the medical firing line.

PSA is a protein secreted exclusively by the prostate to liquefy semen. If the prostate becomes diseased in any one of a variety of ways, PSA production goes up. So by monitoring PSA levels in the blood, a physician can follow the development of prostatic tumors. Since its introduction in late 1991, the PSA test, which measures the amount of prostate-specific antigen in the bloodstream, has proven to be a powerful early predictor of cancer.

Unfortunately, PSA testing is far from foolproof—and by pushing men into surgery may cause some men problems worse than those posed by living with the cancer it detects. This has sparked a heated debate that finds public-health heavyweights split between recommending 1) immediate widespread testing, 2) testing of men most at risk and/or 3) a halt to all PSA screening pending the outcome of further studies.

Among the test's strongest advocates is the American Cancer Society (ACS), which in an unprecedented move as recently as 1993 called for an across-the-board PSA screening program for all men older than 50. The American Urological Association has suggested that testing begin at age 40, while the National Cancer Institute (NCI) warns that all such recommendations are premature and says it will put off making its own until the completion of a sixteen-year study to determine if PSA testing has any positive effect on mortality rates.

According to the latest ACS estimates, 41,000 men nationwide will die yearly of prostate cancer and 250,000 more will be diagnosed with the disease, making it the second most common form of cancer—and the second most deadly to strike American men (lung cancer is first.). For this reason alone, noted urologist William Catalona, M.D., of the Washington University School of Medicine in St. Louis, believes there's no time to waste. "Half a million men will die before the results of the [NCI] study are even known," he says.

Catalona maintains that mass screenings could drastically alter survival rates because the test is capable of detecting prostate cancer in its early stages. "In 70 percent of cases, cancers detected using the rectal exam have already reached an advanced stage and have spread outside the prostate to surrounding tissues," Catalona explains. "However, our research showed that if you use the PSA blood test in conjunction with the rectal exam, you double the number of cancers [found] still confined within the prostate." Catalona's conclusions are based on the assumptions that prostate cancer acts like most other forms of the disease and that early detection will allow physicians to catch it, treat it and cure it before malignant cells spread beyond the walls of the prostate.

Unfortunately, say critics, there's no evidence to support those assumptions. Moreover, while the number of prostate cancers detected has doubled in the past decade and treatments have become more sophisticated, the mortality rate for prostate cancer hasn't changed in twenty-five years. "We don't have any evidence that early detection leads to increased survival," notes William Fair, M.D., chief of urology at Memorial Sloan Kettering Center in New York City. John Gohagan, M.D., chief of NCI's Early Detection Branch, agrees. "A lot of research has been done on PSA," he says, "but one thing the studies don't tell you is if there is any benefit to be gained by screening. They find more disease, but everything after that is [open to] speculation."

Opponents point out that an unknown number of prostate cancer types exist, and few of the known types behave conventionally. In fact, the vast majority of prostate cancers produce no early symptoms and grow so slowly that their victims die of unrelated causes before the malignancy even has a chance to spread.

Prostate cancers fall into two general categories: fast and lethal, and slower than molasses. The quick killers usually strike younger men, spreading rapidly and imperceptibly, often metastasizing to bones and leading to a painful death within a few years. The second variety develops so slowly that it may be forty years before it's large enough to be detected, and by then, for a man in his seventies, the treatment of choice is no treatment at all. So little is known about prostate cancer that physicians aren't even sure how to distinguish the potentially fatal tumors from the "safe" ones.

Another important consideration is PSA's potential for misdiagnosis, which appears to be considerable. According to Elia C. Skinner, M.D., cancer specialist and assistant professor of urology at the

University of Southern California in Los Angeles, when 66 advanced cancer patients at that research center were given PSA tests earlier this year, 25 percent of those whose cancer had spread outside the prostate nonetheless exhibited normal PSA readings. Equally serious is the fact that PSA screenings often indicate a patient has a cancer when there is none, setting off a series of unnecessary and painful diagnostic exams. A high PSA reading can just as easily turn out to be the result of a dormant, nonlethal tumor or even an enlarged prostate.

Furthermore, the PSA test doesn't discriminate between cancer types. "You can't tell from PSA levels what the grade, or stage, of the disease is," explains Gohagan. "The test is like a red flag on a mailbox. All you can do is watch the flag come up, and then you have to go check the mailbox and see if there's anything in there that's of any value. You've got junk mail and you may have good mail. There's no way to discriminate between the two until you go in and perform a biopsy."

Should a biopsy indicate cancer, the prostate is automatically removed in a procedure that carries significant threat to the patient's quality of life. According to Gohagan, studies show that the surgery carries a 2 percent risk of death and leaves 25 percent of patients impotent and up to 18 percent incontinent. Moreover, prostate removal has a less than 50 percent cure rate: Researchers don't even know whether the 45 percent who survive do so because of the type of cancer they had or because of the stage at which it was diagnosed and removed. This is just one of the questions the NCI hopes to answer through its sixteen-year study of 74,000 men, which began in 1993.

At the personal level, the question of whether to get the PSA test isn't easily answered. What *is* clear is that a PSA screening should always be accompanied by a digital exam to limit the chances for misdiagnosis. (Blood should be drawn first, since the rectal exam may cause PSA levels to rise.) The best candidates for screening are men with a family history of prostate cancer, since they stand to benefit most from early detection. Other than that, the question of whether or not to test is pretty much a matter of choice.

Gastrointestinal Problems

Persistent problems of the esophagus, stomach, intestines and colon are among the most debilitating chronic conditions, and can drastically affect the function of other parts of the body and greatly decrease one's quality of life. Digestive diseases affect more than half of all Americans at some point in their lives, and account for more than 200,000 absences from work every day. As many as 32 million Americans may have chronic heartburn, yet 62 percent of those don't consider the problem serious enough to bring up with their doctor. Digestive problems are widely misunderstood, but no one who has ever experienced a serious gastrointestinal (G.I.) complaint will ever write it off as "just a stomachache" again.

The G.I. problem most men experience is an occasional bout of *heartburn*—the painful, burning sensation in the chest that can be severe enough to mimic the symptoms of a heart attack. Heartburn occurs when digestive acids back up, or reflux, from the stomach to the esophagus—the tube that carries food into the stomach. A valve between the stomach and esophagus is supposed to prevent this reflux, but in some it doesn't seal properly. The acidic digestive juices burn the lining of the esophagus, and cause the pain we call heartburn.

Everyone gets heartburn or indigestion sometime; when either occurs on a regular basis, it's time to see a doctor and find out if the pain is a symptom of something more severe. Many men mistake the burning in their G.I. for simple heartburn and try to treat it with antacids only to discover that they actually have an *ulcer*: a raw area in the G.I. tract that is literally being eaten away by the digestive juices.

Ulcers afflict some 10 percent of the population, and for some reason men are particularly susceptible—and not just the high-powered, Type-A's, either. A *peptic* ulcer usually refers either to a gastric ulcer—afflicting the stomach—or a duodenal ulcer, located in the first part of the small intestine. Ulcers are definitely made worse by stress, which can increase the production of stomach acids, but that's probably not the root cause in most people. But increasingly, a common and easily-spread bacterium, *Helicobacter pylori*, is considered the true cause of this disease; it might explain why family members of ulcer patients are three times more likely to be afflicted themselves. Still others think the bacteria enter only after the ulcer is formed. Studies supported by the National Institutes of Health do suggest that treatment combining the standard acid-reduction medications with antibiotics to suppress the bacteria has a success rate of over 96 percent, returning patients to normal within weeks.

If you've experienced persistent pain in your G.I. tract—especially if it's worse at night, when acid production is highest—or if you've noticed blood in your stools, you need diagnosis and treatment from a doctor. If you've had an ulcer, or been told that you might be prone to them, you should avoid aspirin, alcohol, cigarettes, spicy foods and milk (contrary to popular belief, milk stimulates acid production rather than "coats the stomach"). Controlling stress will also help avoid flare-ups, and will augment many other aspects of your life as well (see Chapter Four for more information).

ALTERNATIVE HEALTH

Few dispute the value of traditional Western medicine, especially as practiced in America. (They might take issue with the *business* of Western medicine and the insurance industry, but that's a different discussion.) When it comes to advanced, high-tech diagnostic equipment and heroic surgical procedures, American medicine truly leads the world. But in leading the world, we've also left behind some ancient practices that have been successful for generations, some of which are increasingly proving their worth when put to the rigors of laboratory testing. Many of these techniques fall into the category of Eastern, holistic or alternative medicine, and have provided a wealth of new options to doctors and patients alike. Just as "American cuisine" now includes influences from around the world, American medicine is slowly recognizing and adopting the wealth of knowledge that lies beyond the boundries of Western medicine.

No credible sources claim the alternative techniques are miracle workers. But advocates—and a fair number of conservative, mainstream experts—insist that such methodologies as acupuncture, massage, herbalism, homeopathy, bioenergetics, naturopathy and chiropractic definitely deserve a look, not to mention additional study.

Often missing is the kind of extensive, published research that supports such mainstream techniques as, say, physical therapy or cardiac rehabilitation. So sparse is the published research validating some alternative techniques that advocates have begun to address the problem head-on. For instance, at a meeting in Miami in December 1993, members of the American Chiropractic Association's Sports Council discussed the need for increased research on the benefits of their profession, says Thomas Hyde, a Miami chiropractor and executive director of the council.

Two groups of patients—those with chronic pain and athletes—decided not to wait for the approval of Western medicine and became early proponents of alternative therapies. Those with chronic illness were the most adventurous, looking for ways to cure their pain without a long-term reliance on drugs. Athletes, charmed by promises of quicker rehabilitation, pain reduction and enhanced performance, created a booming cottage industry for such alternative techniques as acupuncture, chiropractic and sports massage. About half of the 3,000 treatments sought by athletes each month at the U.S. Olympic Training Center in Colorado Springs involve at least one of these, says Edward J. Ryan, a certified athletic trainer at the center who has observed a burgeoning interest in alternative approaches in the past five years.

Finding competent practitioners of alternative medicines can be as difficult as locating a good specialist in any field. Often, the best way is to get a referral from a holistic medical doctor. This begs the question, "How do you find an effective holistic healer who's also a practicing M.D.?"

Since the American Medical Association does not recognize a single specialty like "doctor of holistic medicine," open the Yellow Pages and look under "physicians" to check the specialties. See if there's a listing for "nutrition," and give one of them a call. Usually a doctor who thinks nutrition is important enough to advertise it is likely to understand the importance of holistic and complementary medicine. You can also try looking in the Yellow Pages for nutritionists who are M.D.s.

Most alternative-medicine philosophies are strongly rooted in common sense combined with an awareness of self, community and environment. With an emphasis on following a healthy diet and a sensible exercise regime, practitioners recognize the link between one's physical health and one's emotional and spiritual needs. We can look to modern, conventional medical curatives with appreciation and even awe, but ultimately the best cure is simply to stay healthy. Many of these therapies have a better—and more demonstrable—track record than others. With that in mind, take a look yourself. If conventional remedies aren't working for what ails you, then perhaps it's time to try some of the alternatives.

Acupuncture

The theory behind acupuncture stems from the idea that a life force, or "chi," flows through the body along channels called meridians and that trouble erupts when one or more of the meridians are blocked. Practitioners insert slim needles into appropriate acupuncture points to relieve the blockage, sometimes accompanied by a weak electrical current. Proponents say the needles stimulate release of morphine-like substances called endorphins and enkephalins that act as natural painkillers, and block pain circuits in the nerves from sending messages to the brain.

Chinese medical journals overflow with reports about acupuncture; more than 2,500 studies have been published worldwide in the last thirty years. But less than fifty of those articles met the scientific standards set by Western journals. That's likely to change: a number of medical schools including Harvard, Yale, the University of Pennsylvania and UCLA are using acupuncture both for research and as a therapeutic tool. The therapy is thought to be effective for a broad range of conditions, including asthma, bronchitis, osteoarthritis, nausea and even stroke. But the two conditions for which acupuncture has shown great success are chronic pain and addictions.

Acupuncture is one of the very few treatments that seems to reduce the cravings felt by addicts in withdrawal. Some 300 chemical-dependency programs across the U.S. now include acupuncture as part of their therapy, and even some government drug counseling programs are beginning to employ it as well. At least one double-blind study of alcoholics showed a much higher success rate for the acupuncture group than those who received "simulated" acupuncture. Pain control may eventually be the broadest application for this ancient therapy. Research indicates that needles may be more effective than drugs for the long-term control of pain related to angina, diseases of the muscles and skeleton, arthritis and dental problems. Doctors have been particularly impressed with the way the therapy succeeds with chronic pain, which is typically the most difficult type to control.

Both weekend and professional athletes have discovered that acupuncture can reduce the pain of injuries, speed recovery and perhaps even enhance performance. Acupuncturists treat athletes for inflammation stemming from injuries, or stimulate acupuncture points to expand the athlete's range of motion in a specific part of the body. Needling a point below the knee, for example, can increase leg lift for runners, allowing them to increase their pace. Many professional athletes rely on acupuncture to keep themselves injury-free and able to train and compete at their highest level.

For a referral to a physician trained in acupuncture, call the American Academy of Medical Acupuncture at (800) 521-AAMA.

Bioenergetics

Bioenergetics is a unique program combining both psychotherapy and movement therapy. The theory is that the body both stores emotions such as anger and creates negative feelings by becoming tense and rigid. Suppressed emotions are thought to create "armoring" in the form of chronic muscle tension; the armoring drains the energy we need to go about our lives.

In a therapy session you might assume a variety of postures that would help the therapist diagnose your specific areas of tension. The therapist would then try to rid you of the tension using a combination of psychoanalytic "talk therapy," deep breathing, bioenergetic exercises and even massage to release bodily tension and suppressed emotions. You might also be given a series of exercises to do at home to help keep tension from building.

The bioenergetics theory is a modification of the work done by psychiatrist Wilhelm Reich, and is thought to be helpful for those who have a low level of body awareness and extremely repressed emotions.

Chiropractic

The theory of chiropractic postulates that disease results from abnormal nerve function and that manipulation and adjustment of the body's structure can alleviate the problems. Integral to the concept is the fact that our spines are vital to our health. The spine is capable of energizing the nervous system and making the body function normally, the theory goes, and manipulation of the spine makes that happen.

The essence of chiropractic's approach to wellness is that if any of the vertebrae that make up the spine is out of place, it interferes with the brain's ability to communicate with the rest of the body via the spinal nerves. Depending on where they occur, these interruptions can cause various parts of the body to behave erratically. Because the nerves control the function of all body systems, true believers say that chiropractic can cure a remarkably wide array of ills.

Chiropractic does have a good track record with one difficult-to-treat problem: back pain. Published studies in medical journals, some of them chiropractic publications, have found the therapy effective for lower-back pain. In 1992, researchers writing in the *Journal of Manipulative and Physiological Therapeutics* concluded that spinal manipulation is most effective for the treatment of lower-back pain. After comparing twenty-three different studies, the team found that spinal manipulation offered better pain relief than a variety of other standard back-pain treatments, including bed rest, medication and heat. Many people are already voting with their backs: some 7 percent of Americans see a chiropractor regularly, a figure that has doubled in the last twenty years.

As with so many alternative therapies, athletes have been the pioneers of chiropractic. Jim Montgomery, M.D., a Dallas-based orthopedic surgeon who was the head physician for the U.S. Olympic team at the 1992 Summer Games, points out that a chiropractor is an integral part of the Summer Olympics medical team, working alongside a medical doctor, physical therapist, athletic trainer and psychologist. "The whole key [in physical activity] is balance," says Montgomery. "What acupuncture and chiropractic are trying to do is balance the body; chiropractic's role is to assess where you are structurally." Chiropractors are known for taking extensive patient histories to make correct diagnoses. They're able, he says, to assess biomechanical faults that may set athletes up for injuries and to then try to correct those faults with manipulation.

While chiropractic may have a broad range of applications, there are some conditions where it's definitely not indicated. Systemic diseases that affect the entire body, like arthritis, aren't likely candidates. Bone diseases and infections—or a history of steroid use, which can weaken bones—don't lend themselves to manipulation. If you're taking anticoagulant drugs or have a history of heart disease, this isn't the therapy for you. But if you have a recurrent problem that more conventional treatments can't fix, maybe it's time to give chiropractic a try.

Herbalism

Have you ever wondered why restaurant checks often arrive with mint candies? Our after-dinner mint is a distant echo of the ancient practice of chewing mint leaves or sipping mint tea after large meals to prevent indigestion. Do you start your day with coffee, tea or hot chocolate? They all contain caffeine, America's favorite herbal stimulant. If you take a decongestant when you have a cold, the active ingredient is probably pseudoephedrine, a natural decongestant found in a plant called ephedra (one brand, Sudafed, even takes its name from it). That Listerine you gargle with? One of the herbal germ fighters in this mouthwash is thyme oil, which was used widely as a hospital antiseptic until World War II.

The list of botanical medicines we take for granted goes on and on, yet most doctors don't have a clue about how much modern pharmacology relies on plants. Ask physicians if they use herbal medicines, and they reply, no, we use drugs. Few even know that our word drug comes from the Dutch *droog*, meaning "to dry," as in drying medicinal herbs before grinding them up. Most doctors know that codeine and morphine originally came from the opium poppy, and that the original source of aspirin was willow bark, but few realize that an estimated 25 percent of today's pharmaceuticals still come from plants. The latest to be added to that long list is taxol, from the yew tree, which was recently approved to treat certain advanced cancers.

One reason many doctors won't hear of using herbal treatments is that some advocates have been irresponsible in their pronouncements. For example, the notion that "herbs are natural; therefore, they can't hurt you" is wrong. Ephedrine, for instance, which is also used as a stimulant and weight-loss aid, can be dangerous if you have high blood pressure or heart disease.

And, unless you're extremely knowledgeable, foraging for herbs in the wild can get you into trouble. Two young men scouted the woods of Maine for wild ginseng, Asia's most revered (and expensive) herbal stimulant, which is also native to the Northeast. But they dug up and ate the wrong root, water hemlock, the potent natural poison the ancient Greeks used to execute Socrates. One of the men died. The other survived but suffered seizures.

"Medicinal herbs are like pharmaceuticals," says Varro E. Tyler, Ph.D., professor of pharmacognosy (natural products) at Purdue University and author of *The New Honest Herbal.* "If you use them cautiously and responsibly, they can do you good. But if you use them recklessly, you might regret it."

By and large, most herbal medicines are reasonably safe when used cautiously. According to the American Association of Poison Control Centers, legal pharmaceuticals accounted for 6,407 poisonings and 809 fatalities during two recent years. Plants, on the other hand, accounted for just 53 poisonings and 2 deaths, and most of those involved young children munching on poisonous house plants. Most medicinal herbs are less potent than their pharmaceutical counterparts, which means you have to down a good deal to cause harm. In addition, many medicinal herbs taste bitter, which discourages overdosing.

However, pregnant women should steer clear of most medicinal herbs. Nor should they be given to children under two; older kids and the elderly should use reduced-strength preparations. Anyone with a chronic medical condition should consult a physician before using most medicinal herbs.

On the one hand, the Food and Drug Administration prohibits medicinal claims for all but a few herbs (like peppermint and eucalyptus, both of which are FDA-approved decongestants). That's why most medicinal-herb packages make no health claims. On the other hand, the FDA has a hands-off approach to herbal quality control, forcing consumers to rely on marketers' claims.

For many herbs, this is a nonissue: You don't have to be an analytical chemist to recognize garlic, ginger or peppermint. But several of the more expensive and esoteric herbs have lamentable histories of adulteration, among them ginseng, goldenseal and echinacea. The American Herbal Products Association, a trade organization, informally polices its members and has blown the whistle on a few companies whose products were not up to snuff. But the quality of medicinal herbs remains something of a question mark.

Fortunately, the American Botanical Council (ABC) in Austin, Texas, an independent nonprofit education and research organization that's dedicated to promoting the medicinal use of herbs, recently inaugurated its own quality-control initiative by commissioning tests of more than one hundred ginseng products. The results will be published in the ABC's journal, HerbalGram, and the group plans to conduct similar tests of other herbs to persuade any less-than-entirely-honest herb marketers to clean up their acts.

If you'd like to try a few herbs, begin with the ones described here. While they're no substitute for proper medical care, all are readily available and safe even in large amounts.

Ginseng: For athletic performance, try ginseng. Russian, Korean and Chinese studies show that it improves concentration and stamina with a subtle caffeine-like effect. Has also been used for centuries to enhance the sex drive.

Yohimbe: This herb, which comes from the bark of a West African tree, has a long-standing reputation as a booster of male libido. It's available both in approved drugs (called Yocon, Aphrodyne and Yohimex) for impotence and in its natural, herbal form.

Saw Palmetto: Also used as an aphrodisiac, saw palmetto has shown itself to be beneficial in the treatment of benign prostate enlargement.

Valerian: A popular relaxant and sleep aid, used widely in Europe.

Garlic: Has proven to reduce both high blood pressure and high cholesterol—leading risk factors for heart disease. It's also a natural antibiotic.

Echinecea: A potent booster of the immune system, often used to fight or prevent colds and infections. Often combined with goldenseal to enhance strength.

Ginkgo: The oldest surviving variety of tree on earth, ginkgo improves blood flow to the brain to aid in memory. Used in Europe to help stroke victims and those with age-related mental infirmities.

Ginger: Ancient Asian and Greek sailors used it to combat sea sickness; today it's been shown to be more effective than Dramamine in preventing motion sickness. Great for upset stomachs.

Homeopathy

Homeopathy, once popular in the United States and still widely practiced in Europe, is distinctly different from conventional, "allopathic" medicine. It's based on the principle that "like cures like"—that is, a drug that causes a medical symptom will cure an illness that causes the same condition—and strives to bolster the immune system to prevent disease. Homeopaths believe that, as the body reacts to a minute quantity of the drug, its own immune system goes into action, counteracting the illness as well as the drug.

Homeopathic remedies are prescribed in weak solutions called "tinctures," and often in strengths of less than one part active ingredient per million. Skeptics claim the remedies are essentially pure water. Believers cannot always offer rational explanations for their cures but point to empirical evidence of their effectiveness. This might sound a little far-out in the nineties, but homeopathy was a standard part of the American medical landscape until the turn of the century. With the resurgence of alternative medicine in the last twenty years, homeopathy has made a strong comeback.

"Homeopaths provide constitutional care," explains Dana Ullman, founder and president of the Foundation for Homeopathic Education and Research in Berkeley, California. "Diseases tend to run in the family, so we encourage a 'constitutional' treatment that seems to strengthen a person's overall immune and defense system, to not only help prevent symptoms and syndromes but also to help prevent genetic tendencies. We have to understand that genetics always deals with probabilities, and homeopaths find that we can reduce some of these tendencies by strengthening the body's constitution."

The "law of similars" that forms the basis of homeopathic practices doesn't mean that you treat a cold with cold germs, or prescribe two sets of tennis for a knee injury. According to Ullman, "It means you find a substance that, in large doses, would produce the same symptoms that the patient is feeling." A homeopath might perscribe the mild irritant *nux vomica* for indigestion, for example. But beyond that, the homeopath also pays close attention to the kind of patient he has. How do the symptoms strike? What is the patient's lifestyle? Once that is determined, the proper tincture is recommended; 80 percent of the tinctures come from botanical sources, with minerals and animal products each accounting for 10 percent.

American doctors have a tough time with the concept of homeopathy—it goes against virtually everything they learned in medical school. But the practice has remained popular in Europe, with perhaps a third of French physicians using its remedies along with more conventional treatments. Its proponents claim that homeopathy is especially effective against viral infections, allergies, infectious diseases, chronic illness like diabetes and even some addictions. Traumas to bones, ligaments, tendons and muscles are all said to respond well to tinctures, which has caused a number of athletes to turn to homeopaths for help. Homeopathy is cheaper than conventional medicine, and results can occur with surprising speed. A few articles in conventional medical journals have begun to bear-out some of the claims for this treatment. In time, American doctors may once again have this weapon at their disposal.

To find a qualified homeopath near you, contact the National Center for Homeopathy, 801 North Fairfax, Suite 306, Alexandria, VA 22314 (703–548–7790).

Massage

Here's one alternative therapy that nearly everyone endorses—at least everyone who's ever had a massage. Aside from the numerous studies that confirm that this therapy is beneficial for a wide variety of ailments, massage simply feels good. It's a wonderful relaxant—a calmer of both mind and body—with virtually no unwelcome side effects; beyond that, it ranks right up there with sex as one of the most pleasurable activities you can enjoy. (Many couples, in fact, use massage both with and without sex as a way to be more physically intimate.) Aside from the cost of a professional massage, there's no reason not to enjoy this wonderful therapy as often as you want.

Massage has been practiced in Eastern cultures for well over 4,000 years; Swedish massage is only about 100 years old. Both forms seek to stimulate the body into healing itself by stimulating the skin, muscles and connective tissues through the rhythmic rubbing, stretching and kneading of various parts of the body. Eastern massage aims to balance the life-force called "chi" while Western massage has the more straightforward goal of stimulating circulation and improving mobility. Both forms are excellent.

For serious athletes or those who feel the effects of joint injuries, chronic back or neck problems, arthritis or even migraine headaches, massage can be nothing short of a godsend. It can greatly increase mobility for people in all of those categories, and even speed the healing process by increasing blood-flow to injured areas while removing toxins. Recent studies at the University of Miami also confirm that massage can greatly diminish symptoms in illnesses as diverse as asthma, diabetes and arthritis. But the benefits don't stop with the body; massage can be good for your mind, too. It removes stress from tense necks and shoulders, and produces almost meditative mental states in some participants. An added plus is that a massage can be an instructive way to learn where in your body you tend to store stress in the form of muscle tension. That awareness can help you fight stress even when you're off the massage table.

Swedish massage uses five basic strokes to work its wonders, while sports massage typically combines deep muscle massage with stretching to address specific problem areas. Eastern massage like *shiatsu* and *jin shin jyutsu* add a more spiritual element to the bodywork and concentrate on balancing energy within the body. Lymphatic massage encourages the lymph system to drain toxins from the body, while reflexology concentrates solely on the feet. There are other varieties of massage, but no matter what form you try, you're bound to be pleased with the results. Don't wait until you have an injury to indulge in this tried and true alternative therapy.

Naturopathy

Naturopaths are practitioners—often including medical doctors—who embrace both standard medicine as well as a broad range of natural therapies. Naturopathy has a fundamental belief in the body's intrinsic ability to heal itself, and emphasizes preventive measures first and keeps conventional Western medicine as a last resort. Naturopathic practitioners have an impressive number of tools at their disposal: nutrition, herbalism, psychology, homeopathy, traditional Chinese medicine and a number of physical therapies. Perhaps most importantly, naturopathy emphasizes the role that patients themselves can take in their health.

While naturopaths may agree with conventional physicians in a number of areas, they are far less likely to recommend surgery or prescribe drugs to deal with disease or illness. Swelling of the prostate, for example, might be treated with nutritional changes, herbal medicine and perhaps even hydrotherapy (a group of therapies using water a variety of ways to enhance heath) rather than surgical intervention. Although "hydrotherapy" sounds more like a spa treatment than a serious therapy, it comes from the European tradition of "taking the baths." In fact, what we now think of as a spa is based on old naturopathic healing centers in cities like Vichy that have dominated health on the continent for two hundred years.

While a naturopathic cure might not be the wisest choice for a serious illness, the discipline's strong emphasis on preventive medicine makes it appealing to those who want to maximize their wellness and avoid getting sick. A naturopath will spend much more time with you than a conventional doctor explaining diet and lifestyle changes that can greatly improve your health. The doctor-patient relationship is much more of a partnership, with both sides working hard to optimize the proper course of treatment—one that usually emphasizes whole, unrefined foods and pure water as the keys to good health. For essentially healthy patients who want to explore new ways to augment their well-being, naturopathy can be a good choice.

By Fred Hayward

It's a recurring story in the media: Medical research and studies are skewed toward serving male health needs. The implied or direct conclusion is that men get better medical care than women. As much as some people want to believe this is true, it's a conclusion that's hardly supported by the evidence. Despite the fact that all these resources are devoted to our maintenance, here's the unavoidable fact: Women, on average, live about 78.5 years, while we men kick off at 71.8. That's almost seven additional years of life that women get and men don't.

Now, what would happen if these statistics were turned around, and it was announced that the average woman died seven years before, instead of after, the average man? Gender differences in life expectancy would probably be the Number One Equal Rights Issue of our time. Government task forces would be formed. Books would line store windows, updates would be given on the nightly news and talk shows would rack up ratings with topics such as "Gender Genocide—Next on Geraldo." Most of us were taught to "take it like a man"—no matter what that might entail—and so we've also been raised to believe that we should die without complaint.

Thus, increasing men's life expectancy is not much of a priority at all, even in the male bastion of medical research. Indeed, if you were to review the last few times you saw a television news feature or read an article that mentioned the shorter male life expectancy, the story most likely focused on how inconvenient it is for women that men drop dead so soon. Think of the segment titles: "The Shortage of Eligible Men Over 60," or "Poverty Among Widows." The impression we're left with is that dying is just one more way in which men conspire to make life harder for women.

The reason for all this, in my view, is the mind-set among men as well as women that sees medicine as "male dominated." Yes, it's true that most doctors are men. On the other hand, medicine was not created to give job opportunities to the fraction of 1 percent of people who become doctors; rather, medicine exists to give health care to the 100 percent of us who become patients. Viewed from this perspective, medicine is female dominated and getting more so. The majority of people who use medical facilities of any kind across the country are women; the "male-dominated" medical system attends to female patients 37 percent more often than to male patients during any given year.

We have all kinds of outreach programs and clinics specifically geared to women, yet practically none for men, the gender that needs equal time. Women now receive detailed instruction in self-examination for breast cancer; the publicity this disease has received has been widespread and increasingly effective. But very few men know how to examine themselves for testicular cancer, despite the fact that it's the number-one cancer killer among men under 40—partly because men never hear about it. Woman are taught to get regular tests for cervical cancer (Pap smears), while most men do not even know where their prostate gland is until they have to have it removed because of cancer.

So what can we trace our shorter lifespans to, aside from the superior medical care we're given? A study at the UCLA School of Public Health has traced about half of the difference in life expectancy between men and women to seven health habits: Men smoke more, exercise less, drink more, sleep less, eat more snacks between meals, don't eat nutritionally sound breakfasts and are often of a weight that's disproportionate to their height. Men are three times more likely to be victims of homicide and four times more likely to commit suicide. We're also twice as likely to be killed by an automobile and nineteen times more likely to die at work.

The propensity toward death by homicide deserves special attention. While male hormones may play a part, these results of male behavior are more essentially a function of sex roles than biology. We often gravitate toward acts of violence both to protect women directly and to demonstrate to would-be admirers that we can defend them. Why does no one initiate studies in hopes of finding a way to change these roles, and thus these statistics?

Our life span is further shortened by a reluctance to seek medical care. Men are expected to grin and bear it on all fronts.

Men are diverted from concern for their own health by the business of living up to a stereotypical, Duke Wayne image that costs them an average 6.7 years of their lives. Example: While women learn something intelligent about pain (it's your body's way of telling you something's wrong and that you should go to a doctor and find out what it is), men learn something stupid about pain (enduring it is a way to demonstrate your manhood, as in "No pain, no gain").

According to Jean Bonhomme, M.D., director of the Atlanta, Georgia-based National Black Men's Health Network, the ten-year-old kid who learns that brave boys don't cry grows up to be the forty-year-old man who says, "'It's just indigestion,' at the initial signs of a heart attack." Although the medical profession may have a male-dominated veneer, deeply-rooted sexism actually keeps men from seeking its benefits until, says Bonhomme, "We've got one foot in the grave and the other on a banana peel."

There is, of course, a small part of the lifespan differential that results from the special physiological vulnerabilities of the male body. But biology isn't necessarily destiny. Not long ago, for example, women routinely died during childbirth. We didn't shrug our shoulders and say, "Women get pregnant; they take their chances." Rather, we created a pair of sciences, gynecology and obstetrics, to deal with women's special problems.

That concern is ongoing. The director of the National Institutes of Health recently announced that women's medical problems would be a priority of the vast, taxpayer-funded NIH, and there is powerful movement in the medical community, commemorated in a page-one article in *The New York Times*, to establish a medical specialty that deals solely with women's medical issues, separate from obstetrics and gynecology. Our "male-dominated" medical system, however, has yet to see a branch of medicine that deals with specifically male vulnerabilities.

The men's movement is frequently dismissed by the media as being concerned with whiny, silly issues (tom-tom beating, daddy-hatred, fear of women). This is in contrast, of course, to the far more substantive, better-defined women's movement, which takes on serious topics, like the dominance of medicine by males who are concerned only about themselves. Ironically, survival is the one gender issue we can measure objectively. Well, here's our big chance: Men can organize to fight for change—in themselves and in society—to close the lifespan gender gap. Survival, after all, is as good a flag as any to rally 'round.

Men supposedly like fact-based things as a basis for action—car books, tax guides, that sort of thing. The fact is that we get fifty-five seconds of life for every minute enjoyed by women, just as women earn sixty-eight cents for every dollar earned by men. Isn't it time for men to be as justifiably angry as women are with a system and culture that perpetuate these differences? Together, perhaps we can do something about it besides clenching our fists ever tighter.

(Fred Hayward is a California-based lawyer and founder of Men's Rights, Inc., an advocacy group, and the Men's Health Network.)

4

WELLNESS AND THE MIND

As we've seen, men don't have a terrific record when it comes to looking after their physical needs. We avoid doctors and ignore symptoms in the hope that they'll just go away. Do we fare any better with our emotional and psychological health?

The answer is both yes and no. On the plus side, there has been a much greater recognition among men in the last few years that we even *have* an emotional life—an important first step toward building a better one. Our inner lives are just as valid a part of our existence as is our external roles as fathers, providers, lovers or any of the other elements that create the sum of us. There's a much greater sense of freedom for men in getting help with an emotional or psychological problem, too. A man seeking out a therapist was, until recently, seen as somehow suspect and "unmanly." Now we think it strange if someone who needs help doesn't get it, whether that person is a man or a woman.

Men began to pay more attention to their emotional well-being as soon as science linked our feelings to our physical health, steering the subject away from the "soft" science of psychology into the "hard" realm of cardiology. The single topic that caused this transformation was *stress*. Men might not understand emotions, but they understand heart attacks; when the competitive, "type A" men started dying at an early age, the remaining ones began to take notice—and developed a sudden and keen interest in stress and its physical and psychological underpinnings. In fact, the very men who were the least open to "dealing with their emotional lives" were precisely the men who experienced the greatest amounts of stress—and often had their lives shortened because of it.

So stress opened the door for men to explore their emotional health—but it's an entryway that's been largely unused by most men. Unfortu-nately, many of us only get religion about the dangers of stress after something catastrophic happens: a heart attack, a failed marriage, a nervous breakdown, a mid-life crisis. As with our physical health, far too many are willing to ignore emotional and psychological problems until they become so big that we have to address them. But that approach leads to years of needless pain—for ourselves and those we love—and a greatly diminished quality of life. When men do finally deal with the root causes of their unhappiness, they inevitably say, "Why did I wait so long to get help?"

For those who choose not to wait, the best news is that there have never been as many options and opportunities for help as there are today. Short-term "talk" therapies and a host of new psychological drugs (often intended for short-term use) mean that getting help doesn't have to involve years of treatment. For stress reduction and overall enhancement of the quality of life, there's a cornucopia of alternatives—from exercise to yoga to biofeedback—that can make a huge difference in the way you feel every day. As Thoreau wrote in *Walden*, "The mass of men lead lives of quiet desperation. What is called resignation is confirmed desperation." With the breadth of options available today, there is simply no need to resign oneself to suffering—quietly or otherwise.

First we'll examine stress—probably the most pervasive day-to-day emotional problem men face. Everyone feels stress, so pay particular attention to this section. Next we'll look at the "toxic emotions" like anger, hostility and jealousy that most of us suffer from at least occasionally. Then we'll explore the other common behavioral and emotional difficulties some of us face, followed by a range of solutions you can use to combat them. From simple laughter to long-term psychotherapy, there *are* solutions to these problems. Keep that in mind as you read.

STRESS

It's the thrilling edge you need to meet an impossible deadline or reach the finish line of your first marathon. It's also the steady, grinding pressure of being male in the late twentieth century. Stress is part of what keeps you alive—yet if it's too much a part of your life it will kill you.

What is stress? It is the physiological reaction of the body to a perceived threat. When you sense that there is danger about, adrenaline pumps into your system, causing a rise in heart rate, blood pressure and metabolic rate. It's as though someone has rung the "battle stations" alarm in your body, which responds by preparing for a fight. This response is known as the "fight or flight" mechanism because that's how our ancestors reacted to the stresses of their day—by entering into a fight or fleeing the source of the danger. This was a perfect reaction when man still ran into saber-toothed tigers during his workday; today the danger is more likely to be an arrogant boss, and fighting or running away aren't very good options. The undissipated energy—not used by fight or flight—is what we call stress.

The most surprising news about stress is which type does the most harm. It isn't the acute stresses of events like earthquakes or divorce that'll lay you under, but the compounded stresses of those everyday crises—money, work, kids—that eat away at you and destroy your health. Researchers are now more convinced than ever of the links between prolonged mental and emotional stress and life-threatening illness.

In the last fifteen years medical researchers have realized just how destructive stress can be to the body and mind. Stress can lead to high blood pressure, stroke and disturbances in the rhythm of the heartbeat. Chronic, continual stress can cause the blood vessels to "clamp down," further raising blood pressure. Stress can even make the platelets in the blood become more sticky, causing them to adhere to the walls of blood vessels and blocking blood flow; the platelets can even secrete a substance called adenosine triphosphate that can lead to strokes or heart attacks.

Stress can cause headaches and backaches by encouraging muscles to contract; it can also worsen the affects of arthritis and other inflammatory diseases such as lupus. Ulcers and other gastrointestinal diseases are strongly associated with stress, as are eczema, acne and other skin diseases. Animal studies show that stressed-out lab rats actually lose brain cells in the region known as the hippocampus, which controls pituitary secretions and is associated with learning and memory. Stress can also directly affect your sex life by causing testosterone levels to dip and the blood vessels in the penis to contract, making erections difficult to say the least. Stress can make any emotional problem seem much worse, and can indirectly cause people to abuse food, alcohol or drugs.

Perhaps the most pervasive problem related to stress has to do with the functioning of the immune system. Scattered throughout the body in structures like the lymph nodes, bone marrow and spleen, the far-flung cells of the immune system respond in a systemic way to stress. The "fight or flight" response of stress causes the body to activate its defenses too often, so that when a real threat—in the form of a disease—is present, the immune system is too overloaded to respond properly. Chronic stress causes lower levels of white blood cells, the body's first line of defense against illness and disease. This weakened immune response can leave you much more susceptible to every form of illness or disease that plagues man.

The toll of stress is greater than you probably suppose. By some estimates, between 75 and 90 percent of all doctor's visits in the U.S. are for stress-related disorders. Some 72 percent of American workers experience frequent physical or mental conditions related to stress, which greatly increase health-care costs for everyone. The emotional toll on individuals and families is less quantifiable but more profound.

Perhaps the most insidious part of stress is that we bring it on ourselves. After all, the stress reaction is the response to a *perceived* danger; if you don't interpret a situation as being threatening, then your body doesn't undergo profound physiological changes in order to deal with it. Some situations are genuinely threatening—loss of a loved one, a car accident, a hurricane—but most aren't: we only view them as a life-or-death situation. The ironic truth is that, in an actual emergency, those who can control their reactions to the situation are the ones who are best able to deal with it. So learning to take control of stress reactions will not only make them occur less frequently but also leave you better equipped to handle them well when they do happen.

The best way to deal with stress is to change your perception of a pressurized situation, and to practice techniques like biofeedback that can help you deal with the stress when it occurs. We'll examine some of these techniques later in this chapter. Meanwhile, the stress-bombs that modern life hurls at men are falling faster and more frequently than ever, requiring immediate survival strategies. The first step is recognizing the most common sources of stress; then we can learn how to deal with them.

Ten Modern Sources of Stress—and What to Do About Them

1. Role Call

Modern men have had their roles redefined more often and more drastically than any previous generation. When circumstance or economics limited us to killing mastodons or overhauling engines, we didn't have the time or inclination to "get sensitive" and no one thought to ask us to. Our societies needed those mastodons killed and those engines fixed. But with so few of us today doing jobs that require raw courage or brute strength, and with so few acting as sole family breadwinner, all bets are off. "Perhaps the greatest source of stress for men these days is that there are more options and choices than there have ever been in every area of our lives," says Kenneth R. Pelletier, Ph.D., author of *Mind as Healer, Mind as Slayer* and *Sound Mind, Sound Body*.

But men are being pushed and pulled at the same time, caught in a riptide of conflicting pressures. Be soft, but be strong. Look great, but don't preen. Be an animal in bed, but also know how to communicate.

A no-win situation? Not necessarily, says Pelletier. "Role ambiguity can create strain, but it can also challenge us to take the risks that make our lives most meaningful." When you've got options you can be who you really are, and damn the conventional wisdom. Successful men, says Pelletier, "make choices at critical times in their careers and lives that go against the status quo."

2. Social Insecurity Card

A man graduating from college now will, on average, hold eight jobs during his professional life—and lose four of them. "That's a very different contract than my father's generation got," says psychiatrist Don Rosen, M.D., director of the Professionals in Crisis Program at the Menninger Clinic in Topeka, Kansas. "They were often lifers at the first corporation they went to work for." The biggest victims, Rosen says, are guys who fail to diversify their interests and passions. Expand your contacts and skills within your profession. Join professional associations, go to night school, network. Your value to your employers often increases in direct proportion to your ability to leave them.

3. The Clarence Factor

Whatever really happened with Clarence Thomas and Anita Hill, the incident sent men reeling as, practically overnight, new sets of office rules went into effect. Sometimes the rules are explicitly coded. Other times, you only know what they are when you break them.

"The reality is that political correctness exists because gross abuses of power have taken place," Rosen says. "But that doesn't have to be the norm and, of course, men can be subject to harassment too, which is tremendously stressful because there's so little support for men as victims."

Rosen suggests that if you have a good social network outside the workplace, you're more likely to connect with women at work in a smooth manner, whether or not there's romance in the offing. Here's a good standard for casual encounters: Before you pat a female colleague on the back or compliment her on her new hairstyle, think of whether you'd extend the same pleasantries to a male colleague. If the answer is yes, you're not harassing anybody.

As for romance: Don't hope for, pursue or obsess about getting cozy with a woman in your office. You're there to work, not play. That said, if something does arise, there's no reason not to at least consider it. But also consider how you'd want your wife, girlfriend or sister to be treated at work. Better yet, think of how you'd like to be treated by a female coworker who was interested in more than your on-the-job expertise.

4. Labor Pains

Over the long haul, technology which has taken us from a physical-labor-based economy to a mentally driven one has created as many stresses as it has eliminated. "Mental labor," says psychologist and author Bruce Baldwin, Ph.D., "causes forms of fatigue that cannot be slept away. Emotional fatigue, which can take the form of low-level depression, can only be remedied by quality relaxation, the ability to allow oneself to become very deeply involved in any activity simply for the pleasure of it. The deeper the absorption, the more emotional recovery takes place."

A bad way to de-stress is to come home and flick on the tube. Television, says Baldwin, distracts you but doesn't take away that drained feeling. In fact, on one level it reinforces the feeling of alienation many people experience while hunched over computer terminals in their offices. A better approach: Hit the park for a jog around the lake, visit the driving range and whack a bucket of balls, or hike a trail with a friend and watch the sunset.

5. Father's Little Dividend

According to a recent study of dual-income couples funded by the National Institute of Mental Health, kids—more than careers or wives—will predict the degree to which a man suffers such stress-related health problems as insomnia, fatigue and stomach ailments. Those stresses are increasing now that most mothers are employed outside the home.

Compounding the problem, says Rosalind Barnett, author of the study and a professor at Wellesley College in Massachusetts, is the fact that employers don't allow fathers the flextime afforded to working mothers because they haven't caught up with the reality that child care has become an issue for both sexes. "Men need to protest the scheduling of events that conflict with their family time," Barnett says. "If the home life is suffering, the professional performance will also."

6. Her Cheatin' Heart

It used to be that the only fidelity a man had to worry about was his own. Now statistics show that fewer married women are remaining faithful than ever before, and younger women have surpassed men in the speed with which they have extramarital affairs.

W. Terrence Mooney, Ph.D., director of the Stress and Anxiety Clinic at Kamer Psychological Associates in Albany, New York, says that as men rush to fill the growing social and economic demands of modern living, "two of the first things to go are sleep and relationships. Many men still have a lot to learn about their partner's and even their own intimacy requirements."

Though the numbers indicate a closing of the gap between men's and women's attitudes toward relationships, Mooney says he still sees a big difference. "While women talk about how they feel, men still talk about what they think," he says. In other words, if you want your relationship to work, don't cut corners on being warm, close and loving.

7. The Air Down Here

One Los Angeles-based journalist recalls that he lived in Southern California for a month before he realized there was a smog-obscured mountain range a few miles to his north. In many American cities, such intense pollution is routine. According to the EPA, twenty years after passage of the federal Clean Air Act, 76 million people live in areas that don't meet clean-air standards. Contaminated groundwater has been found in every state. "These issues affect our lives and our health even now, whether we know it our not, and they are a source of psychological as well as physical stress," writes Jon Kabat-Zinn, Ph.D., director of the stress-reduction and relaxation program at the University of Massachusetts Medical Center, in his book *Full Catastrophe Living*. Kabat-Zinn suggests that educating yourself about the environmental issues that impact your community and identifying one to work on can increase your sense of power in relation to global problems that might otherwise seem overwhelming.

8. Crime Story

It's no longer just women who look over their shoulders at night. Forty-five percent of men in a national Victim Center Survey report they now limit the places they go by themselves due to fear of crime. Dan Smith, Ph.D., a clinical psychologist at the National Crime Victims Research and Treatment Center at the Medical University of South Carolina, says that the media's intense focus on violent crime has caused public concern about crime to rise at a faster rate than crime itself.

Short of walking around with a bunker mentality, Smith suggests that men can increase their sense of personal security by using some of the crime-protection advice and resources directed at women. If you're going to be working late, make sure you're locked in and notify your building's security staff. Park as close to your building as possible, preferably under a light. Learn how to use and carry pepper spray. If you do fall prey to criminals, don't discount the benefits of short-term therapy or a support group; and don't blame yourself for being targeted.

9. We Trust in Whom?

If you were dragged to church or Sunday school as a child, you may still equate religion with torture. Indeed, there's been a decline in church and synagogue attendance by men in their twenties and thirties. While involvement in a religious community can provide the social support that helps reduce stress, experts agree it's the spiritual aspect of religious commitment—the connection to something beyond the individual—that's most important.

Pelletier says that of the fifty-one highly successful people he interviewed for *Sound Mind, Sound Body*, only three or four were orthodox practitioners of a specific religion, but all described a spiritual element in their lives. "They saw a larger purpose in their lives beyond simply making a movie or a good investment. While they are financially successful people, their definition of success had much more to do with involvement in something they believed to be important."

If your job doesn't provide this type of fulfillment and you're not particularly religious, volunteer work or political activism can add meaning to your life and offer the social network formerly provided by church membership.

10. Fountain of Age

If someone told you you'd be driving your Toyota for the next fifty years, you probably wouldn't skip a single oil change, tune-up or car wash. Well, perhaps you should think the same way about your body, because you're probably going to be living in it for a long time. Thanks to a jump in men's life expectancy during the past 15 years, those who make it to age 65 can expect, on average, to live another 15.2 years.

Joel Posner, M.D., chief of geriatric and rehabilitation medicine at the Medical College of Pennsylvania, says that a life of sound physical (and fiscal) health culminates in a healthy old age free of anxiety and depression.

Financial fitness should complement good health. While men save an average of 5 percent of their income, experts recommend doubling that. At the least, take advantage of tax-deferred retirement programs available through your employer.

SEVEN INSTANT STRESS-BUSTERS

If you're a mess from stress, the first thing you've got to do is realize that it's not your main problem. It's merely a symptom of feeling out of control, of being swept away from yourself by life's momentum. The key to relaxing, says stress-management expert Saki Santorelli, is to "return to yourself periodically during the day." He calls this "mindfulness," and it has to do with becoming more aware of your body and your mind in the midst of all the turbulence. Here are seven simple ways to do it:

- If you watch the clock a lot, then use it to unwind. Stick little colored dots on all your timepieces. Then, whenever you check them, you'll be reminded to devote a few seconds to yourself. Take a deep breath and drop your shoulders. Don't be surprised if you end up giving yourself fifty of these minibreaks a day.
- Instead of leaping for the shower immediately after the alarm clock sounds, lie in bed quietly for a few minutes. Listen to the sounds from outside or gaze through a window.
- Resist the urge to reach for the phone immediately when someone calls. Let the first ring signal you to take a deep breath and relax. Receptionists who started doing this had frequent callers remark how calm they sounded.
- While driving, turn off the radio and tune in to body tension. Sit back, unclench your knuckles on the steering wheel, release the tension from your legs.
- Eat one or two lunches a week by yourself, in silent contemplation.
- Pay attention to the short walk to your car after work. Take your time, breathe deeply, listen.
- Change out of your work clothes when you get home to ease the transition into your next role.

TOXIC EMOTIONS

Jack remembers what was going through his mind the day he got fired from his job. "It had been building for months," he says. "Everything I did, they wanted me to do over. Everything they did, I found myself second-guessing. So when I walked into that meeting on my last day, I was already juiced for a confrontation."

The meeting concerned a project Jack had been developing for his employer, a marketing firm. "The first time they questioned the way I was approaching it, I blew up. I told them the project was an idiotic idea, that it wouldn't make a dime for the client and that my considerable talents were being wasted." Jack acknowledges that his behavior was boneheaded at best, fantastically self-destructive at worst. "I sure wish I would've handled that one differently," he says, his voice trailing off wistfully. "Maybe next time."

For Jack, as for many men, anger has always seemed like a good idea, at least in theory. He remembers his father telling him to "get mad at it" when he wasn't strong enough to loosen a bolt on his bicycle. He also remembers the result of his getting mad: a ruined bicycle. (His solution was to attack the bolt with a hammer.)

And, indeed, male rage—what we call tantrums in childhood, "blowing off steam" in our adult lives—is a glorified commodity in our popular culture. We cheered when John Wayne, in *True Grit*, responded to a personal insult by telling his taunter, "Fill your hands, you son of a bitch!" (With guns, he meant.) We identified with Kurt Russel's violent revenge against Ray Liotta, who, playing a jealousy-consumed cop in *Unlawful Entry*, threatened Russell's life and marriage. And we laughed when Tom Hanks, in *A League of Their Own*, tried to get control of his all-woman baseball team by screaming, "There's no crying in baseball!"

But while explosive emotions may feed the box office, they're often disastrous to men's personal and professional relationships. Among the most troublesome and potentially dangerous emotions for men, experts agree, are anger, hostility (anger's first cousin) and jealousy.

Los Angeles psychologist Harriet B. Braiker calls them "toxic emotions." But Gordon Clanton, who teaches sociology at San Diego State University in California, thinks such labels are unjust. It's not the emotions per se that are negative, Clanton says, but the manner in which they're expressed and to what degree. "Even emotions with bad reputations are useful in their own way," he adds. "They're signals to be interpreted." When men demonstrate these so-called negative emotions appropriately and analyze them properly, Clanton contends, they can actually improve their relationships, their careers, their overall well-being. But when expressed inappropriately, "explosive" emotions can even be physically damaging.

The jealous man who, for instance, obsesses about having what others have or about what other men may be seeking (like his mate or job) often finds relaxation elusive and stress his constant companion. Anger and hostility keep your body in the "fight-or-flight" stance, which can wreak havoc on your entire body. "A person who is angry all the time is prone to medical problems such as hypertension, ulcers, headaches and probably heart disease," says psychologist Thomas Bowlus, chair of mental health in Los Angeles and Orange Counties for FHP, a health maintenance organization.

Indeed, outbursts of anger seem to actually affect the heart's functioning, according to a study published in 1992 in the *American Journal of Cardiology*. When heart patients described past incidents that still infuriated them, the pumping efficiency of their hearts temporarily declined.

Historically, anger had cultural value, allowing our ancestors to fend off enemies, says Houston psychiatrist Kenneth Wetcher. A society without appropriate anger would mean no resistance against attack or monumental injustices. But in modern society, angry responses are often not in reaction to true life-and-death situations but to relatively minor annoyances like sluggish restaurant employees or traffic jams.

The effects of anger aren't just physiological, of course. Angry outbursts can mean the difference between job promotions and firings, between gaining a reputation as a team player or the office hothead. Anger can spoil an evening or an entire relationship.

It's no surprise to Wetcher that men are considered the explosive gender. Part of the problem lies in our upbringing, he says. "Society discourages little boys from expressing feelings like sadness," he explains. Then boys are encouraged to participate in competitive events such as sports. And on the playing field, it's acceptable—even good—to get angry.

Society tolerates angry behavior in boys much more readily than in girls, contends Wetcher, who directs a therapy clinic that specializes in treating men. There's a biological component as well. "Aggression is mediated by male hormones," he says. "After puberty, there is a great propensity to feel that surge of aggression and to express it in an angry way." And when anger is expressed by men, it's more likely to result in violent behavior than when it's displayed by women. According to Braiker, one reason is that society is more likely to give men permission to be angry and violent. "Violence is considered a masculine trait," she says, "and distinctly unfeminine."

Even so, Braiker points out, "Anger is not in and of itself a toxic emotion if it is expressed appropriately." You sometimes need to get angry to make yourself heard, for instance. She distinguishes between demonstrating anger in an assertive way, which can be healthy and proper, and venting it in an aggressive way, which can be counterproductive and sometimes dangerous.

Anger in men is frequently accompanied by hostility, and while the two emotions are often exhibited simultaneously, experts say there's a difference between them. Anger is often a reaction to a specific incident or perceived injustice, such as being cut off on the freeway. "Hostility is a pervasive, free-floating attitude," Braiker says, "the feeling that people are out to get you." Anger, she adds, is often rational, while hostility can seem groundless: "Hostility is connected to cynicism, which is known to be a cardiac poison. You don't trust people; life stinks. And to top it off, you don't expect anything to improve."

The green-eyed monster jealousy often finds an even more powerful expression in men than does hostility, despite the fact that women are often stereotyped as the jealous gender. Researchers find little difference between men and women when it comes to this particular emotion. In men, however, jealousy often masquerades as anger or hostility.

Men deny they're jealous by quickly relabeling their own expression of the feeling as righteous anger, says Clanton, who with Lynn G. Smith wrote the classic academic work on the subject, *Jealousy*. Or, he says, men will bottle up jealousy until they either explode in anger or become increasingly hostile. "Jealousy is an integral part of cynicism," says Braiker. A cynical person basically doesn't trust other people, she adds. "And that's what jealousy is all about, the belief that other people can't be trusted."

Even when men do acknowledge feelings of jealousy, they often refuse to explore them. "The most common male reaction," says Wetcher, "is to say, 'I'm outta here.'" Often a man will terminate a romantic relationship rather than explore the roots of his jealous feelings. In the professional world, jealousy of another man will often take the form of sarcasm about and criticism of a coworker, boss or subordinate. Again, denial of the emotion plays a strong role in its inappropriate expression. In proper perspective, jealousy is an early-warning system that lets people know a relationship they value is threatened in some way or perceived to be threatened, Clanton says. It's an emotion that's often symptomatic of deeper problems, usually a lack of trust.

It's easier to handle powerful emotions if you step back and consider your underlying feelings. What's going on is usually more than simple anger, hostility or jealousy. When it comes to anger, men often feel a lack of control behind the emotion, Bowlus says, whereas jealousy seems to arise from a lack of self-confidence.

Hostility may have at its root helplessness, lack of control or cynicism. "If you can verbalize the real emotions, you can begin to deal with the situation," Braiker says. Communicating so-called negative emotions to the people directly involved can help, too. Honesty might not always have the desired effect of changing the situation—but at least you'll know where you stand and can then seek other outlets for your feelings. It can sometimes also help to visualize the potential physical damage caused by negative emotions in order to dispel them. Braiker tells her anger-prone clients, "Think about what is going on inside your body while you are experiencing all this anger. You are the one who is being damaged most."

Making an effort to talk frequently with other men can help you cope with the "toxic" emotions, Wetcher says. That might require some real changes in the traditional male outlook. "Most men think they communicate better with women. In fact, they do that with lots of ulterior motives; it's not the same way that they would talk with other men," he says.

Wetcher's advice instead is to spend time with other men, not just during traditional male activities like sporting events or poker games, but at leisure, when the focus is on communication rather than an outside activity. "Some men do it formally in a men's group, others casually," he says. "But the more time you spend with other men, the more you'll be able to express your feelings and the more new ways you will learn to deal with potentially harmful emotions."

Therapy can help men unravel and deal with the underlying feelings that lead to harmful expressions of emotion. A technique called cognitive retraining can help you express your emotions more healthfully, Bowlus contends. In a nutshell, that means "looking at the thoughts you have and the behaviors of others and determining if your interpretation of them makes sense."

Treating so-called toxic emotions as a warning sign, not an excuse to become violent or walk out on a relationship or a job, can mean the difference, experts say, between keeping a job and losing it, enjoying an intimate relationship and watching it disintegrate—perhaps even between being healthy and landing in the hospital.

HOW HOSTILE ARE YOU? A QUICK SELF-TEST

According to Duke University professor Redford Williams in his book *The Trusting Heart*, hostility has three particularly toxic aspects:

- cynical beliefs that others are inherently bad, selfish, mean and untrustworthy;
- angry feelings when these negative expectations are frequently fulfilled;

- the overt expression of these angry feelings in aggressive acts directed toward others.

Do any of these apply to you? Look at the following situations and see if you recognize yourself. There's no scoring system; if you answer in the affirmative to more than one, you're hostile.

1. You've pushed the elevator button and the elevator stops two floors above for a bit longer than normal. You think something like, "How dare they carry on a conversation while I'm in a hurry!"
2. You're in the express line at the supermarket, and, after counting the items in everyone's basket and satisfying yourself that no one has more than the limit, you comment to the person next to you that store management always assigns the slowest checker to the express line.
3. You see the light change to yellow as you approach an intersection. You think you can make it, but the car ahead of you stops. You stew, waiting for the light to change; then as soon as it turns green, you honk at the driver ahead of you to get moving.
4. You're on an airplane. The person in the next seat is overweight, and parts of him hang over your armrest. You think that some people just don't have the decency to lose weight and stop inconveniencing others with their flab.
5. Your child spills his food on the floor, and you yell at him to be more careful. When your wife gets mad at you for yelling at the kid, you say to yourself that if she were better at cleaning up after such accidents, you wouldn't worry about them.
6. When someone is driving with his brights on, you turn yours on—and keep them on—to try to get back at him.
7. You read the above list and say to yourself, "But these are the normal ways to react to these situations! If you act any differently, you're either a wimp or you're dead!"

OTHER COMMON BEHAVIORAL AND EMOTIONAL PROBLEMS

Depression

We live in a culture in which men are supposed to be open and honest (you know, *sensitive*), yet tough and silent (like just about every major male movie character, and some recent females, too). So it's no surprise that guys remain pretty unreceptive to topics like depression, even when its incidence, particularly among men, continues to grow steadily.

That tally doesn't refer to random everyday disappointment nor exclusively to major depression, the kind characterized by feelings of doom and hopelessness. Usually, depression is more ambiguous than that, lacking specific boundaries or form. For instance, the mood swings of manic depression can camouflage themselves as mere eccentricity. The emotional lows of seasonal affective disorder (SAD), caused by winter's low light level, may simply seem like potent holiday blues or fatigue. With chronic depression, also called dysthymia, you might just consider the glass perpetually half drained—and yourself perpetually dissatisfied. But you don't have to be.

Half the population still considers depression a personal weakness or character flaw, according to the U.S. Department of Health and Human Services, even though the annual tab for lost productivity, medical expenses and suicides caused by depression is almost $44 billion. As it is, 17.5 million people in the US have been diagnosed with depression, and the rate has been increasing globally since 1915—especially since World War II.

Frederick Goodwin, M.D., former director of the National Institute of Mental Health and now director of the Center on Neuroscience, Behavior and Society at George Washington University, has a good idea why: the steady erosion of our traditional sources of spirituality, connection and stability. "In the same era that we have seen, essentially, the doubling of depression among the young," Goodwin explains, "we've seen a doubling of divorce rates, a sharp decline in net parenting time and a tripling of the mobility rate," or the average number of times a person changes residence. Experts, including Goodwin, also suggest that the steady revision of men's role in society may add to this subtle sense of drift among men.

Knowing exactly what's expected of us as males can cause confusion. Are we brave defenders of women and children, or scared like everybody else? Do we still hold doors open and pick up the check on dates? Are we allowed to show fear and express our vulnerabilities or will doing so make us unattractive to the people whose opinions matter most to us? That's not to say men haven't dropped their guard a bit. "Until recently, women have been much more likely than men to seek help for emotional suffering," says psychiatrist Harold H. Bloomfield, M.D., author of *How to Heal Depression*, "whereas men in general are much more likely to suffer silently." He's watched his own clientele shift from 80 percent women to a 50–50 ratio.

Goodwin notes a similar transformation. "Ted Turner is saying, 'Lithium saved my life.' Dick Cavett is saying, 'I'm only here today because of [shock therapy].'" Goodwin points out that Mike Wallace and Art

Buchwald have publicly discussed their depression as well. Nevertheless, both experts acknowledge that the numbers seem off. After all, twice as many women as men have been diagnosed with depression. (Not long ago, the ratio was three to one.) Yet men are three times as likely as women to develop alcoholism, and males kill themselves at four times the rate as women due to behaviors inextricably linked to depression. The hypothesis: Old habits die hard. Though men have evolved, the stiff upper lip still rules.

To speed evolution along, more than eight million Americans have turned to Prozac, a drug that revolutionized psychopharmacology when it came out about seven years ago. "Too many people," a pharmacist told me during a random opinion poll. "You have regular doctors who aren't psychiatrists prescribing it left and right. People come in all the time asking for it. It's not good." One reason for such mass prescribing is that Prozac, which belongs to a new class of antidepressants called selective serotonin reuptake inhibitors (SSRIs), treats a range of ills, from major depression to dysthymia to excessive shyness to eating disorders. It achieves all this with fewer nasty side effects (such as dizziness and sedation) than its predecessors cause.

The side effects SSRIs can create, though, include initial headache and nausea, as well as trouble reaching orgasm. Eli Lilly, Prozac's manufacturer, estimates that only about 2 percent of users suffer this problem, but Columbia University psychiatrist Ron G. Goldman, M.D., reports that about 5 to 15 percent of his male patients complain of it. Nonetheless, he probably speaks for the majority of psychiatrists when he points out that patients often feel so much better after being relieved of their depression that they gladly sacrifice an easy orgasm; some patients even like taking longer to climax. When no amount of hard work will bring sex to a happy conclusion, however, doctors often turn to a drug called Wellbutrin, which is in a pharmacological class by itself and deals out sexual complications quite sparingly (about 3 percent of users complain of them).

Even newer drugs are on the way. Already, the antidepressant Effexor has made waves because of its mild side effects and dual action, combining benefits of SSRIs and tricyclics (an older, side-effect-ridden class of drugs that block the neurotransmitter norepinephrine). "It's being referred to as Prozac with a boost," Bloomfield says.

For some experts, like William B. Swann Jr., Ph.D., a professor of psychology at the University of Texas at Austin, the solution lies in the interpersonal—listening to what supportive friends and relatives say and seeking therapy to relearn ways of thinking. "I have friends who take [antidepressants], and friends in the clinical psychology community who recommend them strongly, but personally, I'm wary of these drugs," Swann says. In fact, therapy alone works at least half the time. But antidepressants' results are better: They work about 65 to 75 percent of the time. Thus, many experts—backed by solid research—agree that the two treatments should be combined.

And just about all professionals in the field recommend simply eating right and exercising. "I've been in practice for thirty years, and I find that people who change their cholesterol levels and their diets, exercise more, lose weight and stop smoking are happier people generally," says William E. Connor, M.D., professor of medicine at the Oregon Health Sciences University. Connor co-authored the Family Heart Study, in which more than 300 men and women from 233 Portland families were put on cholesterol-lowering diets for five years. By the end, the people who had gone heavy on complex carbohydrates and light on fat showed significant drops in depression *and* hostility. Connor attributes these results to the ego boost that comes with getting healthy, but he also nods at the food-mood connection. "Fat can make you feel sluggish because it takes a long time to digest," he says. Because of this, blood that would otherwise be bathing your brain goes to your abdomen to aid digestion.

Exercise ties right into the whole process: It burns fat, reduces stress and spurs the brain to produce endorphins. Connor notes that you don't have to run long stretches to enjoy the same benefits; any vigorous exercise in which you elevate your heart rate between 20 and 30 percent above your resting heart rate will stir them up. "I ride a bicycle for fifteen minutes," he adds, "and I feel [the endorphins]."

No one's suggesting that the gym alone can replace therapy, just that it can help. So can reconnecting with people and establishing a sense of spirituality. That doesn't mean you have to get religious. "It's about having a sense of purpose, which can provide motivation," Goldman says. "A key aspect of spirituality is the sense that the group is important."

Attending a church service, joining a local twelve-step chapter or just celebrating your family—all offer a brand of spirituality, a chance to reconnect. In a country whose people have begun feeling profoundly disconnected, that's some strong medicine we could all use, depressed or not.

Anxiety Disorders

Anxiety, like stress, is a part of everyday life. But at what point does anxiety become enough of a problem to warrant attention? If determining a level of "normal" anxiety seems hard to you, then pity the psychological researchers; they've been trying to make that determination for years.

For most people anxiety is linked with the cornucopia of life's stresses, and rises and falls in accord with them. When apprehension and worry seem to come out of nowhere, last longer than six months, and greatly affect the quality of life, then it's time to suspect an anxiety disorder.

Anxiety disorders generally fall into five categories, though there can be overlap between them. A *generalized anxiety disorder* is what most people think of as anxiety, but it happens when life's circumstances seem to be good; it's unrelated to traumatic outside events. In *panic disorder*, those affected get panic attacks—sudden, intense periods of fear and discomfort that can be accompanied by dizziness, nausea, a racing pulse, chest pain, and other worrisome symptoms. In *social phobia* the sufferer has fear of certain social situations or activities where he thinks he may be subject to embarrassment or ridicule. Those with *obsessive-compulsive disorder* have the need to repetitively enact certain rituals for up to several hours a day. Finally, *post-traumatic stress disorder* strikes those who have experienced or witnessed cataclysmic events such as war, rape, natural catastrophes or assault.

Generalized anxiety disorder is probably the most common form that falls within the category of "anxiety disorders." For most of us, anxiety is closely related to stressful life events: birth, death, job changes, and the like. The period of anxiety closely follows the timeframe of the event; when the wedding is over, for example, you're no longer stressed about it. In a generalized anxiety disorder the apprehension seems to come from nowhere, and may last for months. As a result you can become fatigued, overwrought and unfocused, and may experience symptoms like headaches, insomnia, shakiness and edginess. It affects both sexes equally, and often strikes in the twenties or thirties. Both pharmaceuticals and short-term "talk" therapy can be used to treat the disorder.

Panic disorder can occur concurrently with other anxiety disorders; some 25 percent of those with panic problems also have a generalized anxiety disorder. It can also affect those with depression. Panic attacks are usually triggered by specific situations that someone finds particularly stressful, but typically at least one of the episodes will simply occur out of the blue. The attacks are accompanied by a number of physical symptoms such as nausea, shortness of breath, trembling, chills, hot flashes, dizziness, rapid heartbeat and chest discomfort. Perhaps the worst symptom is a feeling of dread and impending doom. Some sufferers are convinced at these moments that they are about to either die or go insane.

Panic disorder usually begins in the midtwenties but can strike at any age, and women are affected twice as often as men. As many as 70 percent of those with the disorder also suffer from agoraphobia—the fear of confined spaces. Both pharmaceuticals and short-term "talk" therapy (discussed later in this chapter) can be used to treat the disorder.

Social phobia, as with the other anxieties, is an example of a common feeling of apprehension carried to an abnormal degree. The normal apprehension many people feel before a party or while speaking in public can be amplified so that virtually any social contact—even a phone call—brings on a crippling feeling of anxiety. As a result, that person reacts by withdrawing from social situations that may bring about those feelings. Social phobics often experience a self-fullfilling cycle: they dread a social interaction and once there become so anxious that they end up feeling humiliated—making them even less inclined to go out and interact.

Social phobia affects men more often than women, and may first appear in adolescence. Though it may hang around for years, it seems to decline after mid-life. This anxiety disorder is almost always treated with a form of behavior therapy called "systematic desensitation." Starting with brief exposures—say, walking into a crowded store for five minutes—the therapist helps the patient confront his phobia until he is no longer affected by symptoms.

In *obsessive-compulsive disorders* (OCD), everyday habits become rituals that the sufferer is forced to endlessly repeat—sometimes for hours at a time. The ritual is fueled by obsessive thoughts that drive the behavior. These behaviors are supposed to prevent or produce a future event, even though the rituals themselves may have nothing to do with that event. Cumpulsive washing is a typical example, in this variety of the disorder, one might repeatedly wash one's hands—for up to three hours a day—until the skin is raw and broken. (A high percentage of obsessive-compulsive patients have an inordinate fear of germs.) Others may continually check to see if the stove is off or the doors are locked. The patient usually recognizes that his behavior is compulsive, but is absolutely compelled to undergo his personal ritual. While most of those afflicted show symptoms before age thirty-five, older adults are not immune. (Howard Hughes, whose compulsion caused him to line windows with aluminum foil and save jars of his urine, didn't become demonstrably obsessive-compulsive until late in life.)

The trigger for the behavior is rarely known, and treatment generally takes a hit-or-miss approach with varying degrees of success. Some doctors have focused on behavioral therapies—making patients confront their obsessions and resist them, one minute at a time, until they eventually are free of the ritual. This approach has worked for 60 to 90 percent of those affected. Even antibiotics have helped some patients, leading researchers to suspect a physiological basis to the disorder. Mood-regulating drugs like Prozac and Nardil have also been effective. The syndrome can also simply appear and disappear on its own.

Post-traumatic stress disorder (PTSD) is most closely associated with Vietnam War veterans, but it also strikes civilians who've experienced or witnessed particularly horrible events. The event may have caused physical injury or psychological scarring, but in either case keeps "playing back" in the mind of the afflicted. The person re-experiences the trauma in night-mares, flashbacks, or intrusive thoughts or images of the event. The person might also repress memories of all or part of the actual event.

PTSD causes an extreme sense of removal from life, defined by an emotional numbness and estrangement. Forming or maintaining any sort of relationship may be difficult. Extreme pessimism concerning the future is often present, and a number of anxiety symptoms—sleeplessness, explosive outbursts, or irritability—may also be found. Major depression often accompanies PTSD, as do suicidal tendencies, panic attacks, and substance-abuse problems. PTSD symptoms will often last for years; should they occur for less than one month, then the diagnosis is probably acute-stress disorder.

PTSD can strike anyone, but certain people are more susceptible: the very young, older people with physical problems, and those with other psychological problems or who are without a good social support system of friends and family. Long-term psychotherapy, both with or without phar-maceutical therapy, offers the strongest chance for recovery.

Attention Deficit Disorder

At thirty-seven, Tom should have been hitting his stride, both personally and professionally. And, to all appearances, he had life nailed: a good job, the respect of his co-workers, a solid reputation as the go-to guy, the orga-nization man who knew how to get things done.

What Tom's co-workers couldn't see, however, was a tormented inner life. His moods swung from elation to bitter depression, and if any-one changed any part of his day-to-day routine, he went into a tailspin of anger and resentment. The worse he felt, the harder he worked to maintain a facade of professional competence, and the effort drained his energy, com-promised his health and ruined his relationships.

Without knowing it, Tom was quietly falling victim to attention deficit disorder (ADD), a glitch in the brain's ability to selectively filter informa-tion, discover which is most important and then apply that information promptly and appropriately. Educators and psychologists have long understood how children suffer from ADD; unfortunately, the adult version of ADD is little known and rarely diagnosed.

Adult ADD is often characterized by low energy, high levels of anxiety, poor self-esteem and a chronic inability to sustain any type of regimen—especially in environments of challenge and change.

Joey Lerner, M.D., a Colorado psychiatrist specializing in the treatment of ADD, emphasizes that most people—including many medical professionals—simply don't understand that ADD is a legitimate physiological condition. Without an understanding of ADD's symptoms, a scenario such as Tom's can easily be mistaken for chronic fatigue syndrome, job burnout, obsessive-compulsive disorder, clinical depression or the infamous "mid-life crisis." Like these other conditions, ADD undermines a person's ability to chart a course and sustain it. Unlike them, its treatment can be quick, easy and effective—with dramatic results.

First and foremost, ADD is not a virus that strikes from out of the blue; it has a neurobiological basis that represents a lifelong condition. A person's experience of its symptoms, however, can develop and change over time. While no two people display the same symptoms in the same ways, an ADD sufferer will generally display at least four of the following symptoms:

- Distractibility. Your attention wanders, especially in circumstances that hold little immediate interest or significance for you.
- Restlessness. You tend to fidget, mentally and physically, and are always impatient.
- Impulsiveness. You make quick mental leaps that others have a hard time following. You feel burdened by routine, facts and details and prefer to act on your instincts.
- Moodiness. Friends and co-workers approach you with caution; they've seen your mood swings and test the waters with each new encounter.
- Disorganization. You frequently misplace things; it's difficult to maintain order and routine in your home, work area and thoughts.
- Low tolerance for stress. The smallest complications disrupt your uneasy truce with the world. You avoid committing yourself to specific deadlines or expectations, and change—any change—can throw you into a tailspin.
- Suppressed rage. Your deep reservoir of frustration, discontentment, anger and defensiveness emerges when you—and others—least expect it. Or your rage is buried so deeply that you never express any emotions at all; rather, you display a resentful, pessimistic view of life.
- Low energy. Since you're wary and mistrustful of outcomes, you begin to put forth less and less effort. Physically and mentally, you maintain a

low-arousal state that insulates you from immediate demands and expectations.

Of course, not everybody who experiences the symptoms of adult ADD necessarily has ADD. The distinguishing factor is the degree: How often, how severely and how persistently do the symptoms present themselves? This questioning process challenges you to initiate the process of diagnosis and treatment. If you think four or more of the listed symptoms are so chronic that they're creating significant stress and dysfunction in your life, it's time to talk with someone.

Start with your family physician. Ask what he or she knows about ADD in adults. Ask if there is a colleague who might know more, or a specialist he or she might recommend. Don't be put off by assurances that "there's really nothing wrong that a little more rest and relaxation can't fix." You can also contact a national organization such as the Attention Deficit Disorder Association. There are calls you can make and people you can talk to no matter where you live. If it seems difficult and you can't bring yourself to sustain a search (which is a natural extension of the symptoms), enlist the help of a friend or spouse.

Since so much is known about childhood ADD, there's no shortage of treatments available, and researchers are discovering that many of these work for adults, too. Resources include the following:

Medications such as methylphenidate (Ritalin) or dextroamphetamine (Dexedrine) that act on the brain's neurotransmitters. By stimulating brain activity, patients frequently realize an improved ability to focus on, filter and respond to external stimuli.

Emerging biofeedback technologies that allow an individual to monitor and control his own brain waves, helping to shape emotional and physiological responses to the world.

Nutrition therapies (especially involving amino acids such as tyrosine) that show a link between nutrients and brain activity.

Support groups, books and articles can help the ADD-affected adult turn the corner toward a more enjoyable life.

Because adults carry a lifetime of habits developed in response to ADD, it is often important to couple any medical or nutritional therapy with counseling and behavioral conditioning. The need may not be immediately apparent, but it's essential to recognize the complexity of the human system and not trivialize the changes you're able to make with the attitude that "all I needed was a quick tune-up."

Since ADD often runs in families, it may be helpful to determine whether parents, siblings or children are affected by the same condition and work as a team to encourage and coach each other through its challenges. The changed dynamics in your family relationships can be especially rewarding.

With a combined treatment of low-dosage medication and periodic counseling, Tom's good humor has returned. He's rediscovering the little joys in daily life. He makes time for his wife and children. And, for the first time in his life, he has established—and sustained—a regular routine of weight training and cardiovascular conditioning. He has lost twelve pounds and begun playing outdoors again. In short, he's healthy, energized and excited about life.

For some, like Tom, medical intervention can have an immediate, dramatic effect. For others, success depends on a comprehensive program of counseling and behavioral conditioning. While no single therapy can guarantee success, psychiatrist Lerner emphasizes, "It's important to start somewhere." In any case, the most immediate benefit of treatment is often hope. And from there, anything is possible.

For more information, contact the Attention Deficit Disorder Association at (800) 487–2282.

THERAPEUTIC APPROACHES

Therapy for Guys (AKA: Short-Term Action Therapy)

Let's face it—almost any man would rather eat dirt than talk to someone about his problems, especially a therapist. He hates finding himself in a one-down position where he doesn't know something, isn't in control or, worse, might be made to look bad. What could be more disconcerting than sitting in front of some annoyingly soft-spoken counselor and being asked such questions as " . . . and how do you feel about that?" In fact, the typical gut reaction of most men to counseling is that it's something that was invented for women, and they want nothing to do with it.

If you've ever found yourself caught between counseling and a hard place, there's good news. Thanks to insurance cutbacks, managed care, a growing impatience with psychobabble, an increased appreciation of gender differences and probably a host of other forces, there's a whole new trend in psychotherapy these days that's right up a man's alley. It's called short-term action therapy, and instead of being talk- and feeling-oriented ("gal" therapy), it's task- and results-oriented.

It goes by many other names: solution-focused brief therapy, goal-oriented therapy, present-focused therapy, crisis counseling, behavior therapy, problem-solving therapy, cognitive therapy, reality therapy. They all have a number of things in common: a focus on brevity, an emphasis on taking specific actions, helping clients realize they already know how to solve their own problems, and requiring that clients become active participants in the therapeutic process.

People don't need insights in order to change. They don't need to know why they do, feel or fear something in order to overcome it. "It's useless to ask male patients how they feel or why they feel that way," says Mark Mitchell of Playa del Rey, California, a marriage and family counselor specializing in solution-focused brief therapy. "The typical man will say, 'Give me something to do and I'll try it,' so what you do with men in therapy is give them a problem to solve."

Mitchell finds this therapy appropriate for all kinds of men, from teamsters to executives. And the approach appears helpful in dealing with problems in many areas—anxieties, phobias, fathering, marriage, work, addiction, creativity, impulse control, communication, depression and sex.

The short-term therapist is different, too. Unlike the traditional counselor who maintains distance behind the so-called "blank screen," he or she is likely to be more interactive; you can expect interaction, feedback, personal insights and even advice. The therapist may skip over past-oriented questions and get right to the problem: "What brings you in here? What needs to be fixed?" After that, you move on to future-oriented questions like, "What actions can you take today to resolve your problem?"

The premise behind short-term therapy is that while insight is interesting, it rarely changes anything. What does change people is action, doing something. It's not that talking has no value; it does. But it's not a substitute for action. In psychotherapy, it's too easy for patients to fall into the age-old trap of thinking that just because they're "in therapy" they're doing something about their problem.

But the fact that therapy is quick doesn't mean it's a one-shot process. You can always go back for a tune-up. After all, as your grandfather probably told you, you are what you do. Action will always speak louder than words.

When your job's on the line, your love relationship ends or a parent dies, calling a therapist just makes good sense. But what about when your problems are much less dramatic, when you feel you really have no right to complain? Your job is going well, for instance, but you're discontented. Your relationship with a lover is good, but you know it could be better. Are these times to see a counselor?

Absolutely, says Mark S. Goulston, M.D., a psychiatrist at the University of California, Los Angeles, who firmly believes in such "noncrisis intervention." There's a big difference, he says, between therapy during a crisis and therapy during a less tumultuous time of life. "A crisis pushes people to the point of changing," he says. "The problem is, as soon as the crisis passes, you often don't sustain the change. The reality is this: The best time to make changes that endure is when desire—not fear—is pushing you toward the changes."

Here, Goulston elaborates on the theory and practice of "noncrisis" therapy. Call it, if you will, therapy for the undisturbed.

Men's Fitness: What are some of the reasons men come in for "noncrisis" therapy?

Mark S. Goulston, M.D.: One common scenario is that a man who has established his career begins to doubt whether he should continue scratching his way up the career ladder. Often I hear this from men: "I know how to achieve and I know how to accomplish, but it doesn't make me any happier. Yet it's all I know how to do." People frequently confuse job security and achievement with fulfillment and happiness. Men often have a sense of disappointment because achievement and accomplishment can become hollow experiences.

Often, too, they tell me it's just tough to make life choices. Men don't always know what will make them happy in terms of a career, a hobby, a relationship. In therapy, we confront the illusion that a man will miraculously find his passion—in work, life, a relationship. Many men have an idea that the answer will suddenly burst upon them. They don't realize that this is highly unlikely. You are more likely to discover what you want to do while you are active and doing many things. Many men tend to think too much, to overanalyze, further incapacitating themselves.

MF: Can therapy help improve creative problem-solving skills?

MG: I think so. I remember a writer who was having problems with his work. He had had early success and felt pressured to keep producing better work. At one point I suggested a topic, just meaning to be helpful. He got very competitive with me. Something inside him seemed to say, "He's a therapist; I'm the writer. I can do better than that." He got fired up. I think he might have lost that competitiveness along the way and, in the process, some of his creativity.

MF: What other everyday dilemmas might therapy help you solve?

MG: You can gain insight into characteristics that impede your work or relationships. Procrastinators, for instance, are not necessarily lazy. Often they are lonely and just don't want to go off and work on a project alone—solitude can reawaken memories of when you were lonely, home alone, or otherwise felt anxiety. Therapy can also help you deal with difficult people in ways you might never have dreamed possible. Let's say you have a manager or boss who is very scattered and keeps changing assignments on you. He has an idea a minute, gives you instructions, then is onto something else.

You might think you have to simply find a way to please him or risk losing your job. Not so. Talk to your boss, in this case about your desire to produce for the company. Say something like this: "I'm having a problem. I like to follow through on assignments, but they change so frequently it is difficult to do so. So I propose a choice: I can put a little effort into all the assignments you give me, or we can put more initial thought into assignments so fewer get ditched."

The message you're giving your boss is that you want to work hard, you want to do right by the company. It would be difficult for the boss to take this personally. You might have to explain or give an example of how he changes his mind—invite him to your office to see the pile of unfinished projects, for instance. What would be the usual—and wrong—way to handle this? You get frustrated, you "stuff" your feelings out of fear of risking your job. You get depressed, take out your frustration and depression on your relationships outside work, turn to alcohol or drugs. Eventually you lose your productivity, all because you didn't think you could hold your boss accountable.

MF: What time frame are you talking about for therapy of this nature?

MG: Generally it's short-term, sometimes a matter of a few sessions. The more a person is ready to change, the quicker the therapy.

MF: Besides the usual advice to be on time for sessions and to ponder the feedback your therapist offers, are there ways to minimize the time you spend in therapy while maximizing the benefits?

MG: I have been suggesting for years that patients tape our sessions and listen to them later. About 60 percent of my clients do so. Listening to the tape after the session can serve many useful purposes. For one thing, it helps distinguish between relief and resolution. The tape doesn't lie. I have suggested this technique to couples in therapy and ask that they listen separately, or together if they promise not to get defensive and interrupt. One man listened to himself on tape and confessed he heard a Neanderthal who grunts and often doesn't finish his sentences when talking to his wife. His mate realized that she interrupts every other word her husband speaks. Some patients who get discouraged in therapy go back and listen to the initial tape and can feel good about the progress they have made.

MF: How much therapy is too much?

MG: It's a difficult question. I've seen some people once or twice, and they would say I've "cured" them. I have seen other people for eleven years. The difference is this: Long-term therapy is for healing broken people. Healing such people requires that a therapist be there with a client until the person feels strong enough to stand on his own feet. He has to heal before he's ready to change. Healthy people are *already* ready to change.

Behavior Therapy

You learned your bad behaviors at some point in your life, so this theory goes, therefore you can also unlearn them. The behavior therapist is more focused on present-tense conflicts and problems than the Freudian morass of early childhood. The behaviorist assumes that any childhood problems have mutated and taken on new forms in the present, and that those are the issues that should be dealt with.

Not surprisingly, behavior therapy is more short-term than traditional psychoanalysis, and has a good track record in addressing specific problems such as phobias. Behaviorists also offer instruction in techniques like relaxation, assertiveness training and communication skills in order to improve the day-to-day functioning of their patients.

Cognitive Therapy

This therapy focuses on the recurrent negative thoughts, images or a generally pessimistic worldview that can that can produce depression, phobias, obsessions, social isolation or other unenviable states of mind. Cognitive therapists help patients recognize negative thought patterns and help them analyze their source. Some also combine both cognitive and behavioral approaches to help break these thought patterns.

Once patients understand that their pessimistic vision of life is largely a creation of their own mind—not to mention a self-fulfilling prophesy—they are often able to eliminate these thought patterns and greatly improve their quality of life. Cognitive therapy is generally a short-term affair.

Jungian Analysis

Named for the psychotherapist Carl Jung, who was perhaps Freud's most gifted and insightful student, Jungian analysis looks at life's journey through the mythical archetypes that occur in different cultures around the world and make up what is called the "collective unconscious." The

Robin Williams character in the movie "The Fisher King" was obsessed with a delusional battle against a dark knight—a classic retelling of a myth that is as old as man. Jungians concentrate on dreams as a way of understanding one's own personal mythology, and to help patients understand the course of their own lives.

Jungian analysis takes a long time; it's usually a once weekly commitment that can last for up to seven years. It's thought to be particularly effective for those going through a major transition in their lives, especially the dreaded "mid-life crisis." It's also a good approach for grappling with larger, open-ended questions. If you're particularly interested in the mythological aspects of life and can handle the commitment of time and money, then you may find Jungian analysis a particularly enlightening form of therapy.

Family and Marital Therapy

What these therapies share is a similar focus on relationships, whether between family members or married couples. The couple or family meets together with the therapist, and their interaction is the primary focus of the work that goes on in the sessions. Problems dealt with in this type of therapy range from estrangement and lack of communication to incest and domestic violence.

In family therapy, a child's behavior is often the impetus for seeking help. Yet quite often the behavior of the child is a reflection of some unhealthy dynamic taking place within the family. Family therapy is effective in revealing these dynamics—as long as all family members are willing to participate. Marital (or couples) therapy is similarly effective for partnerships that have reached an unsatisfying stasis, or in relationships in which one or both members are frustrated or unhappy. Marital therapy doesn't always save marriages, but it often resolves them. Even if the couple divorces, they should have a better understanding of the patterns that resulted in the end of the marriage. These therapies are often short-term, and the therapist may try to schedule more than one session per week to more quickly resolve issues.

Freudian Psychoanalysis

This is what most think of when they hear the word "therapy." Though Freud's patients did indeed lie on a couch, psychoanalysis can assume a variety of forms. Some patients prefer to make eye contact with the analyst, and some analysts are more forthcoming with their own opinions—making the therapy seem less one-sided. What all varieties have in common is an emphasis on the unconscious as the root of psychological difficulties.

Dreams, fantasies and everyday occurrences and conflicts are the grist in the psychoanalytic mill. Patients talk about whatever is on their minds, and the analysts help them make connections between the current session and the issues that have previously revealed themselves. The process is both time- and labor-intensive. Patients may come in from one to five times per week, and the relationship usually lasts for years. Freudians hope that patients will create their own insights and epiphanies, resulting in restructuring of the personality on the deepest level. In this way, problems are addressed at their root causes, and patients are better equipped to handle the events of their lives in the future.

FITNESS AND MENTAL WELL-BEING

While many first approach exercise for its demonstrable cardiovascular benefits and overall ability to improve health, the psychological advantages of working out are what often help people stay with their regimen. Exercise is a wonderful mood-enhancer, and has been shown beneficial for disorders as serious as depression. Best of all, the good vibes we get from working out keep us psyched about going to the gym—which in turn helps lower stress and enhance self-image. The buzz we get from exercise fuels our desire to stay with the program.

While athletes have long promoted the "runner's high" and made other anecdotal claims for the benefits of exercise, research now clearly confirms them. Students in a swimming class at Brooklyn College in New York were compared to a control group; after 30 to 60 minutes per day in the pool, they were found to have significantly lower levels of depression, tension and anger—and higher energy. Overweight, sedentary students at California's Loma Linda University reported a similar increase in energy when they began a walking program of 45-minute sessions five times a week.

These benefits last for hours after a workout, and as you settle into an exercise regimen these psychological improvements can become part of your make-up. Dr. David Neiman, who authored the walking study, found that his walkers were significantly less stressed than the sedentary subjects after the six-week course of the study. Best of all, the walkers wanted to keep walking even after the study was over.

Exercise can also help creativity and slow the decline in mental functioning as we age. A study at New York's Baruch College found that those who engaged in regular aerobic exercise scored significantly higher on aptitude tests for creativity than nonexercisers. (Indeed, many creative types experience a breakthrough or an insight while they are exercising.) While no one claims that exercise actually raises IQ, the increased blood flow to the brain and the reduction in stress probably do help overall cognitive functioning. Perhaps more importantly, workouts help keep whatever level of brain power you have. A study of 300 active and sedentary men and women over age fifty-five at California's Scripps College found that the exercisers scored higher on tests of reaction time, short-term memory and reasoning than did the nonactive. Study author Dr. Alan Hartley notes, "By becoming active when you're young, you're guarding against the mental deterioration that can occur with age and inactivity. "

Exercise releases a pharmacopoeia of the body's own drugs into the bloodstream that both boost calmness and increase alertness. The endorphins released by the body during and after exercise are the source of the "runner's high," and the elevated mood that many enjoy in the hours following aerobic work. Brain levels of the neurotransmitters dopamine, serotonin and norepinephrine also increase, further reducing tension and boosting mood. Exercise seems to be as effective as meditation and group therapy in counteracting the effects of depression and anxiety. In fact, the repetitive body movements of sports like swimming, running and cycling may help induce the mind to fall into a meditative state. An additional neurotransmitter, epinephrine, works with norepinephrine to raise the ability of the brain cells to transmit information—and so increases alertness.

Exercise also trains your body to react less intensely to stress by causing the "stress hormones" to release in a more controlled manner. In fact, a short workout is one of the best ways to deal with the first signs of stress or depression. If your boss is getting you down or you feel yourself going into a funk, exercise can be just what the doctor ordered.

SELF-HEALING STRATEGIES

We don't laugh because we are happy. We are happy because we laugh.

—William James

Humor

A funny thing happened on the way to the hospital. Joel Goodman was visiting his father, who had been suddenly struck with a grave illness, and he found himself boarding a courtesy van with other visitors from a nearby hotel. The atmosphere in the van was heavy with sadness, stress and anxiety. Then Alvin, the van driver, took the helm, telling jokes and doing tricks. Within minutes, he'd magically lifted the spirits of his passengers, some of whom actually laughed for the first time in days.

This was in 1977. With Alvin's magic fresh in mind, Goodman, a lecturer, consultant and motivational speaker, founded The Humor Project that same year. Based in Saratoga Springs, New York, the group has given grants to more than two hundred hospitals, schools and businesses to study the practical applications of humor.

Giving his cause a major boost was Norman Cousins's groundbreaking 1979 book, *Anatomy of an Illness.* In it, Cousins described how he overcame a serious and painful disease with the help of daily doses of the Marx Brothers and "Candid Camera." Since then, all manner of health-care providers have researched humor, finding that laughter really is the best medicine. Psychologists and family practitioners have preached the power of humor in interpersonal relationships—and even promoted it as exercise.

William F. Fry, M.D., a psychiatrist and emeritus professor at Stanford University Medical School, has been studying humor and physiology (a science known as gelotology, in case you ever get on "Jeopardy!") since the 1950s. He's found that a good belly laugh is a lot like strenuous exercise, and equally beneficial. "Laughing is no different from rowing or tennis," he says. "The length of time is shorter, but you do it more often." He contends that one hundred laughs a day is equivalent to ten minutes on the rowing machine. "Mirthful laughter," he adds, "is a total-body experience."

Cousins called laughter "jogging for the innards." It gets the heart pumping, the blood flowing and increases respiration. Such a workout helps oxygenate tissues, stimulates the endocrine system, reduces swelling, circulates such immunity-enhancing substances as lymph and phagocytes, and improves the vitality of infection-fighting white blood cells. It also clears the lungs of mucus as much as it clears the mind of cobwebs.

Indeed, there's evidence that laughter raises levels of catecholamine—a chemical that increases mental alertness and memory while decreasing pain, which researchers suspect might have something to do with the production of endorphins. When laughing subsides, cardiopulmonary rates often decrease to below-normal rates, inducing the same feeling of relaxation a good workout creates. (Cousins reported that laughing for twenty minutes let him sleep, pain free, for hours.)

Holistic physicians such as Deepak Chopra, M.D., have long maintained that laughter also counters the impact negative emotions have on the body. (He reports, for instance, that the tears of laughter differ chemically from the tears of sorrow.) But until data recently began accumulating, Western medicine was virtually closed to even considering the topic.

Fry points to the three basic negative emotions: anger, fear and depression. Anger, he explains, has been proven to impair heart and circulatory system functioning. Fear often triggers gastrointestinal ailments. "Depression is much more complicated," he says. But most of us know that when we're feeling blue we're more likely to contract colds and other nagging ailments. Humor can assuage these negative feelings. "If you get angry, shift to the ridiculous aspect of your anger," Fry suggests, and literally laugh away the heartache. That's why many hospitals around the country now offer patients "comedy carts," stocked with movies, books, games and toys.

Of course, you don't have to be hospitalized to need humor. The stresses of daily life are more than enough. Take relationships . . .please. Why is it that at the top of most people's wish list of attributes for a mate, often ahead of looks and money, is a sense of humor? "There is no better way than humor to come together with people, to deal with the inevitable conflicts," says Goodman. "[Comedic pianist] Victor Borge says a smile is the shortest distance between two people. It is a way of making us more approachable, more human and humane. Conflict happens in any relationship, and humor is a great conflict resolver. It helps us communicate a message that otherwise wouldn't get in the front door. "

That's why flexing your funny bone at work can be such a help. The *Washington Post* reported a Cornell University study that showed how people who had watched a comedy were better able to solve problems than others who had either exercised or watched a film about mathematics. Goodman calls it the connection between "ha-ha," "a-ha" and "ah!" and notes that when a Chicago job-placement firm surveyed 737 CEOs, 98 percent of them said that they'd rather hire someone with a good sense of humor than without. Students of the business world as disparate as John Cleese and Tom Peters sing humor's praises. Cleese, the former Monty Python member who has built a successful career as a corporate trainer, bases his whole approach on the fact that, as he says, "humor is not a luxury." When you have a serious job to do, Cleese says, humor can help.

Humor is tricky, though, especially in this era of hypersensitivity and political correctness. To be safe, think more Jerry Seinfeld, less Howard Stern. You can still have a sense of humor without being especially risky. "I have what I call the AT&T test," says Goodman. "Is it appropriate, timely and tasteful? If not, it might backfire." Likewise, don't expect much good from nastiness cloaked in humor. The kind that does a body good is the kind that brings people together.

Humans have been hard-wired for humor—anthropologists like Jane Goodall have found practical joking among chimps and other primates. But as Goodman points out, for many of us, it fades over the years: "Studies show that kids laugh, on average, 400 times a day, but adults laugh only 15 times a day." But even the humor-impared among us can overcome. "Unlike other natural resources," Goodman says, "the more you use humor, the more you have it."

Meditation

The Western mind tends to believe that logical thought can produce the solution to every problem. But increasingly, athletes, doctors and alternative-medicine proponents are advocating the periodic suspension of normal mental processes as one key to better health and a more productive life.

Meditation, which temporarily clears your mind of conscious, logical thoughts, can be practiced in any number of ways: by chanting a seemingly nonsensical phrase, called a mantra; by staring at an object, such as a candle or flower; by praying or chanting in a religious context; or by practicing such "secular" forms of focusing as yoga, the relaxation response, transcendental meditation (TM) and visualization. The goal of each is the same: to improve your physical and mental health and performance by lowering tension levels and eliminating the effects of stress.

Meditation in Western culture has gone by many names; in fact, meditation is probably the least often used. In 1954, when British runner Roger Bannister broke the four-minute-mile barrier, he acknowledged the role of meditation in his accomplishment. He told reporters that he would go to a place where he could completely relax and then picture himself running the race in perfect form.

Similar meditation techniques have since caught on with other athletes, Greg Louganis and Kareem Abdul-Jabbar among them. No one's sure just how or why it works, but researchers say meditation causes the production of serotonin, a mood-enhancing brain chemical, or the alteration of normal brain-wave activity.

Currently, the main focus for meditation researchers is on the science of mind-body healing called, for lack of a shorter word, psychoneuroimmunology, or PNI. Proponents of PNI believe that meditation plays a strong part in maintaining and restoring overall wellness and, increasingly, some in the traditional medical community agree.

Giving PNI legitimacy is a host of studies crediting various forms of meditation with lowering blood pressure, reducing anxiety and depression, easing the grip of addictions and helping us stay young. Claims have even been made that meditation hinders the action of free radicals—the blood-borne particles blamed for everything from cancer to wrinkles to aging.

Men with cardiovascular disease may be the primary beneficiaries of meditation. Research by Dean Ornish, M.D., showed that a regimen of yoga, meditation, group support, exercise and diet could actually reverse the course of heart disease. At the University of Massachusetts Medical Center, Jon Kabat-Zinn, Ph.D., director of its stress-reduction clinic, has been using a meditation technique he's dubbed "mindfulness" for the past thirteen years with male patients, many of whom have chronic pain or heart conditions.

"Meditation is nonjudgmentally paying attention from moment to moment in the interest of self-understanding," Kabat-Zinn says. His program has participants focus on everyday sensations—eating, breathing, sitting, walking. "This is no New Age clinic," he says. "The goal of the program is to let go of expectations and practice being aware." Paying deep attention to physical or emotional pain often helps people conquer it, he says. As with most meditation programs, "mindfulness" relies on repetition of particular phrases chosen by Kabat-Zinn.

Other sources in the traditional medical community are also lending support to the notion of meditation as medicine. For example, in a 1991 study published in the *Journal of Asthma*, forty-six asthmatics found significant relief through daily yoga training. At the end of the forty-day study, the participants showed a significant increase in lung and exercise capacity.

Research published in the March, 1990 *Journal of Addictions* concluded that 90 percent of the members of a group trying to quit smoking either succeeded or drastically curtailed their habit after they started meditating twice a day. And a study of senior citizens who began regular meditation showed they scored lower than average on tests of depression and anxiety.

In certain circumstances, though, meditation is less a cure for modern ills than a dose of old-fashioned religion. "For some people, meditation is more comfortable and effective if they incorporate their religious faith," says Herbert Benson, M.D., associate professor of medicine at Harvard Medical School. Benson's research on meditation has found that, when given a choice of mantras (the sound or word that gives a person the feeling of stillness), many participants chose words relating to their religion—

"Jesus" is particularly popular. Men who used such words, Benson found, tended to stay with the program longer and achieve better health-related results. He calls this the "faith factor."

Still, 80 percent of his participants chose a classic Eastern mantra — "om" as the perennial favorite—and indeed, many "traditional" meditators shudder at the thought of bringing Western religion into the picture. In either case, meditation works the same way: Practitioners focus, eyes open, on a particular object (a lit candle set a few feet away is a popular choice, but anything will do) in a quiet environment. They then repeat their mantra over and over for twenty to forty minutes, banishing all other thoughts from their minds.

Intramural squabbling aside, all proponents agree that anyone can meditate. It's as simple as closing your eyes and repeating a mantra. There are complete instructional programs, though, which aim to let you maximize the benefits of meditation, whether you're trying to crank your mental or physical performance up to the next level or to improve your health. Finding such a program is as easy as looking under "meditation" in your local bookstore or Yellow Pages or calling a college or university psychology department.

No matter what method suits you, the point of them all is the same: Put those stress-producing thoughts out of your mind and allow the power of relaxation to work its magic.

YOGIC MEDITATION

The basic yoga technique incorporates aspects of yoga and meditation, which, when combined, are an excellent way to clear the mind whenever the need arises. In order to ensure that you will be able to devote yourself totally to the meditation process, it is important that you create an atmosphere without distractions. Therefore, it is suggested that you do it at a time when your children and pets are not in the room and your telephone can be turned off.

Begin your practice by positioning yourself on the floor or bed, on a blanket or towel. Keep your head flat in order to keep your spine straight; however, if you must use a pillow for medical reasons, make sure it is small. If you must support your lower back, take a few pillows and place them under your thighs to alleviate the pressure on your lower back. While in the meditative state your body temperature will drop somewhat as a result of your heartbeat and respiration slowing down. Therefore, it is suggested that you cover yourself and wear socks to keep your feet warm. You'll enjoy the feeling of security being covered gives you while meditating.

Begin to totally relax your body, keeping your arms at your sides, hands turned upward, fingers relaxed. Now, beginning with your forehead, close your eyes and concentrate on relaxing each part of your body, first focusing on that part, letting it completely relax, then moving on to the next part. As you picture your forehead in your mind, concentrate on letting the lines of your brow relax, removing any tension from the forehead and eyebrow area, then move down with your mind's eye. Keeping your eyes closed, now focus on your eyes, as if you were staring directly into a mirror at them. Now, as the image in your mind fades, let your eyes and the muscles around them come to rest. Next, let your face feel that total sense of relaxation, just feel the tautness fall away as you envision your facial muscles, jaw, teeth, nose and mouth just hanging loosely. Let your mouth drop open as the sense of relaxation spreads down your face. Now move down to your neck and shoulders, and as you envision every part of these areas, let them rest. When you get to your shoulders, let your arms drop a little farther. Then relax your upper arms, your elbows, your forearms, your wrists, and lastly, your hands and your fingers. Continue gradually to work your way down, relaxing each part as you move along. When you get to your chest, relax your heart and lungs too, breathing in slowly, exhaling and relaxing at the same time. Breathe normally now as you move down to your stomach muscles and internal organs. You are now letting your hips, legs and feet feel the tension leave them, and as that happens, your legs will open slightly and your feet will slacken. Now turn your attention to your spine. Slowly move up your back, visualizing every vertebra, then letting it go, completely releasing any tension in your spine as you let it rest on the floor. Let your waist relax, then your shoulder blades, your upper back and your neck. Finally, when you reach the top of your spinal cord, let it relax and then let your brain rest, let your thoughts go into a peaceful state as you prepare to meditate.

Your meditaiton will begin with a mantra, a type of chant that has been used in the practice of yoga for thousands of years to acheive calmness or other effects. The most frequently used mantra is "OM," traditionally used prior to meditation, and you can begin by repeating it to yourself several times, concentrating on that sound and nothing else. As you do this, let all other thoughts leave your mind as you seek that sense of total peace and stillness from within. Your body is totally relaxed, your mind is totally relaxed, and now, as you recite "OM" over and over again, let that become the only thought you have. Eventually let the sound "OM" also recede so your mind can become completely still. If your mind seems to race at first, let it; soon the thoughts will quietly slip away, and you will experience the silence that you seek. It wil not come to you right away—just let it happen. If something comes to mind that worries you, let it pass, move on. You might feel sleepy, or fall asleep; this is not uncommon for beginning practitioners. Eventually you will be able to relax completely and remain awake. Remember to leave yourself enough time to meditate before going out—do not put undue pressure on yourself.

Your yogic meditation session is over, and you feel wonderful. Before you get up to resume your day, reflect on how you felt during that period. Try to recapture the feeling in your mind so that, if ned be, you can recall it during the day as you feel the need.

For more general information about meditation and yoga, contact the American Yoga Association, 513 South Orange Avenue, Sarasota, Florida 34236, or call (800) 226-5859.

Biofeedback

If you're sure you've never used anything as sophisticated as biofeedback to change your behavior or emotional state, consider this: You probably use it every day, starting with your morning shave. That's because the simplest biofeedback device of all is a mirror.

Despite its high-tech, even "out there" image, all biofeedback does is measure small, subtle physiological changes and relay them—feed them back—to your brain via visual or auditory images. With proper guidance, you can then learn, with increasing skill and subtlety, to use your mind to control body functions generally regarded as involuntary. These include heart rate, blood pressure, muscle tension and brainwave frequency.

"When I happened to glance in the mirror this morning while I was combing my hair, I could see whether there was tension along my forehead or if my jaw was clenched," says Wes Sime, a biofeedback "coach" who works with professional baseball teams. Those physical cues, Sime says, enabled him to gauge his emotional state, then use his mind to calm himself down. In the same basic way, but using more sophisticated technology than a bathroom mirror, researchers hope to allow athletes, students and anyone else who's concerned with his mental or physical performance to use subtle physical cues to improve that performance.

Formerly controversial and often regarded as a fringe therapy, biofeedback is now fully credible in the eyes of many doctors and scientists. "Physical therapists taking their boards have to know about it," says Lieutenant Colonel Richard Sherman, Ph.D., a rehab specialist with the U.S. Army. "Rehabilitation-medicine physicians are being trained in it. Biofeedback is slowly entering the mainstream."

When undergoing biofeedback, you usually sit comfortably attached to electrodes that measure muscle tension, blood pressure, perspiration, heart rate and sometimes brain waves. (Polygraphs, or lie detectors, use the same technology.) The information is represented on a computer screen, typically as a growing or shrinking circle or bar; it can also be manifested as a tone that changes in pitch or, in some more sophisticated machines, a digital picture. A therapist then guides you toward a mental image (a soothing sunset, for example, or the sensation that your hands are immersed in warm water). By watching the effects on the screen change, you learn to control what are seemingly involuntary physiological changes.

Biofeedback has been tried with some 250 conditions and is widely used to treat stress-related ailments, such as some skin and gastrointestinal conditions, migraine and tension headaches, anxiety, hypertension, muscle tension, neck and shoulder pain and the phantom-limb pain commonly suffered by amputees. A new trial expected to involve some 4,000 volunteers focuses on lower-back pain.

Some patients—recovering stroke and accident victims, for example—use biofeedback to exercise atrophied muscles. In many cases, limbs that may seem completely paralyzed are actually capable of minor movements; capturing them on a screen gives the patient a means to re-create those movements and thus rehabilitate the limb. "Biofeedback can pick up tiny movements that are much smaller than you can feel," Sherman explains. Other muscles may atrophy because they're difficult to access and exercise. For example, many cases of incontinence (which primarily affects older people) result when the sphincter muscles controlling urine flow lose their tone.

Not all biofeedback applications strengthen the mind's control over the body. Some are designed to improve brain function itself. Attention deficit disorder (ADD) and alcohol and drug abuse may be mitigated by biofeedback that involves learning to control brain waves. "Some people with ADD get stuck in a [state of] slow-brainwave production," says Steven Fahrion, Ph.D., a biofeedback specialist with the Life Sciences Institute of Mind-Body Health in Topeka, Kansas. "They get very day-dreamy and have trouble focusing their attention, so we try to increase their production of faster rhythms. When you're dealing with substance abuse, you go the other way, because addictive people often are stuck in a fast rhythm associated with constant craving." A large body of studies supports biofeedback for ADD; a few small studies show promise with substance abuse.

A form of biofeedback based on this idea of "stuck" rhythms has been tried with stroke patients, depressives and people with post-traumatic stress disorder. "We use the person's own brain waves to [control] the frequency of strobe lights," says Len Ochs, Ph.D., a psychologist in private practice in Walnut Creek, California, who has performed very preliminary studies of this technique. "This is custom-tailored to the individual's brain activity. He can be sleeping, awake, thinking about what he's going to have for dinner." According to Ochs's theory, a variable strobe gently but continually pulls the subject's brain waves out of their stuck rhythm, restoring some flexibility to his brain functioning. "This is really preliminary," he admits, "but their symptoms just vaporize. It's the most startling thing in the world to witness."

But succeeding with biofeedback is only half the battle, points out Steve Wolf, Ph.D., of the Emory University School of Medicine in Atlanta. "Biofeedback certainly shows that someone is able to interact with the machine," Wolf says. "But for the interaction to be truly successful, he must be capable of achieving those same [results] without the machine."

To learn more about biofeedback or to get the name of a practitioner near you, write or call the Association of Applied Psychophysiology and Biofeedback, 10200 West 44th Ave., Suite 304, Wheat Ridge, CO 80033; (800) 477–8892.

Yoga

Yoga, which in Sanskrit means "union of body, mind and spirit" is a system of exercises and postures designed to promote health and well-being. The process is twofold. The physical side of yoga—the workout—is designed to enhance circulation, flexibility and respiration while regulating the heart rate and lowering blood pressure. The spiritual side reduces stress and increases mental focus and energy. Yoga's twisted history began thousands of years ago in India as a system of preventive medicine. Now many doctors who practice traditional Western medicine pay homage to the preventive powers of yoga.

If yoga's roots sound esoteric, its benefits are straightforward. It's simple exercises are an excellent way to relieve stress and to improve overall conditioning. Many think that yoga is simply a systematized method of stretching, but properly done it increases both strength and flexibility—and is perfectly safe for people of all ages and fitness levels. Best of all, it can be practiced anywhere. Just using its breathing techniques can greatly combat stress in practically any situation.

Rudolph Ballentine, M.D., who runs the Center for Holistic Medicine in New York City, is one who has jumped on the yoga bandwagon. "Yoga helps people develop a better sense of self-awareness so they can recognize disorders before they develop into diseases," he says. "Too often, before conventional medicine can diagnose disease, people are already too far down the path. Then, at best, they can only manage the disease instead of restoring health."

Government healthcare researchers recently asked Ballentine for his suggestions on improving the delivery of medical services in the United States. His response was succinct: "I told them that if you develop a good program for patient self-awareness, you can prevent expenditures and suffering. The basic premise of yoga, which deals with uniting the body, breath, and mind, is not a patented technique—it's what you naturally do."

Practicing yoga is also a method of improving your chameleonlike ability to respond to external pressures. "Yoga increases our adaptive powers in dealing with the environment," says Rajashree Choudhury, one of the head instructors at the Yoga College of India in Beverly Hills. Choudhury has teamed with her husband, Bikram, to attract a legion of celebrities to this mecca for yoga. The Choudhurys apply yoga techniques to help people with illness ranging from migraines to cancer. Many students use yoga to rid themselves of addictions and to manage stress.

"Yoga relaxes me," says Jerry Seinfeld. "Tension tends to build up in the spine—the target area for many of the exercises. I'll assume a pose, completely still, my muscles trembling from maintaining the position. But when I release it, the stress abates as well. The muscles in my spine become stronger and more flexible from bearing the strain. It's like going through a wringer. Believe me, the sensation is totally unique."

You don't need a hit series to release tension during a yoga workout; yoga is distinctly noncompetitive. It doesn't discriminate on the basis of age or fitness level, and it's offered in many forms. Hatha yoga, which translates to mean "union of the sun and moon" (a balancing of opposites), is by far the most popular. Several systems operate under the Hatha umbrella, which emphasizes poses and breathing technique.

As the noted social critic Seinfeld puts this Eastern discipline into a day-to-day Western context: "Why do I do yoga? Try limitless energy. Hey, with my work schedule, I'm just trying to stay alive. I'm going nonstop 12 to 14 hours a day, and there's no way I could sustain this crazy schedule without the yoga. It makes my life better, and to me, that's what exercise is all about."

Affirmations

An affirmation is the best kind of self-fulfilling prophesy. It's a positive belief that you tell yourself, which in turn sets up a beneficial chain of events: the belief creates action, the action creates result, and the result confirms belief. This is how self-fulfilling prophecies become reality.

Throughout history there have been stories of people who, despite all odds, succeeded in achieving their dreams. The strength of their beliefs seemed to carry them through impenetrable obstacles. If beliefs can have such a powerful effect over physical realities, it is hardly surprising that our beliefs can also affect our minds and the way we perceive things. Our beliefs about ourselves and the world alter our energy, health, mood, actions, relationships and eventually our external circumstances. If we see how we do this, we can then create positive self-fulfilling prophecies based on unlimited beliefs.

Positive affirmations were first brought to notice in the Western medical world by Emile Coué, a 19th-century French pharmacist who noticed that several of his patients improved when they focused on positive health rather than the negative fears and imaginings of illness.

However, affirmations may be really difficult to believe, which is why positive-thinking techniques are sometimes restricted in effect. In many of them, an exclusive focus on the positive can result in a sense of unreality. For example, if you have a strong inner belief that you are ugly and the world is a bad place, telling yourself that you and the world are beautiful is not going to work. It is often necessary to recognize and challenge the negative before the positive can be effective.

Affirmation is really a form of positive brainwashing. We've been brainwashing ourselves for years with limiting beliefs, such as "I'm a bad person." When you substitute an opposite, unlimiting belief, such as "I love myself," you're deliberately washing your brain with what seems at first to be an artificial construct but which you hope to be able to believe.

The artificiality may be a problem at first. For example, the affirmation that "It is my natural state to be happy—I am free from my past" can sound pretty ridiculous if you're feeling unhappy and angry about something that's happened in the past. The trick is to play with the new belief as if it were true. Our minds cannot yet accept a belief that contradicts the old limits, but it can accept a kind of imaginary game in which we play with the new belief as if it were reality. It's through the play and the practice that the new belief gradually becomes more believable.

Putting the new belief into outward action confirms and strengthens it. What you are really doing is acting on faith. You hope that your new belief can be reality and so you act as if it is. At first you do this in a very small way, setting easily attainable goals. After the act, the very fact that you did it feeds your belief. And life will change, in its own way and in its own time.

When we see that whatever we believe becomes manifest in our lives, we might as well believe the very best. We learn to believe the best of ourselves and of others, not out of blindness to faults but out of well-founded hope in creating the most positive self-fulfilling prophecies. Truly, as we change our minds, we change our world.

HOW TO MAKE AFFIRMATIONS WORK
1. Understand and accept that the old belief isn't reality.
2. Have a genuine desire to change.
3. Substitute the old belief with the new affirmation.
4. Combine the affirmation with positive action.

Visualization

Imagination is a powerful tool in your efforts to achieve your personal best, whatever of life's endeavors you choose to undertake. The technique of visualization, widely used by athletes to improve their performances, marshals the incredible forces of your mind and the neurological system that connects it to the rest of your body. In a real sense, you *are* what you think.

A few years ago, a couple of cybernetics experts (people who study automatic control systems, such as computers and the human brain) decided to investigate what goes on in the brain when a person experiences a variety of stimuli. They hooked up a number of people to an electroencephalograph (EEG) so their brain waves could be recorded. While the volunteers sat wired up in the lab, the researchers exposed them to various experiences: a gunshot, a woman's scream, a dog running across the room. After each, the experts checked the EEG reading to see how the brain responded.

The study participants were then asked to simply imagine the dog, the gunshot and the woman screaming. When the brainwaves recorded during the imagined experiences were compared with those evoked by the real things, they were found to be identical. It appears that, drawing upon past experiences, your imagined experiences are just as much conditioners of responses as your actual experiences are.

Not only does a visualized experience condition the human brain, but it will also program the human body. This mind-body connection brought about by visualization is known as the ideomotor concept: As your brain conceives of an act, it generates impulses that prompt neurons to "perform" the movement being imagined by transmitting those impulses from the brain to the muscles. According to this concept, if you close your eyes and visualize yourself doing something, your body's actions are programmed in exactly the same manner as if you actually did them.

If you were to picture yourself bench pressing, someone observing you would see no muscle movement in your chest or arms. However, if he attached your chest and arms to an electromyograph (EMG)—which records the electrical activity associated with skeletal muscles—he would not only get a reading but also would actually be able to tell which muscle groups were coming into play during the "lift." (Of course, the strength of the impulse wouldn't be as strong as one generated through actual physical performance.)

But visualization's greatest benefits happen outside the gym. A form of visualization called "guided imagery" is used by patients with serious illness such as cancer to help marshal the body's defenses against the disease. A cancer patient might create a mental image of their antibodies successfully fighting back against malignant cells—and there is at least some evidence that such imagery increases the likelihood of recovery. (At the very least, it does no harm and helps the patient feel he is actively trying to get well.) Guided imagery has also shown success in treating those with depression or addictions.

For the healthy man, visualization is a way to codify what you want to have happen in your life, and to begin to take the steps to achieve it. Once you visualize what you want in your mind's eye, you have already taken the largest step toward reaching it.

Prayer

A New Jersey chiropractor bows his head and prays as he stands outside an examining room, a ritual he follows before he meets a new patient. A Los Angeles dentist admits he occasionally prays for patients for whom he feels special concern. And in Denver, an osteopath suggests to a chronic sinus sufferer that he include prayer, which the doctor calls "spiritual exercise," in his treatment regimen.

Prayer as part of a healthcare program may sound strange, regardless of your religious orientation. But even some of the most conservative M.D.s are taking a fresh look at this ancient approach to wellness, as recent research shows that prayer actually can improve health.

The connection between faith and healing is very old. From the dawn of history, medicine men and shamans have known that trust in the healing power of spirits, rituals or incantations could effect cure. The earliest physicians were aware of the "placebo effect," a phenomenon that sees one-fourth to one-third of patients show improvement if they believe they are taking an effective medicine, even when the pill or potion contains no active ingredients.

Incidents occurring at revival meetings and religious shrines, such as Lourdes, and the activities of faith healers, including Aimee Semple McPherson, Kathryn Kuhlman, Mary Baker Eddy and Oral Roberts, have provided anecdotal testimony to the power of faith in physical healing. The medical establishment in this century has discounted "miracle cures" as spontaneous remissions or the result of suggestion, but in recent years medical science has begun a search for clinical evidence of the spirit's effect on the body.

As mentioned earlier in this chapter, Norman Cousins's *Anatomy of an Illness* helped promote the idea that belief is more than a state of mind;

rather, he said, it's a physiological reality. He complained that when doctors focused only on the body's five major systems—circulatory, digestive, endocrine, nervous and immune—they neglected two that were just as important: the healing system and the belief system. New research on the biochemistry of emotions has found that when a patient prays, what Cousins called "the biology of hope" kicks in.

Cousins based much of his work on the research of cardiologist Herbert Benson, an associate professor at Harvard Medical School, who proved that psychological states could affect physical well-being. About thirty years ago, Benson asked people to meditate using a mantra, a single word or syllable with no meaning, such as "om." Repetition of the mantra resulted in a lower metabolic rate and blood pressure, and a slower heart and respiration rate. Benson observed that this "relaxation response" had always existed in religious teachings, especially in Eastern cultures. He noted that the response was the opposite of the stress reaction known as "fight-or-flight" on which much modern disease is blamed.

Well, cynics might say, transcendental meditation might have cooled out some hippies back in the sixties, but what about your average American Joe? It happens that Joe has a long history of cooling out with prayer, the standard Western form of meditation. About 75 percent of Americans claim to pray at least once a week, and 52 percent say they pray at least once a day. Sociologist Andrew Greeley estimates that close to 20 million Americans report having mystical experiences, including healing. A statewide poll in Virginia showed that 14.3 percent of adults said they had been healed either by prayer or a divine source.

Benson next studied the physiology of practicing Christians and Jews. He asked subjects to pray regularly using short repetitive phrases. Catholics were to repeat, "Hail Mary, full of grace"; Jews, "Shalom" or "Echad" (meaning "one"); and Protestants, "Our Father, who art in heaven" or "The Lord is my shepherd." Again Benson found the relaxation response. Since 1988, Benson and psychologist Jared Kass have been investigating the health implications of prayer at Boston's New England Deaconess Hospital. They measured feelings of spirituality before and after prayer and found that people high in spirituality had fewer stress-related symptoms and the sharpest drop in pain.

Prayer apparently works best when practiced as part of a belief or trust in a higher power, not when undertaken solely for its beneficial side effects. Benson has taught scores of clergy how to achieve the relaxation response through prayer. Other researchers are coming to some startling conclusions about prayer. Meyer Friedman, one of two researchers who first described the Type-A behavior seen in people prone to heart attacks, believes people who are excessively driven to succeed have unfulfilled spiritual needs. Gerontologist Kenneth Pelletier found that the executives under severe stress who avoid heart attacks have a deeper spiritual dimension. Lake Placid, New York, psychiatrist Arthur Kornhaber told *Newsweek*, "To exclude God from psychiatric consultation is a form of malpractice for some patients."

Spirituality appears to have beneficial effects whether a person prays for himself or is the subject of someone else's request. Research also indicates that people who are prayed for benefit whether or not they themselves are believers. In a 1988 double-blind study at the University of California, San Francisco, 393 hospitalized heart patients were divided randomly into two groups, one of which was prayed for by Christians. Cardiologist Randolf Byrd found that the patients who were the subjects of others' prayers had a lower incidence of pulmonary edema and less need for two kinds of medical intervention.

As creatures of the scientific method, doctors have been slow to acknowledge prayer as a therapeutic tool. The American Medical Association takes no position but apparently worries that patients will endanger their health by turning to prayer in place of medicine: In December 1990, the AMA adopted an action that said, in part, "Prayer as therapy should not delay access to traditional medical care."

Nevertheless, the new medical discipline of psychoneuroimmunology, which deals with the interplay between the mind, the brain and the immune system, has encouraged physicians to acknowledge the connection between faith and healing. "The medical profession is increasingly aware that love and joy and hope can strengthen the immune system," says Carl Hammerschlag, M.D., author of *The Dancing Healers: A Doctor's Journal of Healing with Native Americans.* "Maybe a younger doctor would be reticent to say prayer works," says Karlan, who is a member of the AMA's prestigious Council on Scientific Affairs, "but I've practiced surgery for more than thirty years and I can say it does. I've seen it work."

The Flow

We have all been there. Reggie Jackson has, when he hit four home runs in a single World Series game. So was Albert Einstein, when the theory of relativity revealed itself to him as he rode a trolley through the streets of Vienna. You've been there too, while cutting firewood, designing a computer program, scaling a rockface or playing with your children. "There" refers not to a specific place but to a state of mind called "flow." According to the psychiatrist who first named this state, the ability to induce flow is what separates the happy from the unhappy—and a fulfilled life from an unfulfilled one.

The concept is simple enough: when you're engaged in an activity that commands all of your attention, your concentration becomes so intense that the rest of the world seems to drop away, and you have a feeling of effortless control. Your actions become spontaneous and automatic; you almost *become* the thing you are doing—and nothing else seems to matter. Hours can pass like minutes, and the anxieties and distractions of the self and of everyday life dissolve. You have a sense of focus, clarity, profound satisfaction and increased self-esteem that stays with you after the activity is over. This "flow state" is what most people would describe as happiness, and it happens most often while at work, not at play.

A psychologist and former department chairman at the University of Chicago named Mihaly Csikszentmihalyi (pronounced "chick-sent-me-*high*") came upon the concept of flow as part of his thirty-year research into the nature of happiness, and he published his findings in a book called *Flow: The Psychology of Optimal Experience.* Though it sounds like self-help, it isn't "a popular book that gives insider tips on being happy," as the author says. Rather, it's a cogent and well-researched investigation into the nature of work, happiness and enjoyment. "Work" might at first seem an unlikely component of happiness, but as Csikszentmihalyi discovered, "work is often the most enjoyable part of life"—provided that one's work gives the opportunity to learn and grow.

Csikszentmihalyi's theory is at odds with one of the central goals of the industrialized world: the creation of leisure time. Leisure is what we are all supposedly working for, whether it's a few slack hours on the weekend or the indolent retirement we fantasize about for our "golden years." But as Csikszentmihalyi's research has shown, passive leisure doesn't really seem to make people *happy*.

Csikszentmihalyi discovered this when he and his colleagues in Canada, Germany, Japan, Italy and Australia interviewed some 8,000 people worldwide using a unique research method. They had their subjects wear a pager for a week; the pager was activated by radio signal eight times a day in a random fashion. Whenever their pager sounded, the subjects where supposed to record their moods, thoughts and activities for that moment. Each interviewee, from Navajo sheepherder to Alpine farmer to Midwestern industrial worker, provided "snapshots" of their lives that linked their moods to what they were doing at a given moment. To date, Csikszentmihalyi has collected over 100,000 of these snapshots, which he calls "cross-sections of experience."

The researchers found that their subjects experienced moments of intense concentration, happiness and satisfaction—flow, in other words—when they were actively engaged in something, not when they were passively pursuing "leisure." When the interview subjects recorded their feelings while at work, as many as 54 percent reported experiencing flow: they used words like "strong," "active," "creative" and "motivated" to describe their moods. When their beepers went off while they were watching TV, dining out or having friends over, only 18 percent indicated that they were in flow. Although the mind prefers the challenges and goals of work to the dubious pleasures of chilling out Csikszentmihalyi notes that, paradoxically, "even when people feel good about working, they say they would prefer not to be working."

Yet those who can find new challenges and goals in even the most mundane of jobs report that work is "like play" for them, and that money or job security are secondary to the enjoyment they get from it. "It contradicts a ruling theory of behavioral psychology, in which work is something you do for the reward you get afterward," says Csikszentmihalyi. With flow, "the experience *itself* is so enjoyable that people will do it for the sheer sake of doing it." This is a defining characteristic of flow: its value is in the doing.

But "work" and "play" can be confusing terms. If your leisure activities call upon new skills and challenges—work, in other words—you're liable to experience flow during them. But as Csikszentmihalyi points out, "In our culture the aversion to work is so ingrained that, even though it provides the most complex and gratifying experiences, people still prefer having more free time—although a great deal of free time is in fact boring and depressing."

The key element to creating flow in any activity—work or play—is complexity. Flow comes when you're challenged by something, are able to meet the challenge, and can then set more advanced goals that can inspire you to further develop. For example, piloting the Concorde is complex, but wouldn't be enjoyable if the skills called for were too advanced for your level of experience. Learning to fly the Concorde would be possible, and enjoyable, if seen as a series of discrete challenges—from taking flying lessons to getting a pilot's license to becoming a commercial aviator—that systematically developed your skills. "When we choose a goal and invest ourselves in it, whatever we do will be enjoyable," says Csikszentmihalyi. "And once we've tasted this joy, we will redouble our efforts to taste it again."

Perhaps the most appealing aspect of Csikszentmihalyi's theory is its universality; even in the most awful of life's circumstances, there are opportunities to create flow. Csikszentmihalyi recalls the story of how

Alexander Solzhenitsyn dealt with his imprisonment in Siberia by composing poetry in his head. As Solzhenitsyn later wrote: "Sometimes, while standing in a column of dejected prisoners, amidst the shouts of guards with machine guns, I felt such a rush of rhymes and images that I seemed to be wafted overhead . . . I was both free and happy . . . The head count of the prisoners remained unchanged but I was actually away on a distant flight." As Csikszentmihalyi's groundbreaking work indicates, that flight is available to anyone who can learn to flow.

GOING WITH THE FLOW

Though most people tend to experience flow only randomly, it can be developed as surely as muscle strength. Here are a few pointers to help you get in the flow.

- Recognize flow. Identify activities you're already immersed in, and transfer that absorption to other areas. "Once you begin to recognize flow," says Csikszentmihalyi, "it kind of grows by itself."
- Develop attention. The ability to focus is key to becoming immersed in an activity. Meditation is an ideal way to develop attention, as are yoga or any of the martial arts.
- Get complex. Complexity doesn't mean complication; it means enjoying new skills and experiences. Acquiring a new skill—chess, a musical instrument, rock climbing—can give you the same sense of satisfaction that learning did in childhood.
- Go beyond the self. Find a group that shares your goals—from the Cub Scouts to a political organization—and work with them. Active participation with others in a cause makes you feel more in control of your world.
- Develop a life theme. Any legitimate theme, such as "I want to make a safer world for my children," will create a set of new goals, call for new skills, pull you beyond the self and give meaning—and flow—to your experiences.

5

BODY IMAGE

A man's body does not betray its tenant as rapidly as a woman's. Never as fine and lovely, it has less distance to fall; what rugged beauty it has is wrinkle-proof.

—JOHN UPDIKE

THE "NEW" MALE VANITY

When you were a kid, could you picture your dad getting a nose job? Your Uncle Bob having his hair colored? How about grandpa drumming in the woods, howling at the moon with a group of other men? Doubtful. "Not for me," they'd snort; vanity after all, is feminine, maybe even sinful. But what may not have been acceptable when baby boomers were growing up in the sixties is increasingly acceptable to men today. They're nipping, tucking and pumping their bodies, while at the same time contemplating their navels as never before. The trend may signal male insecurity as well as male vanity, according to leading figures in the self-absorption business. And to these trendsetters and watchers, that's not necessarily a bad thing.

When it comes to social commentary, few media psychologists have been giving it as long as Dr. Joyce Brothers. She thinks men are, if not vain, more concerned about their appearance, and that it's a healthy thing. "If a man has a job that involves dealing with people in any way, he's going to want to look vigorous and younger," Brothers says. "And let's not forget that the methods and techniques are better. Twenty years ago, if someone—man or woman—had a face-lift, it was pretty obvious." But Brothers thinks the majority of men will draw the line when they get to the point of total artifice: "I don't think we will see large numbers of men going to salons to have their hair permed anytime soon."

The men plunking down the big bucks at the José Eber Salon on Beverly Hills's Rodeo Drive might disagree. The salon is a temple of vanity, a mecca to ambitious egos. A white marble spiral staircase rises from street level to a black lacquered desk where beautiful, poised women funnel the well-heeled and often-celebrated clientele to services ranging from haircuts (the base cost is over $75, though $200 bills are common) to ultraviolet scalp massages. It's the type of place where men have always pictured women spending their money.

But a glance around the cutting floor (there are about thirty pairs of shears at work) shows a good portion of the clientele to be male—and two of them are in buttoned-down Brooks Brothers shirts. "I guess you could say I'm a regular," says Jack, a thirty-five-year-old who manages to look relatively conservative despite the fact that his hair is wrapped in little Christmas-tree shaped cones made of tinfoil. "I come once a month for a facial and to have my hair colored and cut."

And what does Eber think of the waiting room full of male clients? "It's terrific that men want to look better and aren't satisfied with looking like someone took a steak knife to their hair," he says, then adds with a sigh, "even though there will always be guys who want a $10 cut."

For the man who's not satisfied with purified pores and a haircut that matches his personality, there's always the plastic surgery card to play—which, it appears, is becoming as popular as foreign cars among appearance-conscious men of all ages.

"Back in the sixties," says Alan Matarasso, M.D., a Park Avenue plastic surgeon who's seen a 20 percent increase in the number of male patients he has served over the last few years, "medical textbooks used to instruct doctors not to do nose jobs on men, for the most part. Something about a phallic fixation. So men didn't have much done. But all that's changed over the last five years or so. These days I get everyone from construction workers to actors to CEOs. They want face-lifts, liposuctions, facial contouring—you name it, they want to improve it."

To what does this leader in physical reconstruction attribute the change in attitude? "A lot of men tell me it's because of competition from younger guys. But that's only part of it, because younger guys are getting it done, too," Matarasso says. "I think men in general are more willing to admit they want to look better. And they're just as demanding as the women. More so, in some cases. Some men can go overboard. I had one patient who had midsection liposuction, an eye job, pectoral implants, chin implants, cheekbone implants and a facial skin peel. I don't think this patient existed five years ago. But then, neither did a lot of the procedures we do."

All this newfound appearance-consciousness among men didn't spring from empty space. Admen, not satisfied with emptying women's purses, have decided to make a grab for the male wallet by using the same methods that have been used on women since the dawn of billboards. "I think the big change in selling to men came about fifteen years ago," says Donald Ziccardi, president and CEO of Sussman/Ziccardi, a major New York advertising firm that handles male-oriented fashion accounts like IZOD-Lacoste shirts. "That's when the Calvin Klein campaign aimed directly at men was launched, emphasizing the male form."

And what does he think of the male image in recent campaigns, like the pouty-looking men in Calvin Klein ads? "Those ads are doing something that's been done for a long time—they sell a sexual image to men," Ziccardi says. "The way we now sell to men is the same way we've always sold to women. We look for images that convey happiness and health, which all men want. It's a pretty simple formula. There is one difference, though. Because men in their thirties and forties are more conscious of their looks these days, what we do is place an older man in a younger setting—at the beach, for example."

Externals like shopping for a new face, better hair and a sculpted body aside, few things could be more self-absorbed, individually and collectively, than the men's movement. Their meetings, at which men vent their feelings about their own inadequacies or those of others (fathers are a favorite target, followed by ex-wives), have been described by some as a kind of male mental masturbation. Joyce Brothers thinks the men's movement may not exist at all, except in the cameras and pens of television crews and magazine editors. "I'm not sure to what extent this may be a phenomenon created by the media," she says.

Not so, says Warren Farrell, Ph.D., a founder of the movement's political arm and author of *Why Men Are the Way They Are*. Farrell says that just a few years ago even he couldn't imagine thousands of men attending men's movement meetings. "I think men are searching . . . to reexamine their relationships with their mothers and fathers. In many ways, the men's movement is about men undergoing true personal transformation." And the forest drumming sessions? "That will remain a small part of the whole picture," Farrell says.

The sometimes cantankerous author of *Real Men Don't Eat Quiche* and *Real Men Don't Bond*, Bruce Feirstein, thinks men were just fine before someone decided we needed a collective face-lift, and he doesn't think much of the men who've hooked onto the latest trend. "These terminally insecure guys were into est ten years ago, rolfing five years ago and now they're into the Course in Miracles. They used to be worried about being vulnerable and sensitive. Now they're worried about being masculine and powerful," he says.

And as sales of skin products for men soar and the famed Canyon Ranch Spa offers a "Men's Week" (at several thousand dollars a pop), how do the experts on male behavior think the new male peacock streak will develop? Will men go anorexic? Will male CEOs hold up traffic applying Man-Tan from compacts? Robert L. Green says he doesn't think it will go that far, but he believes that men will grow increasingly concerned about maintaining a healthy appearance.

Joyce Brothers is less certain about the direction the modern male is going to take. "I don't think we're going to see a surge in sales of rouge and mascara to men," she says. "Men have limits. After all, it's been proven that you can sell boys' toys to girls, but not girls' toys to boys."

RETURN OF THE BIONIC MAN— SURGICAL OPTIONS

Think men aren't vain? Face up to these numbers. According to the American Society of Plastic and Reconstructive Surgury (ASPRS), about 400,000 elective "cosmetic" surgeries are performed every year. Fully 12 percent of the patients for these procedures are men. What are the most popular operations? Here's a list based on ASPRS statistics. Prices are approximate and based on national averages.

PROCEDURE	COST
Nose Reshaping	$3,200
Eyelid Surgery	2,700 (uppers and lowers)
Liposuction	1,700 (per site)
Breast Reduction	2,300
Face-lift	4,300
Scalp Reduction	varies by procedure
Ear Surgery	2,200
Dermabrasion	1,500
Chemical peel	1,500
Chin augmentation	1,200–2,000

THE HIGH PRICE OF A PERFECT BODY

If you are one of those men who devotes much of your time and energy to developing the perfect body, welcome to the nineties. You're the New Male, and research shows your numbers are legion.

However, an unhealthy self-interest in image has its price: "Who am I as a man, and how do I make a difference in the world?" gives way to "How do I look, and what image should I project?" Your true self, which is composed of your values, feelings, thoughts, familial and societal roles, and how you define yourself as a man, ends up buried and unexpressed. You need an authentic sense of identity.

A case in point is a thirty-four-year-old patient named Ted who was being treated for exercise addiction. He told his doctor, "I thought if I made a lot of money, bought a Porsche, perfected my body and controlled my eating, it would make me feel less out of control. I would feel better about my marriage, get close to others without feeling suffocated and feel more powerful."

In seeking external control, he began to feel desperate and out of control. He focused on the wrong problem—his body—without really looking inside, getting to know himself and developing skills that would give him control of his life. Sure, he looked good, but he found himself drinking too much and constantly comparing himself to others, generating feelings of inferiority.

Ted's father raised him to be strong and silent, to regard his body as something to be either mastered or ignored. Ted's code of masculinity prevented him from developing skills to connect with other people or to express, even recognize, his feelings. He was to perform, regardless of his physical state.

In therapy, Ted began to work on his low self-esteem and deteriorating marriage. He realized that his physical ideal (full chest, thin waist, with a look of strength and agility) could never vanquish the powerlessness he felt inside.

He struggled with his definition of what it means to be a man. He sifted the characteristics of traditional manhood that he valued logical thinking, assertiveness, perseverance—from those he didn't: invulnerability, fear of closeness, a predisposition toward anger, rage and violence. He worked to modify such facets of himself and to be more human and realistic. He found himself becoming more open to others and developing a healthier connection to his body, heeding and respecting it rather than sculpting it. He ate more healthful foods, exercised moderately and spent more time relaxing and having fun with other people.

When you accept the cultural message that your body is an "it" to be changed and controlled, a "machine" rather than an "I," you become disconnected from yourself and from people around you. The less you pay attention to the messages your body gives you, the more vulnerable you are to physical and emotional disorders. You end up alienated from your feelings—numb, desensitized, out of control.

The solution is greater "embodiment." This means developing an awareness of and responsiveness to bodily sensations that lead to a stronger sense of self, a deeper connection with others and an empowered state of being. How can you do this?

1. Begin to recognize your body as the home of yourself. Every negative thought about your body contains a negative thought about yourself. Keep track of when you have these thoughts, where you are, whom you're with and what is going on. Your goal is to learn what body loathing may be distracting you from.
2. Try exercises such as meditation and yoga that let you slow down and reconnect with your body.
3. Keep an emotional-response log. Record tensions in your body (stomach upsets, backaches, racing heartbeats). What goes on between you and others during these times? What are you feeling when such discomforts arise? Do they camouflage emotions you are unable to identify or express? Develop a vocabulary to describe your emotions, especially the tender, more vulnerable ones.

By allowing yourself to experience your body more fully, you come to know and express your true self. With the body as a guide and mentor, you can be enriched by connecting with yourself and others. True power doesn't come from running the extra mile when your body is exhausted, but from listening to your body, responding to it and letting it guide your reaction to the world.

WHAT MAKES A GOOD-LOOKING MAN?

We each have an image in our mind's eye of what we'd like to change about our looks in order to be more aesthetically pleasing to ourselves and others.

Maybe a little more hair on top, a little less in the nostrils, straighter teeth, wider shoulders, eyes a little less beady, bigger pecs . . . the list can be endless. But when you're thinking about your looks and how to improve them, it's important that you determine whether you're trying to please yourself or buying into someone else's (perhaps an advertiser's) idea of how a man should look.

The mesomorph—the wide-shouldered, square-jawed type—dominates our concept of male good looks. Mesomorphs have a more athletic musculature than their endomorphic (round-shouldered and wider at the hips than at the shoulders) and ectomorphic (narrow-shouldered, narrow-hipped, minimally muscled) brethren. Mesomorphs tend to dominate adolescent sports, which, of course, gives them an early, well-developed sense of self-confidence. That bravado usually carries over into their adult lives, in both a personal and a professional sense.

Although they by no means have a lock on success (Henry Kissinger is a classic short, round endomorph who got both the tall blond and the President's ear), there are inordinate numbers of mesomorphs among the highly visible men in our society. Just look at the bulk of professional athletes and entertainers—precisely those men who shape other men's ideas about how they should look.

And so the cycle continues: Nonmesomorphic men become convinced there's a link between the character strengths and the good looks they see in the Arnold Schwarzeneggers (and even the Ronald Reagans) of the world. They believe that the same mental qualities they admire—high professional and sexual self-confidence with a touch of fearlessness—would be theirs if they only possessed the same physical characteristics as these role models.

But is anatomy really destiny? "*Charisma* would be a good word to describe what I'm talking about," says Joy Davidson, Ph.D., a Los Angeles-based psychotherapist. "And from what I've observed in male behavior patterns, it's as important as physical good looks in determining how others view you. But it's something of a catch–22: Having good looks and an athletic, well-developed body gives you a greater jump on developing self-confidence than do skinny arms and a paunch."

Some therapists credit healthy childhood development as well as good genes for the aura of self-confidence that successful, attractive men seem to exude. Mark Tollefson, a busy New York commercial model, says the natural energy (not to mention the physical attributes) that makes him a favorite of casting agents springs from a completely supportive home environment when he was a kid: "That early self-confidence," he says, "lets any negative energy I get as an adult roll right off my back." But if, as men's-movement guru Robert Bly says, "Ninety percent of us grew up in dysfunctional families," the looming question is: Can the internal security and external energy that are the hallmarks of "attractive" men in our society be acquired by the average Joe?

You can also develop the inner man. Psychologist Davidson advises men who lack self-confidence to take public-speaking classes or voice and diction lessons. "Of course, self-esteem problems caused by physical or emotional abuse in childhood make things more complicated, and men who suffer from extremely low self-esteem, no matter what they look like, should seek some form of professional therapy."

Once you have a grounded sense of self, there's nothing wrong with correcting a few physical flaws. "Dermabrading acne scars, straightening teeth or fixing the hook nose you always hated is fine," says Alan Matarasso, M.D., a Manhattan plastic surgeon. The problem comes when you keep going back for more plastic surgery because no matter what you do, you still don't feel attractive.

So while having Paul Newman's eyes, Kurt Russell's jawline and Patrick Swayze's grace couldn't hurt, it's not all that attracts others to us. And although the path of that most envied of men, the good-looking mesomorph, seems to be paved more smoothly than the rest of ours, not being born an Adonis doesn't by any means condemn you to sitting out life on the sidelines. Turn your attention instead to developing the inner man who makes the outer man magnetic.

WHAT'S YOUR BODY TYPE?

Are you a Clint Eastwood type of man—long, lean and tall in the saddle? An Arnold Schwarzenegger clone, with gigantic muscles protruding from every inch of your physique? Or perhaps your big hips and prodigious thighs conjure up images of actor John Goodman, working-class hero and enemy of buffet tables everywhere?

These three men exemplify the three basic body types. "But few men are entirely one type," notes exercise physiologist Daniel Kosich. "Most of us are a blend of different body types, with a tendency toward one profile or another." The following list details the basic body types as well as the recreational activities for which each type is best suited.

Ectomorphs (Clint):

This type has a long, narrow trunk with long, thin limbs and face. Many distance runners have this build. They are lean, wiry, fat-burning machines who—because of their speedy metabolism—often have trouble building muscle size. The best sports for ectomorphs are long-distance running, volleyball, skating, cross-country skiing and basketball.

Mesomorphs (Arnold):

This type has strong muscles, big shoulders, a broad trunk and well-proportioned limbs. He has lean body mass and an uncanny ability to make quick gains through weight training. Mesomorphs should focus on middle-distance running, tennis, mountain climbing, skating and basketball to take the best advantage of their body type.

Endomorphs (John):

This type has a broad trunk, relatively short limbs and a round face. They generally carry a higher percentage of their weight as body fat, and usually need to increase the amount of aerobic work in their routine in order to burn more calories. Good sports for endomorphs include swimming, cross-country skiing, paddling sports, cycling and golf.

WHAT DO WOMEN THINK ABOUT MEN'S BODIES?

There's never been any doubt that women look at men just as much as men look at women. What has changed in the last few years is that men have become nearly as objectified as women. Advertising in particular has employed the masculine physique as never before. Men now have a taste of what it's like to walk down the street and be surrounded by public advertising that uses the male body to sell products. The upshot is that men's bodies—how they should look, how they *shouldn't* look, and which parts might be more significant than the whole— have never been the subject of so much public scrutiny.

What do women really think about the male figure? Writer Jill Neimark of *Psychology Today* examined the results of a survey on that subject commissioned by the magazine, and came away with some surprising conclusions. Two-thirds of the 1,500 respondents were female, demonstrating

women's keen interest in the subject. The answers reveal a fascinating discrepancy between the sexes when it comes to men's bodies:

- Men think their appearance is more important to women than women themselves actually acknowledge. From hairline to penis size, men believe their specific physical features strongly influence their personal acceptability by women.
- Even though their "ideal male" may be different, women are quite willing to adapt to their own mate's appearance, accepting features such as baldness or extra weight. Women tend to like what they've got—whether he is bearded, uncircumcised, short, or otherwise "off " the norm.
- A new subset of women who are financially independent and rate themselves as physically attractive place a high value on male appearance. This vocal minority

unabashedly declares a strong preference for better-looking men. They also care more about penis size, both width and length.

- Personality wins hands down, for both men and women: it's what men believe women seek, and indeed, what women say is most important in choosing a partner.
- That said, men still care about their own looks. Men may still give top priority to their sense of humor and intelligence, but a nice face is a close third, and a good build is not far behind. Women give an overall lower significance to men's physical appearance, but height is still an important turn-on for women.
- Men fear losing their hair, but women are more accepting of baldness in a mate than men realize. Both men and women currently prefer clean-shaven men.

- Men are less worried about being overweight than are most women, but more concerned about muscle mass—reflecting our cultural ideals of thin women and powerful men. The muscle-bound body build was highly rated by men, while women preferred a medium, lightly muscled build in their ideal males (think Harrison Ford, not Arnold).

Curiously enough, there seems to be emerging a single standard of beauty for men today: a hypermasculine, muscled, powerfully shaped body—*homo Soloflexo*. It will be interesting to see if that standard will become as widely accepted—and as punishing—for men as has women's superthin archetype. In the nineties, for good or ill, the bottom line is: everybody is a sex object.

GROOMING: THE BASICS

Shaving

The first shave a man attempts, the one done with half a can of shaving cream and a bladeless razor his dad fixed up, is often the best one of his life. After that, it's all downhill.

Think about it: It's probably been a while since you had such a perfectly painless shaving experience. Cuts, stings, nicks, bumps and ingrown hairs are all daily realities for many men. For the most tormented, growing a beard and getting electrolysis are options. However, you can avoid such extreme measures by making some simple adjustments to your daily ritual. Incorporate some of the following tips, and you can probably save your shave.

Most problems begin before a blade ever cuts a hair. "Think spaghetti," says Kirk Merchant, a barber and owner of Truefitt & Hill barber shop in Chicago. "If you try to eat uncooked spaghetti, it will crack between your teeth. However, if you boil it for a few minutes, it becomes soft. Hair is the same way once you get some water in it." And, therefore, it's easier to shave. Merchant uses hot towels to soften up his clients' beards. At home, the best time to shave is during or after your shower. The heat and steam will soften your beard, and the wash will remove the night's accumulation of oil. (You can also use a preshave lotion, but proper preparation invariably makes those unnecessary.)

Next, apply a shaving cream, foam or gel. Which type or brand you choose isn't important: it's how you use it that counts. Merchant suggests applying it with a shaving brush, not your fingertips. "Each beard hair has an outer layer of cuticle, which the brush opens so more moisture can be absorbed," he says. Wait a few minutes to let the moisture penetrate the hair before shaving. Also, avoid putting anything cold on your face. If your shave cream is cold, immerse the container in hot water.

No matter how well you prepare your beard, a dull razor is going to tear up your face. As long as they're sharp, both razors with changeable blades and disposable razors do the job. A changeable is a bit sturdier for thicker beards, provided you replace your blade as often as necessary. If you have a heavy beard, you may want to change blades after every shave; you can use it for up to a week on a fine beard. "But if the razor starts to tug and doesn't take the beard off like butter, it's time to change," Merchant says. For best results, use razors with stainless steel blades, pivoting heads and lubricating strips.

Properly prepared, begin your shave at the top of your cheek near your sideburns. Use short strokes in the same direction your hair grows. Shaving with the grain of your beard lessens your chances of razor burn and ingrown hairs. Do your neck next, saving the areas around your mouth and below your chin for the end. This gives these whiskers—the thickest on your face—more time to soften. Don't apply too much pressure with the razor, no matter how heavy your beard is. You're begging for a bout of razor burn, the result of a too-close shave.

If you do get a burn, soothe your skin with a hydrocortisone ointment. Forget blotting any cuts with toilet paper; use styptic instead. Be careful, though; styptic won't come off clothing.

Men with specific skin or beard problems should take additional steps to get a smooth shave. One option, according to Vincent DeLeo, M.D., associate professor of dermatology at Columbia Presbyterian Medical Center in New York City, is an electric razor. But if you just can't bring yourself to plug in, here's what you need to do:

Dry Skin: Use a cream-based soap like Basis or Dove and a shaving cream for dry or sensitive skin. Afterward, use a moisturizer with glycolic acid. "It softens up the outer layer of skin so you don't look like an onion," says Jenny Bluestein, a cosmetologist and registered nurse in St. Louis.

Oily Skin: Use soap and water to tighten pores and remove traces of oil before and after a shave.

Sensitive Skin: Try fragrance-free products or those designed for sensitive skin.

Acne: Wash your blade with hot water or dip it in alcohol to prevent bacterial growth. Stay away from oil-based products as well. Acne is one case in which an electric razor is recommended.

Thick Beard: Rinse your razor more frequently and change the blade often.

Men like to stretch their skin to get a closer shave. But while stretching will enable you to cut the hair farther down the shaft, that hair will sometimes slip farther under the skin when you release your grip. When it grows back, it may not be able to find its way out of your skin. These ingrown hairs cause *pseudofolliculitis barbae*, or shaving bumps, and it's a common problem for African-American men and others with curly hair. If you want a closer cut and are prone to these irritations, try shaving twice. Or, as many men do, grow a beard.

To avoid this and all the other aforementioned problems, begin preparing for tomorrow's shave as soon as you're done with today's. Rinse your razor and shake it dry to eliminate stubble and foam. Wash your face to get rid of dead skin. If you like aftershave, choose witch hazel over any alcohol-based product to avoid irritating or drying your skin. Other options are alcohol-free balms or moisturizers. Follow these guidelines and your face will feel like new. Until tomorrow, that is.

GOING ELECTRIC

Do you hit the snooze button so many times that, when you finally wake up, it's either shave or be late for work? If you're consistently faced with this dilemma, try an electric razor. Most are quick and easy to use, and some are portable.

But convenience isn't the only benefit. They're probably the best option if you tend to get shaving bumps, razor burn or acne. "Your skin is more likely to be irritated by shaving creams and the blade than by anything else," says dermatology professor Vincent DeLeo, M.D., of Columbia Presbyterian Medical Center in New York City. Two types, foil and rotary, are on the market. They're both good for problem skin because neither type shaves hairs below skin level. The tradeoff with electric shavers: Because they don't cut hairs below the skin, your shave is less smooth.

If you choose an electric, keep these tips in mind:

- Keep your face dry. Wash your face to remove oils accumulated overnight but make sure to let your skin dry for five minutes prior to shaving.
- Don't use too much pressure. A light, gliding motion works best. Stay too long in one area, and your skin will get as irritated as it does with a conventional razor.

Hair

Aside from the dreaded male pattern baldness (which will be covered later in this section), most complaints about hair focus on dandruff and seborrhea—the flaking scalp condition that can afflict men from puberty through old age. Though many assume that the conditions are the result of scalp dryness, the opposite is true; the oils produced by the scalp cause the normally invisible dead cells of the scalp to clump together, producing flakes.

In seborrhea the skin cells multiply (and die) too rapidly, causing an abundance of flakes when they mix with oils from the sebaceous glands. Daily washing with regular shampoo is often enough to keep dandruff at bay, but seborrhea should be combated with shampoos containing zinc pyrithonate, selenium sulfate or tar; try each variety for a couple of weeks to see what works best for you. If you use a selenium shampoo for several months and find it's no longer working, try one with tar or zinc. Your scalp can adapt to the medication after a while, and using a different agent for a few weeks can help get your flakes back under control. Funguses may play a role in seborrhea, and your dermatologist may want to prescribe a shampoo containing an antifungal ingredient.

In terms of hair care, less is more. Shampoo enough to keep your scalp from getting too oily and to keep your flakes down, but not so often that you risk drying it out. If you shampoo in the morning and shower again later in the day after a workout, water alone should be enough to clean your scalp and hair—and you might need a light conditioner. Blow drying, coloring, relaxing, waving or perming the hair might well cause or exacerbate problems by exposing the scalp to chemicals or excessive heat. You might keep that in mind when deciding what vanity to inflict on that clump of dead cells atop your head.

Teeth

Most men find time to at least guide a toothbrush around their mouths on a fairly regular basis. Where most fall short is on flossing. You should floss every day; it's the only way to free up the debris that your brush can't reach, and it's the best way to clean in between the teeth and along the gumline. Regular bleeding during flossing or vigorous brushing is a sign that there is already some inflammation in the gums, and your teeth might already be endangered. If you haven't flossed in awhile and you're getting back in the habit, a little bleeding isn't unusual and will probably stop as your long-neglected gums get used to the attention.

An antiplaque rinse, used after flossing and before brushing, can also be a great help. If your gums have already receded somewhat, your dentist might want to prescribe a fluoride treatment to protect the newly exposed enamel. Brushes with soft bristles are the way to go; ask your hygienist to refresh you on the best brushing motion and the amount of time you should spend on different parts of your mouth. Also, ask his or her opinion of electric toothbrushes; the Braun Oral-B is highly rated by dentists and consumer groups, and some men—ever searching for another power gadget—are more motivated to brush when they use an electric.

Aside from the obvious payoff in the form of pain-avoidance and smaller dental bills, good oral hygiene has another benefit: good breath. Bad breath—or halitosis—is primarily caused by bacteria, which find the mouth to be a perfect breeding ground. A secondary cause of halitosis can be a systemic disorder like kidney disease or diabetes. Most bad-breath problems are related to the overall health of the mouth, and disappear when your teeth and gums are functioning well. If you find you're constantly battling bad breath, it's probably an indication that there is something wrong with your gums—and that you should see your dentist as soon as possible.

In addition to seeing the dentist, try a few of these tips. They're simple and effective when done regularly:

- Scrape your mouth gently. Use a spoon at the back of the tongue and sides of the mouth, areas where bacteria like to hide.
- Brush and floss regularly. "Do it at least two times a day," says Scott Tamura, D.M.D., a dentist in Marina Del Rey, California. "Keep a toothbrush and floss at work, too." You'll get rid of food particles, keep your gums healthy and prevent plaque buildup. If your gums bleed often, that's a sign that your oral hygiene may not be adequate.
- Brush your tongue, too. Again, bacteria like to hide there.
- Avoid foods like onions and garlic.
- Don't smoke. It stimulates the production of proteins in the mouth on which bacteria like to feed.
- Avoid drinking alcohol. It dries out the mouth, making it easier for bacteria to grow.
- Eat breakfast. When you wake up in the morning, your mouth is as dry as a desert. Eating and drinking help get saliva flowing.

Nails

Most nail care focuses around simply trimming them and keeping the area under the tips of your nails clean. For care of the cuticle—the area where flesh and nail meet—get a manicure from a professional, and pay attention. You might find the buffing a little fussy, but manicurists are experts at caring for the cuticle and grooming nails.

If you have cracked or brittle nails, you might try the vitamin biotin; one Swiss study found that a daily dose of 2,500 micrograms resulted in nails that were 25 percent thicker, and less prone to split. Nails take about seven months to grow out fully, so you might have to follow this regimen for quite a while before you see results.

YOUR SKIN AND THE SUN

The High Price of a "Healthy Tan"

We know, we know, we know. Physicians, researchers and your Great Aunt Mary have for years been exhorting you that the sun is the skin's worst enemy. It can cause irritations, premature aging and cancer. There's even new evidence that prolonged sun exposure can inhibit the infection-fighting power of the immune system.

You probably already knew that. But did you know that, according to Nelson Lee Novick, M.D., associate clinical professor of dermatology at Mount Sinai School of Medicine in New York City, of the 80 percent of Americans who are aware sun exposure is unhealthy, only half are taking steps to protect themselves? Apparently, all the advice and evidence in the world won't change the fact that a suntan is still considered fashionable. And neither is anything likely to change the fact that there's never been such a thing as a safe suntan. "It's an oxymoron. A little tan still means skin damage," says Novick.

Sun damage comes from both ultraviolet B (UV-B) and ultraviolet A (UV-A) rays. The former, thought to be the most dangerous type, lead to sunburn and later to skin cancer. (The sun and skin cancer will be addressed later in this chapter.) The second type penetrates deeper, disrupting the collagen and elastin structures that support the skin and keep it resilient. That means the UV-A bulbs in tanning beds are also dangerous— and it's why patrons must sign waivers absolving salon owners of any responsibility for short- or long-term health problems. It is also one of the reasons why the Food and Drug Administration now requires salons to affix warning labels on their machines. According to Baltimore dermatologist Warwick Morison, M.D., tanning beds are more threatening than the sun because they encourage year-round exposure.

Experts agree there's only one way to achieve a safe golden glow: tanning or bronzing lotions. But if you're still convinced you have to go outside, be as sun-safe as possible:

- Avoid sun exposure between 10 A.M. and 3 P.M., when the rays are most damaging.
- Wear sunscreen. Novick recommends starting the tanning process with a high SPF sunscreen, at least 25. As you acquire color over the course of a few days, cut back to lower-SPF products until you get the tan you desire. Then move back up to a high SPF for maintenance.
- If you burn at all, your product's SPF isn't high enough. SPF 15 is the absolute minimum level of protection.
- Apply sunscreen at least fifteen minutes before you go outside so it can dry. Don't forget the tops of the ears and feet, and the backs of knees.
- Use a water- and sweat-proof sunscreen when you're exercising. Coppertone, Aramis, Neutrogena, Borghese and Polo Sport all have options in a wide range of SPFs.
- Swimmers should use sunscreen on all parts of the body. Ultraviolet light can penetrate up to three feet of water.

- Reapply sunscreen every two hours and after every time you take a dip in the water.
- Buy new sunscreen every couple of years. The active ingredients are effective only for a limited time.
- If you're on medication, check with your doctor before spending any time in the sun. Certain drugs like tetracycline can increase sun sensitivity.

What Suncreen Can and Can't Do

What would you think if someone said that sunscreens not only prevent skin damage, but possibly reverse it as well? That's what one group of scientists discovered in 1993. Australian researchers found that sunscreens with an SPF of 17 helped prevent pre-cancerous skin growths called solar keratoses and even partially restored sun-damaged skin to a healthier state.

It's hard to appreciate the importance of sunscreen without understanding the havoc wreaked upon skin when you decide to get "a little color." First, when the sun's ultraviolet rays collide with your body, they trigger the release of melanin, a natural pigment agent that is meant to ward off further damage. In other words, your tan isn't a sign of health; it's a sign of injury.

As previously mentioned, the sun's UV-A rays affect collagen in the skin over the long term, resulting in coarsening, wrinkling and other symptoms associated with aging. At the same time, UV-B rays put up an assault that may damage your DNA and impair your body's immune system. Both processes contribute to skin cancer—but that's not the only concern. Dr. Peyton Weary, a professor of dermatology at the University of Virginia, notes that, "We already know a lot about the relationship between sunlight and skin cancer. But beyond that, I think that there's a lot of things we don't know about the connection between immune suppression and sunlight."

Your appearance may be the least of your worries. The rate of melanoma, the sun-related cancer than can quickly spread from the skin to the internal organs, is growing faster than any other type of cancer in the country. The National Cancer Institute found that the number of melanoma cases jumped 90 percent between 1973 and 1990. The probability that an individual would get this cancer in the 1930s was 1 in 1,500. Today, you have a 1 in 80 chance of developing melanoma at some point in your life.

Researchers say a number of factors may be responsible for the sharp rise: increased leisure time, decreased clothing cover and our relatively newborn love for the deep, dark tan. The depletion of the ozone layer, which protects the earth from UV radiation, may also be a factor.

For years dermatologists have been counseling patients to decrease their risk of skin damage by using sunscreen, but no study has ever firmly shown its value—until now. The breakthrough came in Australia, which has the worst rate of ozone depletion and highest skin cancer incidence in the world. In 1992, researchers there began focusing on the effect of sunscreens on solar keratoses—small, tannish, wart-like growths that are rough and scaly and result from cumulative sun exposure. Keratoses are generally harmless. In fact, they often disappear on their own, especially with reduced exposure to sunlight. But they can be harbingers of skin cancer.

The researchers chose 588 people who had keratosis lesions. (One-quarter of them also had a history of skin cancer.) Roughly half received a sunscreen that was "broad spectrum" (meaning it blocks both UV-A and UV-B), with an SPF of 17. The other half received a placebo cream with no sun-blocking ingredients. All the subjects were also told to avoid the sun during midday and were required to wear hats and other protective clothing whenever they went outdoors. After seven months, 25 percent of the sunscreen users' growths had vanished compared to only 18 percent of the placebo users'. In addition, the study found that the sunscreen users were better protected against new lesions than the control group.

The findings are significant for two reasons. First, this was the first proof that using sunscreen actually does prevent skin damage and skin cancer in humans. "It confirms what dermatologists have been telling their patients for more than two decades," says Robin Marks, M.D., a senior lecturer in dermatology at the University of Melbourne and one of the study's researchers.

Even more exciting is the news that using sunscreen today may compensate for previous years spent soaking up rays. Says Barbara Gilchrest, M.D., chairman of the Department of Dermatology at Boston University School of Medicine, "These were older individuals with considerable skin damage. But after only seven months, they were able to partially reverse decades' worth of exposure. One wonders what would happen if you applied the sunscreen for five or ten years or if you began using it earlier." The researchers also found that people get more benefit by using more generous amounts.

Does all of this mean you can tan now and slather later? Absolutely not, Marks says. "A tan is like a total-body callus. To classify [it] as an indication of beauty is very bizarre." Of course, the point isn't to avoid the sun totally but to be cautious. "You don't have to completely change your lifestyle and become a hermit," Starr says. "Just be careful."

HOW TO READ YOUR SKIN

Some identifying characteristics to help you separate the bad from the simply ugly:

Solar keratoses, which are noncancerous growths, are usually small, tan or reddish-tan, rough and scaly.

Non-melanoma skin cancers are generally not fatal, although they can become disfiguring if neglected. There are two main types. *Basal-cell carcinomas* are small, pearly, pimple-like growths that sometimes ulcerate or grow crusty. *Squamous-cell carcinomas* are reddish and scaly, and they tend to grow much faster. Combined cases in this country are about 800,000 annually, according to the American Cancer Society.

Malignant melanomas often have irregular borders. They may start out flat and brown or black and may turn shades of red, blue and white while becoming crusty and bleeding. They often develop from or near existing moles and are most commonly found on the upper backs of men and women, and on the chest, abdomen and legs of women. See a doctor immediately if you have or develop a mole with these characteristics.

Darrell Rigel, M.D., a clinical associate professor of dermatology at New York University, has identified six risk factors for melanoma:

- more than three blistering sunburns by adolescence;
- blond or red hair with freckling on the upper back;
- the existence of keratoses;
- family members with melanoma;
- three-plus years of outdoor summer jobs as a teenager.

COMMON SKIN PROBLEMS

Adult Acne

It's a problem you expect to leave behind once you're out of high school, and certainly by the time you've finished college, established a decent credit rating and celebrated your thirtieth birthday. But life's full of surprises, and adult acne is, for many men, one of the least pleasant. "Zits—at my age?" is their usual reaction. For them, a dueling scar would be preferable to looking like the gawky teenaged boy they thought they'd long left behind.

Adult acne tends to hit men much harder than women. It's usually more severe in men, for one thing. And, of course, it's harder to disguise, since even the most liberated male is apt to balk at using tinted medicines or anything that resembles makeup, despite the perverse fact that the biggest blemishes often strike in tandem with life's golden opportunities—an important job interview, a promising first date. Dermatologists haven't agreed on why they're seeing more male patients with the problem. It may be that for some reason adult acne is more common these days, or perhaps men have simply grown more aware of their appearance and the availability of new remedies.

But you have plenty to be positive about if you're suffering from adult acne. What the doctors do agree on is that the outlook for clear-ups has never looked better. There are new medicines, new techniques and, just as important, the growing realization that to be effective, treatment must be tailored to the patient's unique needs.

By far, the most common variety of acne among adult men is *acne vulgaris*, which occurs when the oil glands on the face and upper body become clogged and inflamed. While it may have been easy a few years ago to blame your acne on raging hormones, that's not usually the cause with adult acne. "The vast majority of people who develop acne have normal hormone levels," says Alexander Miller, M.D., a Yorba Linda, California, dermatologist and assistant clinical professor of dermatology at UC Irvine School of Medicine. But he doesn't rule out hormones altogether. Acne-prone skin, in fact, may be especially sensitive to the effects of hormones, he explains. Likewise, heredity may be a factor in some cases, but though acne can run in families, there's no single cause. "The trigger mechanisms for acne are complex," Miller points out.

If steroids come into the picture, however, finding the acne source isn't so tough. On this one point everyone agrees: Men who use anabolic steroids long enough are likely to develop acne. Steroid-induced cases are easily detected, says Seth L. Matarasso, M.D., a San Francisco dermatologic surgeon and clinical instructor at UC San Francisco School of Medicine. "The bumps are all nearly the same size, and they occur most often on the shoulders and trunk," he explains.

Most dermatologists also agree that people should give self-treatment a try before beginning a regimen of doctor-prescribed acne medication. You can start by picking up some over-the-counter acne-fighting soaps and treatments at the neighborhood drugstore. (Since some have been repackaged with adults in mind, you don't even have to act as if you're buying it for your younger siblings or offspring.) Give these self-help remedies about two months to work. If they don't, or if your acne gets worse, head to a dermatologist's office.

You should expect a dermatologist to give your face as well as any other affected areas a thorough examination. "First, a physician has to determine if this is a new case of acne or a sudden worsening of a previously existing adult-acne condition," says Robert Stern, M.D., associate professor of dermatology at Harvard Medical School and Beth Israel Hospital in Boston. "Sometimes lifestyle changes, such as an increase in stress, can worsen, but not cause, acne," Stern says. "It's also important to assess environmental causes before prescribing treatment."

Once your dermatologist has taken a comprehensive history and a close look at your pimple problem, it's possible to rule out less common forms of acne, such as *acne rosacea*, a chronic skin disorder marked by flushing and acnelike pimples that commonly springs up during cold weather.

The next step is for the doctor to decide upon treatment. "If the acne consists mostly of whiteheads and blackheads, I recommend a combination of old and new treatments, topical preparations like Retin-A or benzoyl peroxide, salicylic acid washes or prescription sulfur-containing preparations," says Miller. What if you have the standard red, irritated, painful-to-the-touch pimples instead? "These respond well to Retin-A and benzoyl peroxide but usually require an antibiotic as well, either oral or topical," Miller adds.

Commonly used topical antibiotics these days are erythromycin and clindamycin. Tetracycline, doxycycline, minocycline or ampicillin are pre scribed orally, either by themselves or to complement a topical medicine. "It takes four to twelve weeks to see a peak level of improvement," Miller warns. "The goal is to phase out the oral antibiotics over several months and maintain the topical treatments for whatever time period is necessary. "

Miller estimates that given enough time, the tailormade-treatment approach, using new and old medicines in combination, helps about 80 percent of male adult-acne patients. But if all else fails, some—not all—doctors will prescribe isotretinoin, or Accutane, a synthetic derivative of vitamin A developed in the early 1980s.

"A twenty-week course of Accutane treatment is typical, and 90 percent of patients taking it will get rid of their acne," Miller says. "And 90 percent of those will remain free of severe outbreaks." But most dermatologists consider this oral drug a last-resort option because its long-term effects are still a mystery and because it produces many side effects. The more common ones include dry mouth, skin and eyes as well as hair loss, sore gums and nosebleeds. Accutane also causes sore joints (a point of concern for active men) and, in men, elevated levels of triglycerides and serum cholesterol. Less common but serious potential side effects include temporary yellowing of the skin, buildup of fluid on the brain and development of bone spurs. The drug has also been known to cause catastrophic birth defects in babies born to women who took it during pregnancy. Close medical supervision, including regular blood tests, while taking the drug is mandatory.

Many men who tough out Accutane treatment are happy they did. One of Matarasso's patients, for instance, a man whose public-relations job requires frequent contact with clients and the media, had to undergo two regimens of the drug before his acne cleared up. But he says he'd do it again in a minute.

For acne or its aftermath, the array of treatment options is ever-expanding. The following top the list:

- Zinc/erythromycin. Some doctors have begun trying a combination of zinc and topical erythromycin after a recent University of Florida study found that a pairing of the two proved superior to erythromycin alone.
- Collagen and silicone. Men who have been left with acne scars and pits whether from an adult- or teenage-era bout can now improve their appearance, too. "We can inject collagen or silicone to help smooth out the peaks and valleys, with very good results. But the injections only work effectively on the face," says Matarasso. Researchers have yet to produce a viable cosmetic remedy for severe acne scars on the chest, back or neck; the pitting in these areas is often so extensive that there's no level surrounding skin to match the "filler" to.
- Dermabrasion is another scar-minimizing option. It entails removing the top layer of skin with chemicals or by "sanding" it. "Dermabrasion works best on light skin," Matarasso notes. The darker the complexion, he finds, the less well it works. And, as with collagen and silicone injections, dermabrasion is viable only for facial scarring.
- Lasers. Lasers are now being used to eliminate superficial acne scars; they're not used on acne itself. This use is still being debated among dermatologists, most of whom prefer dermabrasion as a first choice.
- Lifestyle advice. As they become more familiar with adult acne, doctors also find themselves questioning patients about habits that may contribute to an acne problem and that medicine alone won't solve. The practices mentioned most by dermatologists include not showering after a heavy workout, using irritating hair gels, scrubbing the face too vigorously or letting stress get the upper hand.

Regardless of what approach is used, when acne treatment is successful, dermatologists and their patients notice more than physical changes.

"Many men with acne or acne scars become reclusive 'acne hermits,'" Matarasso says. He reports that he's seen many men blossom after treatment, both professionally and socially: "After all, you're literally looking at the world with a new face."

Other Skin Problems

Acne isn't the only skin problem that men face. To find out what to look for, and how to handle them, *Men's Fitness* consulted a trio of dermatologists: Jerome Litt, M.D., a Cleveland dermatologist in private practice; Nelson Lee Novick, M.D., associate clinical professor of dermatology at Mount Sinai School of Medicine in New York City; and Andrew Scheman, M.D., a dermatologist in private practice in Evanston, Illinois. They agreed on the following ways to deal with four of the most common adult skin ailments.

1. Problem: Dry skin

What it is: Skin is itchy and flaky.

Why? After age forty, dry skin occurs naturally because the thickness of the dermis (the skin's middle layer) decreases by about 1 percent a year, making it less efficient at retaining moisture. Otherwise, dry skin is caused by taking showers and baths that are too long or too hot, and by using harsh deodorant soaps. Spending a lot of time outdoors, especially in winter, is another cause.

Solutions: Take short, lukewarm baths or showers using mild soaps or skin cleansers such as Lowlia Cake and Cetaphil lotion. Pat yourself dry, then apply a moisturizer with glycerin to lock in moisture. Use a humidifier at home, keeping the humidity level no lower than 40 percent. If you're getting shocked by static electricity, the humidity is too low.

2. Problem: Seborrheic dermatitis ("dandruff of the skin")

What it is: A chronic red, scaly, itchy rash that shows up around the scalp and facial hair, behind the ears, on the sides of the nose and on parts of the cheeks—all places where the oil-secreting sebaceous glands are most dense.

Why? The cause is unclear, but stress can aggravate the problem.

Solutions: Shampoo daily using anti-dandruff products. Leave on your scalp for at least five minutes so it can take effect. Use mild soaps and hydrocortisone preparations such as Cort-Aid ointment on other areas.

3. Problem: Rosacea

What it is: Resembles acne, except you don't get blackheads or white-heads. Characterized by spidery broken blood vessels, flushed and over-grown oil glands that can make your face look like W.C. Fields' nose.

Why? Unclear, but unlike acne it can by affected by your diet.

Solutions: Avoid spicy foods, pork products, alcohol and caffeine. In mild cases, over-the-counter acne products may work, but most likely you'll need a dermatologist's help. The doctor will prescribe topical and oral medications, or use special electrical instruments to close off broken blood vessels and shrink enlarged oil glands.

4. Problem: Cold sores

What it is: Irritating and highly contagious blisters that most often appear on the lips and in the mouth. Why? They're caused by the herpes simplex 1 virus, and there is no known cure. Factors that can trigger an outbreak include stress, sun exposure and colds. The virus is easily transmitted from person to person via eating utensils, towels and direct contact.

Solutions: You can reduce the discomfort by applying ice to the infected spot when you first feel an outbreak coming on (tingling and itch-ing are common early symptoms). Over-the-counter preparations such as Campho-Phenique Liquid Gel and Blistex Medicated Ointment can help, too, if used early enough. Also, use lip balm and sunscreen when you go outside.

WELL FED, WELL GROOMED

Let's say you noticed a big spot of rust on your car. Chances are, you probably wouldn't just paint over it, especially if you plan to keep the car for a while; you know the rust will be back in a matter of months. Yet that's how many of us approach grooming, masking rather than repairing and preserving. We tend to forget that our exteriors are an extension of our interiors. And no matter how much time and money you spend on hair- and skin-care products, if you're not giving equal attention to the nutrients you put into your body, you can't really look your best.

Researchers have learned that the first signs of a number of nutritional problems can show up in your appearance. Some of the most dramatic:

• B-vitamin deficiency can result in red blotches on the face, cracks at the corners of the mouth and enlarged pores on the nose.

- Vitamin A insufficiency can make the skin dry and rough.
- Insufficiency of vitamin C and bioflavinoids is associated with easy bruising.
- Lack of folic acid, other B vitamins and vitamin C can lead to unhealthy gums.
- Zinc deficiency may be indicated by dull, dry, brittle hair.

A number of micronutrients (so called because they're essential, but only in very small amounts) are vital to our appearance. They help the skin preserve and repair itself and maintain a barrier against harmful bacteria, viruses and chemicals. Vitamin C, for instance, is critical to the formation of collagen, a protein that, along with elastin, makes up the connective tissues of the skin. Other nutrients important to maintaining healthy skin.

Essential fatty acids help protect the skin from dryness problems like eczema. With names like linoleic acid, linolenic acid and eicosapentaenoic acid (EPA), they're found in oil from such foods as soy, flax and cold-water fish (virtually the sole source of EPA), among others. In one study reported in *The Lancet*, an English medical journal, eczema sufferers found relief when they took supplements of gamma linolenic acid, which is derived from primrose oil.

Magnesium works with essential fats to promote skin integrity, and magnesium deficiency appears to be widespread. Recent studies sponsored by the U.S. Department of Agriculture found that many people's diets fall short of the RDA of between 280 and 400 milligrams of magnesium daily. Foods with the highest magnesium levels include organ meats (liver and sweetbreads) and organically grown whole grains. (Nonorganic soils often contain fertilizers that deplete their magnesium content.) Dark-green leafy vegetables are also good sources.

Zinc, an essential trace mineral, not only helps maintain healthy skin, but also boosts resistance to infection and helps damaged skin heal properly. We need about the same amount of zinc as iron (10 to 15 milligrams). Food processing often ends up removing both minerals, but whereas iron is added back as a "fortified" nutrient, zinc is not. As a result, government nutrition surveys have called zinc a "problem nutrient" for some people. The highest amounts of zinc are found in relatively expensive, unprocessed foods like lean-muscle meats, lean sirloin, beef-stew cuts, lean game, round steak, chicken or turkey breast and whole grains.

Vitamin E, or tocopherol, is last on this list but certainly not least important. Several recently published studies describe how vitamin E helps prevent damage to the body by molecular time bombs called free radicals. These chemical substances develop in the body from exposure to radiation, ultraviolet light from the sun, air pollution, cigarette smoke, rancid fats, drugs or alcohol and from inflammation.

Considered "promiscuous" molecules, free radicals aren't too choosy about which part of the body to target. When produced in the skin, for example, they react with collagen in the connective tissue to produce "cross-links." Once enough cross-links form in a specific area, a wrinkle develops. That's why protecting your skin from free-radical damage combats skin aging.

Many studies have shown that smokers

are much more susceptible to wrinkling than nonsmokers. Others have demonstrated that prolonged exposure of unprotected skin to the sun's ultraviolet rays hastens its aging. When we have enough vitamin E in our diet, this important antioxidant thwarts free radicals before they can wreak their havoc. Unprocessed oils, such as soy or wheat germ oils, are the richest vitamin E sources.

In defending the skin and other organs against free radicals, vitamin E works in concert with carotenes. Found in the orange pigment of such fruits and vegetables as carrots, cantaloupe and squash, carotenes (the best known is beta-carotene) are vitamin A precursors, meaning they're converted to vitamin A in the body. However, their beneficial effects extend beyond those of vitamin A.

As a society, we spend hundreds of millions of dollars annually on skin-care products and cosmetic surgery, all in pursuit of a healthy, attractive appearance. We often forget how finely balanced and generous nature is: It only makes sense that good nutrition leads to good health and a good, healthy look. What cosmetic product or surgical procedure can make both those claims?

CARING FOR YOUR HAIR

To some extent, your hair also mirrors the quality of your diet. No matter what products you use in the shower, the luster, color and thickness of your hair will suffer if you're not well nourished.

Like fingernails, hair is made up of the protein keratin, whose formation depends upon a plentiful supply of the essential amino acid cysteine. "Essential" here means that your body cannot make cysteine from available materials and that it must come from the diet via high-quality protein foods.

Healthy hair also depends on zinc, copper and the B-complex vitamin biotin, all of which should be supplied by a balanced diet. Egg whites are a great source of cysteine-rich protein, as are low-fat cheeses. You can use them both in vegetable omelets and get other nutrients important to your hair's health at the same time.

For an oily scalp or serious dandruff problems, you might find relief in a diet lower in saturated fat, with more hair- and skin-supportive vitamins, minerals and essential fats—mostly from vegetable, grain and bean sources. A well-balanced diet that meets all your daily requirements can do a great deal to improve your hair and skin, although some men have special needs. If you think you do, consider seeing a nutrition-oriented health practitioner to assess your diet.

Hair-Loss Solutions

Coping with hair loss isn't easy. Just ask nearly any of the 35 million American men with *androgenetic alopecia*, or, in plain English, male pattern baldness. Balding arouses considerable anxiety in most men, living as they do in a society that nicknames them "chrome dome" and "cueball," not to mention many far-less-charitable euphemisms. Some settle into a good-humored acceptance of their lot; others experience a certain "follicle envy," casting covetous glances at full-maned men.

For men who are agitated by their hair loss, remedies to combat baldness—some proven, some experimental—probably have never been more plentiful. Certainly, they've come a long way since 420 B.C., when Hippocrates tried to solve his hair-loss problem by applying a potion of opium, pigeon excrement, spices and other aromatic ingredients to his exposed scalp.

The plethora of baldness treatments springs partly from the fact that there is no consensus among experts on the cause of baldness and, hence, the best "cure." But most do agree that male pattern baldness is influenced by a genetic predisposition, age and hormone activity on the scalp. During the balding process, the hair follicle shrinks in volume, leaving a hair shaft that grows progressively thinner in diameter. Eventually, growth stops or is limited to tiny, weak, barely visible hairs.

The key to remedying baldness, some experts say, is to block conversion of testosterone to one of its derivatives that actually causes the shrinkage of hair follicles. And the trick is to block this conversion only in the scalp area. Others say the solution is to stimulate new blood vessel growth in the scalp. A lifetime of treatment might be the only way to ensure continued coverage, others argue. The following is a rundown of ways, some new and unproven, others old but improved, to cover or recover your crown—along with the perspectives of some balding men who think simply looking on the bright side of baldness is the best solution.

- One testosterone-fighting drug now being tried as a baldness remedy is oral finasteride. It inhibits the enzyme that transforms testosterone into the dihydrotestosterone (DHT) form responsible for hair loss. Blocking the action of DHT seems to stimulate growth of stronger, thicker and more pigmented hair. In one Canadian study, 200 males aged 18 to 35 with distinct baldness had a one-inch circle of scalp shaved and periodically examined for hair growth. The report states that men taking 5 mg per day of oral finasteride had significantly increased hair growth. Side effects—which include impotence, loss of libido and reduced sperm counts—affected about 3 percent of those studied and often decreased with time. Ideal candidates should have already fathered all the children they wish, as the use of the drug might be lifelong and might harm any child conceived while taking it.

- Another dihydrotestosterone-inhibitor now being tested is a derivative of hyaluronic acid, the chemical at the tip of sperm that aids penetration of the egg's membrane. Massaged into the scalp, this substance apparently blocks the androgenic action that causes hair loss, but more research is needed before its efficacy and safety are established.

- A drug called Cyoctol looked promising in studies conducted at UCLA, say some experts. Ten of the twelve men who used a higher strength of the drug twice a day for about a year showed hair regrowth, according to Chantal Burnison, chief executive officer and president of Chantal Pharmaceutical, the West Los Angeles firm that hopes to bring the drug to market. Five of nine men who used a lower-strength Cyoctol also had hair regrowth.The drug works by preventing male hormones—testosterone in particular—from binding with receptors in the scalp's hair follicle cells. It thus keeps follicle production up and running. It's this binding that somehow results in baldness, according to some hair-loss experts, but they don't know exactly how or why. As for when Cyoctol may be available, it's difficult to say. It's presently in the second stage of trials mandated by the FDA, but Burnison won't be pinned down to a date: "It won't be tomorrow," she says.

- Another drug, PCIO31, or Tricomin, can produce a 35 percent increase in the number of new hair follicles, according to the Procyte Corporation, which reported the results of an eighteen-man French study at a professional meeting in this country recently. In the nine-month study, 83 percent of the men receiving the higher dose of two formulas tested reported "significant" hair growth as early as two months after beginning the treatment, according to the drug's developer. The product is in first-stage FDA trials, but Procyte spokespeople say they have no idea when it will be approved for general use.

- Other researchers are investigating the possibility that an enzyme deficiency causes baldness and that correcting it will stem the tide of hair loss. In one study, balding men had lower levels of aromatase, an enzyme that helps govern male-hormone balance in the hair follicles. Again, testosterone control may play a role.

- Full FDA trials are underway for diazoxide, a drug used to treat hyperglycemia (high blood sugar). It causes hair to grow all over the body.

- Although treatments like electrical stimulation could be years away from the market, experts do cite a number of advances and refinements in established approaches. Hair transplants or plugs, for example, no longer deserve their bad reputation, say doctors who specialize in this approach. Hair follicles from the lower fringe of the scalp, where hair continues to grow even on balding men, are transplanted to the top of the scalp where hair has fallen out. The number of sessions required depends on the extent of the baldness.

In the past, men who underwent this approach often ended up with a scalp full of hair that looked an awful lot like doll's hair or rows of corn. No longer—at least not in skilled hands, says L. Lee Bosley, M.D., founder and director of The Bosley Medical Group in Beverly Hills, which specializes in the approach.

When skillful transplants are combined with scalp reduction—a technique that cuts down on the surface area of bald scalp—the results can be very natural looking, Bosley says. The trick to avoiding the "picket fence" look is to use hair of the appropriate thickness and to place it properly. Often, Bosley contends, the observer is unaware of an extremely good transplant job. "You see some of my patients on television every week," says Bosley, declining to name famous names.

- Houston hair-transplant specialist Carlos Puig agrees that the key is artful placement and a natural-looking "plug," or graft. Instead of a pie-shaped plug, he uses one that's elliptical. "The shape and taper of the plug make it look very natural," he says, adding that men who got bad results with transplants years ago might consider going in for a "fix-up" session involving some new grafts. Transplantation is also becoming less painful, say Puig. He has developed a method of delivering local anesthetic to the scalp via low-level electrical current rather than a needle. "Patients don't feel it," he says.

- Another alternative is "flap" surgery, in which a section of hair-bearing scalp is separated from the surrounding skin and later rotated to cover the bald area, explains Richard W. Fleming, M.D., a Beverly Hills surgeon who pioneered the technique with his partner, Toby G. Mayer, M.D. The technique requires a light general anesthetic. The "donor" area is closed by stretching together the sections of hair-bearing scalp. A man with extensive baldness might require two flaps, Fleming says, but the results, he contends, appear more natural than other methods can achieve.

- Although hardly the miracle cure its manufacturer first made it out to be, minoxidil (trademarked as Rogaine) has proven effective in some cases. It's also better understood than it was when it debuted as a hair-loss remedy in 1988.

Originally developed to treat high blood pressure, minoxidil works best on men in their twenties and thirties who have just begun to lose their hair, says Laura Harwin, spokeswoman for The Upjohn Company, the manufacturer. Summing up the results of clinical studies of minoxidil on more than 2,000 men, Harwin says about half the men saw moderate hair regrowth; 36 percent saw minimal hair regrowth and 16 percent saw none. "It is not going to grow hair on someone with a head like a billiard ball," she says.

- The most exciting recent development in the battle against baldness is gene therapy. A California biotechnology company has found a way to fire genetic "bullets" at dormant hair follicles, inducing them to produce hair. The genes are encased in man-made spheres of fatty material called liposomes, then applied to the skin containing the non-producing follicles. During experiments, hair growth soon resumed. Now the bad news: the technique has only been tried on lab mice, and any human application is years away.

Today's balding men can be thankful they didn't live around A.D. 100, when the Church pronounced it a mortal sin to wear someone else's hair. Men now have such nonsurgical options as toupees and weaves, both of which have seen great improvement, says Mike Mahoney, spokesman for the American Hair Loss Council, a Texas-based nonprofit organization of dermatologists and hair-replacement specialists.

Today's better toupees look natural and, properly fitted, even stay put in a stiff breeze. Hair weaves involve sewing the man's own hair onto artificial braids to give a fuller look. The real hair continues to grow, so the braids must be tightened periodically. A newer option, Mahoney says, is using an adhesive to bond existing hair to the hair addition without the use of braids. This creates less tension between the artificial and existing hair so there's less chance of breakage. There's also less bulk, so the hair feels and looks more lifelike, he says.

The Cost of a Cure

Deciding on a baldness remedy isn't easy, partly because doctors who specialize in hair replacement don't agree on the best approach, with some calling others' techniques controversial, ineffective or even dangerous. Asks one doctor who specializes in transplants, "Have you ever seen a good flap?" Which is, of course, a rhetorical question, because if you can see it, it's not good.

"We advise consumers to be careful," says Mahoney, who is especially wary of over-the-counter remedies that lack scientific backup. Men spend about $2 billion a year on such hair-replacement products and procedures, he says. Beware of exaggerated claims, and take before-and-after pictures with a grain of salt. Contact your state department of consumer affairs and see if any complaints have been filed against a doctor or manufacturer you might be considering. Don't be embarrassed to shop around, and try to choose a method, product or practitioner based on word-of-mouth rather than advertising claims or a sales pitch.

Choosing the best "cure" for baldness is further complicated by the range of fees. Depending on the practitioner, the geographic region and the method, costs run the gamut. But the American Hair Loss Council often sites average figures, advising consumers that fees in metropolitan areas are usually higher than those in less populated areas.

The average yearly cost of hair additions, such as weaving and bonding, is about $1,200, according to the council, compared to about $600 for minoxidil. The price of surgical hair replacement, generally a one-time fee, is about $6,000, Mahoney says. Transplants take place over an extended period and can cost more than $2,500.

Even the best hair-loss expert can't help everyone. Richard Fleming, the Beverly Hills hair-flap expert, is a case in point. He explains his own receding hairline to patients day after day. He simply doesn't have enough donor hair, he says, to warrant undergoing the flap procedure.

There is also a growing understanding that a single treatment won't work for everyone, however skilled the provider or perfected the technique. For some men, temporary solutions can serve as stopgaps while they decide about costlier, more permanent remedies. For instance, some stylists specialize in curling and coloring to create the illusion of a fuller head of hair, Mahoney says. Dyes work by minimizing the color difference between hair and bare scalp.

Paralleling the explosion of baldness treatments has come a real understanding that hair loss truly disturbs many men. It's a stressful process, says Thomas Cash, a psychologist at Old Dominion University in Norfolk, Virginia, who recently surveyed 145 men, two-thirds of them bald or balding. Balding men have a "tendency to compensate in other areas," says Cash, by such actions as growing beards or working out to extremes.

Though baldness continues to provide fodder for comedians, few men see hair loss as funny. Still, some do manage to retain a sense of humor about it. Take the Bald Headed Men of America, a group headquartered in Morehead (get it?) City, North Carolina. The founder and president, John T. Capps III, has a simple motto: "No drugs, no rugs, no plugs." Then there's Professor Cueball's Bald Club for Men, a new San Francisco-based organization. It was founded by Kirk Malley, whose hairline is only slightly receding, after a very balding coworker complained about all the teasing he endures.

Soon after his club made headlines, Malley recalls, he received numerous calls on his toll-free line. "We got about twenty phone messages from women saying they think bald men are sexy," Malley says. His personal favorite? The woman who ended her call with an apology for not leaving her name. "My husband has a very full head of hair," she whispered quickly before hanging up.

Another top body-image complaint concerns weight. Unlike the self-esteem problems that can come from baldness, being overweight also carries a societal value judgment. No one holds baldness against a man, yet someone who carries too much fat might be seen as lazy or gluttonous. But worse than any snide remarks is the toll being overweight can take on a man's self-image—not too mention the profound health risks associated with an abundant waist. Losing weight isn't easy, but it can be done.

WHAT TO DO ABOUT UNWANTED WEIGHT

In our efforts to lose weight, we Americans spend a corpulent $30 *billion* a year on diet programs, videos, foods, pills, powders, devices and elective surgery. Ironically, we're only getting fatter despite this huge outlay. During the "health decade" of the eighties when more people than ever claimed to be watching their diet and working out regularly, the number of obese Americans actually increased by 8 percent. Our knowledge concerning fat has never been greater—and we've never been fatter.

Paradoxically, one of the primary reasons that we are gaining weight as a nation is diets themselves. After decades of investigation, researchers are now convinced that many reduction-diet programs actually backfire, not only causing additional weight gain once the diet is over but perhaps also increasing the chances for heart disease and even early death. The concensus is clear: weight-loss diets don't work. At best they are a short-term solution to a long-term problem. At worse, they can greatly diminish both the quality and quantity of your life.

The problem isn't so much losing weight in the first place as much as it is sustaining the loss. Weight loss is easy. You can cut calories, cut fat, burn more of both, take appetite suppressants, even check yourself into a hospital for a supervised fast or a stomach-stapling procedure. Even the diets recommended by doctors in books (and celebrities in supermarket tabloids) will make you lose weight for a short period of time.

But most pounds return. On average, people who lose weight gain back between 33 and 66 percent of it within one year. A *Consumer Reports* survey of 19,000 men and women who used commercial weight-loss programs—from the Diet Center to Weight Watchers—found that people stayed on the program for about six months, lost 10 to 20 percent of their body weight, then regained almost half of it six months after quitting. Two years later, they'd regained two-thirds of it. A favorite figure cited by diet critics comes from a study demonstrating that 95 percent of dieters put back all their lost weight within five years.

Adding to the case against dieting have been reports that repeatedly gaining, losing, then regaining weight—yo-yo dieting—predisposes a person to weight gain and upper-body obesity (the worst kind for your health) and even increases the risk of death from heart disease. But other studies don't show those effects, and the issue remains unresolved. People often gain weight with age, too, so weight increases among long-term dieters may simply come from getting older.

No one has ever studied whether people whose weight yo-yoed were actually dieting. They could have been sick, depressed, indigent, addicted to drugs or saddled with any number of problems that can hinder health. A 1994 National Institutes of Health task force concluded that the evidence doesn't prove yo-yo dieting promotes weight gain or harms health. Says NIH obesity researcher Susan Z. Yanovski, M.D., "We don't have the answers." However, she adds, "If you are not overweight but are aiming for the perfect body, you need to know that weight stability is the most healthful state." She notes that remaining at a fairly stable, normal weight is associated with less illness and longer life than either gaining or losing weight or doing both repeatedly.

So if statistics show that diets don't work, are you back to square one? Well, those statistics aren't altogether reliable. For instance, the oft-cited study showing that 95 percent of dieters fail was done back in 1959. Moreover, diet-failure statistics are culled from people who volunteer for medical school studies, and they're often the hard-core obese, not people trying to shave a few pounds. "These figures may not represent overweight people as a whole," Yanovski says. "We don't know how many people have lost weight and kept it off on their own."

Anne Fletcher, author of *Thin for Life*, knows at least 160 such people. Her book chronicles the successful strategies of men and women who lost a minimum of twenty pounds and kept them off for three or more years. "Obesity's reputation for intractability is exaggerated," she says. The *Consumer Reports* survey, for instance, found 76,000 people who lost an average of ten pounds on their own. And Fletcher's own research for her book revealed a similar trend. "About half the people I interviewed lost weight on their own, half through some organized group," she says.

"Many threw out all the diets and just started to eat healthier, cut fat and exercised more, but others needed to cut calories. About a third accepted a weight that was higher than their original goal. Most took six to eight months to lose the weight; some took years. Some are still losing."

The recent discovery of an obesity gene in mice has given weight to the argument that heavy people are programmed, and therefore destined to be that way. Though that may be true for some people, it's pretty unlikely that it applies to the full one-third of the U.S. population that's obese. It's believed that genes determine about 60 percent of weight and behavior accounts for the rest. Wayne Callaway, M.D., associate clinical professor of medicine at George Washington University in Washington, D.C., estimates that as many as 50 to 60 genetic determinants may affect a man's size, ranging from metabolic rate to muscle mass to fat-storing efficiency.

But genes aren't destiny. Even identical twins (who tend to be closer in weight than fraternal twins, no matter where they live or what they do) sometimes differ by twenty or more pounds. Being fat remains largely a lifestyle disease, one that is greatly affected by what we eat and whether we work out. To mangle the Bard, the culprit is not in our genes but on our shelves.

"I've yet to have anyone tell me, 'I'm eating low-fat and continuing to exercise, yet the weight just came back,'" Yanovski says. "What I hear is, 'I got very busy at work and stopped the exercise program.' When weight is gained back, people have changed the behaviors that helped get it off in the first place." Much weight gain stems from lack of physical activity and the resulting loss of lean body mass (that's muscle to you).

Experts have very little enthusiasm for over-the-counter diet products. Meal replacements won't by themselves enable you to lose weight. What they will do is confine you to an inflexible, hence nonsustainable, diet. And over-the-counter diet pills suppress appetite but can lead to dependency, dehydration, high blood pressure and poor nutrient absorption.

For the intractably obese, there's the option of drug therapy, possibly for the rest of your life. The popular antidepressant Prozac may help control binge eating; FDA approval for that use is pending. In an ongoing study of another antidepressant, Sibutramine, the highest doses given resulted in a twenty-pound weight loss in six months. Another drug under study, Orlistat, minimizes the amount of fat your body absorbs from food, letting about a third of the fat you eat pass through undigested. And there's a new generation of prescription appetite suppressants that don't have amphetamine-like effects. At the moment, however, none has a long safety history. In fact, some experts charge that fenfluramine, probably the biggest name among these new drugs, is toxic.

For other people, old-fashioned low-fat eating is enough. One Vanderbilt University study compared two groups of overweight volunteers. Both groups cut their daily fat intakes to no more than 30 grams, but only one also restricted calories. Because fat is so calorie laden, even the "non-dieters" wound up cutting out about 400 calories a day; the dieters eliminated 600 to 800 calories. Although the dieters lost more weight initially, the difference between the groups a year later was statistically insignificant. The dieters had regained much of their lost weight, while the low-fat folks kept off most of the weight they lost. (Fat will be discussed in more detail in the next chapter.)

Others, however, believe that what really matters is how many calories you burn. "If you've had trouble with losing and regaining weight, exercise is no guarantee, but it's the best hope we have at the moment," says Steven Blair, a physical-activity epidemiologist with the Cooper Aerobics Institute in Dallas. As to how vigorous the exercise should be, don't sweat the details—at least initially. "There's no persuasive evidence that it makes any difference whether the exercise is strenuous or moderate, all at once or in many bouts," Blair says. "What is important is expending the calories." He recommends a balance of aerobic, strength and flexibility training. The best rule of thumb is: do something active every day.

If you want to lose weight, set realistic goals, focusing more on the eating and exercise habits you can change than on the scale. Better yet, get rid of the scale and have your body fat measured (your doctor or health club can do this for you). It's a much more accurate yardstick of your progress. Try to lose five or ten pounds and keep them off for six months before losing more. "We need to get away from the idea of losing large amounts of weight to reach some ideal, and toward losing more modest amounts, which can be maintained," Paul Thomas says.

And remember that behavioral habits are hard to change in a moment of resolution. "I call it the Oral Roberts treatment: sudden enlightenment. It doesn't work," says Dr. Wayne Callaway of George Washington University. In other words, hang in there, even when your enthusiasm wanes.

You might think you're too fat when you have to buckle your belt on a looser notch. Or maybe you swear by the scale: If you don't weigh any more than the height-weight tables at the doctor's office, you figure you're not too fat. Unfortunately, both suppositions are wrong.

The only accurate way to know if you're too fat is to get a measurement of your body composition, an analysis of how much of it is fat and how much is muscle, bone or other lean tissue. You can look slender and have unacceptably high body fat. Or you can tip the scale way beyond what's acceptable on a height-weight table and simply be muscle-bound—but lean.

There's more to the question of body-fat ratios than vanity. If your body-fat level is ideal, you reduce the risk of high blood pressure, stroke, heart attack and diabetes. Monitoring body fat can also help you track progress on a weight-reduction program, to help you be sure you're losing mostly fat instead of muscle. It can help tell you if your exercise program is really adding muscle. Last but not least, knowledge of your body composition can help your physician determine your optimum dose of medications and, should it be necessary, anesthesia.

Once you're convinced that your bathroom scale, your belt or the tried-but-not true method of standing naked in front of the mirror won't tell the truth about how fat you are, you can choose from a host of ways to analyze your muscle-to-fat ratio. The gold standard—underwater or hydrostatic weighing—has been joined in recent years by several other methods. Experts say that, in terms of accuracy, some of these come close. Here's what you need to know.

- Underwater weighing in a tank of water is still the most accurate method of body-composition analysis, provided it's done correctly, says Covert Bailey, author of *Smart Exercise.* Clad in swim trunks, you slowly immerse your entire body, including your head, for about thirty seconds. The premise is simple: The amount of water displaced is directly proportional to your body's volume. Fat floats, and so displaces less water; muscle is heavier and displaces more. The only trick is to expel air from your lungs before the test. Underwater weighing for body-composition analysis is now offered at many sports-medicine clinics and at some community hospitals.
- Almost as good is the calipers method. An instrument called a calipers gently pinches and measures your skin-fold thicknesses at various locations on your body. The best four sites, says Polin, are the triceps, biceps, base of the shoulder blade and below the waist. "Calipers measurement is cheap, easy and relatively accurate," he says. Calipers measurements are sometimes available at health fairs or community hospitals as well as many health clubs. But for the shy or modest, there's a new at-home skin-fold measuring device.
- Yet another method to assess body fat is based on bioelectrical impedance. You lie down as small electrodes are attached to your wrist and ankle. Next, a very low

level of electrical current is passed through your body. "Fat is a poor conductor of electricity," explains Polin. "Apply electrical current to a piece of fat, and nothing will happen. Muscle, though is a good conductor." The impedance unit works on the principle that the lower the electrical resistance, the more lean tissue (and less fat) a person has. Impedance measurements, available at some sports-medicine clinics and health clubs, are accurate if done properly, experts say. Some research suggests that the calipers method was judged superior—probably because it's easier to use.

Once you have your results, how do you know how you stack up? What's a healthy body-fat percentage? Experts agree

that a healthy man should have less body fat than a woman. "Anything below 20 percent is acceptable for a man," Polin says, but others say even that's too permissive.

In general, men should strive for a body-fat measurement of 15 to 18 percent, says Philip Walker of the Cooper Institute for Aerobics Research in Dallas. Men under 30 should try for about 13 percent, he contends, adding that a small increase is acceptable with age. Men from 30 to 39 should target about 16.5 percent; 40 to 49, up to 19 percent; 50 and over, 20 percent.

When you go for a follow-up test, try to use the same method and the same technician to ensure accuracy. If you really need to know your measurement is correct, have it done first by one method and then by another, then take an average of the two.

FIGHTING BODY FAT

The problem of fat is actually two problems. There's the fat you eat and the fat you wear. These issues are related, of course. Dietary fat is the prime source of body fat because it is stored more easily than carbohydrates or protein. Though related, food fat and body fat deserve to be examined separately. This chapter will concentrate on the fat you wear, and the best strategies for getting rid of it. In the next chapter, we'll discuss fat's role in the diet as part of the general guidelines for healthy eating.

For all the guilt-ridden time, attention and energy many of us devote to it each day, fat may as well be the eighth deadly sin. Yet we're still confused about the stuff. Whereas one man's idea of limiting his fat intake is turning down that third double cheeseburger, another's is eating only whole grains, fruits and vegetables—hold the oil, please. One man takes his daily jog slow because he's heard that's the way to shed his gut, while another sends his heart rate through the roof because he thinks that's the best way to burn the fat off.

Exercise: How Intense?

When your body is at rest, stored carbohydrates will cover about 40 percent of your energy needs, while fat provides for the other 60 percent. "As the intensity of exercise increases," says Jack Wilmore, Ph.D., a professor of kinesiology at the University of Texas in Austin, "the percentage of calories coming from carbohydrates increases and that from fat decreases. In an all-out sprint, for example, you would draw almost entirely from your carb stores."

You'd think, then, that to lose body fat, you'd want to exercise at lower intensity. You'd be right—and wrong. This is one of the most controversial areas in exercise physiology and weight loss. Covert Bailey, the exercise guru with an in-depth knowledge of nutrition, chemistry and exercise physiology, says slow is definitely the way to go. Exercising at the lower end of the aerobic zone (but for a longer duration—at least thirty minutes) allows the body to burn more body fat as fuel, he maintains. Working at a more intense level causes the body to burn more blood sugar (or glycogen) than body fat as its fuel, and that results in less fat loss. His books *Fit or Fat* and *Smart Exercise* are well-researched odes to the concept of low-intensity workouts.

Wrong, say James Wilmore. "The fallacy of this theory, were you to take it to its logical extreme, is that you'd burn fat better just lying in bed," Wilmore says. The best way to burn fat and lose weight, he advises, is to exercise regularly at high intensity. "The total grams of fat used will be about the same or more as during a lower-intensity workout," he says, "but the total calories are considerably greater."

What's the solution to this dilemma? Which method works best for an individual may depend on the amount of his body fat, lean-body mass, and his overall level of fitness. Highly fit people with a few pounds to lose may do better with higher-intensity exercise. Less-fit people with more weight to lose often have more success with the longer, lower-intensity route and adding more sessions per week. Try both the Bailey and Wilmore methods for a couple of weeks and see which works best for you.

So should you focus on aerobics and skip the bench presses? Hardly. A pound of muscle consumes 30 to 50 calories per day just to maintain itself, whereas a pound of fat can hang around for a measly 2 calories. In a recent study conducted by Wayne Westcott, Ph.D., national strength-training consultant for the YMCA, people who combined resistance work with a half hour of aerobic exercise lost 2.5 times more fat than those who did the same amount of aerobic exercise alone.

Despite the claims of diet gurus, there is nothing too complicated about losing weight. Consistent exercise and longterm diet modification will make your body lose fat. The trick is to make your mind understand that it is worth the effort to stay with the regimen through thick and thin.

The Role of Metabolism

"I had a patient a while ago," says Jerry C. Sutkamp, M.D., a weight-loss specialist based in Ft. Thomas, Kentucky, "who knew he was thirty pounds overweight but refused to take action. 'Gosh, doc,' he'd say, there's nothing I can do—it's my metabolism.' I don't even think he knew what *metabolism* meant, but he was ready to blame it for his failure."

Don't blame your metabolism without first knowing what it's all about. Your basal, or resting, metabolic rate (BMR) can actually determine whether your weight-loss program succeeds or fails. "Your metabolic rate," says Peter Vash, M.D., author of *The Dieter's Dictionary*, "is your body's rate of heat production, measured in specific units—usually calories per hour." Food is the fuel that stokes this corporal furnace, and every chemical reaction in your body contributes to its output. "This heat can be measured as it escapes your body, and that measurement is your metabolic rate," Vash says.

Calories burned per hour is, of course, a handy indicator for anyone looking to shed pounds, as burning calories is essential to losing weight. Sutkamp throws up a red flag, though, when it comes to blindly cutting down on calories without considering the effect on your BMR.

"After a couple of days [of reducing daily calories], your BMR will start slowing down," says Sutkamp. "Your brain thinks your body is being starved and slows down the BMR to make the most of what food is coming in." After a couple of weeks of dieting, your BMR can drop as much as 20 percent, and your weight loss will be minimal because your body is not converting as much food into heat energy; instead, it's trying to store as much as possible.

So what's the point of cutting out the Twinkies if your BMR slows down to accommodate less food? Sutkamp says you have to pursue a two-pronged weight-loss strategy incorporating the right foods and exercise if you're going to be successful in raising your BMR to the level where you can begin losing weight again.

First, he says, you have to reduce the fat content in your daily diet; 10 to 15 percent of total calories from fat is ideal, though other experts find that figure too low and recommend up to 30 percent. Sutkamp recommends replacing the lost fat with complex carbohydrates, which elevate BMR through their rapid conversion to heat energy. " Your body," Sutkamp says, "prefers to store fat around your waistline, but it will put complex carbs, like pasta, right to work as energy. "

A fat-to-carbs change is important, says Sutkamp, but when it comes to BMR it's exercise that makes the difference. The good news is that it doesn't need to be excessive. "You don't have to run a marathon to get your BMR up to weight-loss speed," he says. "If you walk at a moderate pace for just twenty or thirty minutes three times a week, your BMR will rise and you'll continue losing weight."

Good news for the overweight man who often points to his "slow" metabolism as the source of his woes. In most cases, says Sutkamp, there is very little difference between the BMR of a mildly obese man (20 percent over ideal body weight) and that of a skinny-as-a-rail triathlete—except that the heavy man will convince himself that his BMR is the sole reason he's fat. (There's a greater BMR disparity, of course, when the heavyweight is extremely obese.)

A recent study conducted at St. Luke's-Roosevelt Hospital Center in New York City found that diet-resistant people—those who believed they couldn't lose weight—actually consumed twice as many calories as they thought they took in and burned about a quarter less through exercise than they imagined. The researchers, publishing in *The New England Journal of Medicine*, say the results indicate that an underactive metabolism is much rarer than self-delusion.

One other metabolic issue is the benefit of adding lean muscle mass to replace excess body fat; people with a high ratio of muscle to fat tend to have higher metabolic rates. The reason? Muscle tissue is metabolically more active than fat tissue, according to Peter M. Miller, Ph.D., the man behind *The Hilton Head Metabolism Diet*. "It takes more body energy for muscle to function; fat is relatively inactive, while muscle cells are extremely active, even when you are resting," Miller explains.

Both Vash and Sutkamp agree that an exact metabolism measurement is needed only in cases of extreme obesity. As Sutkamp says, "You're better off simply knowing what BMR is and how you can best manage yours for successful weight loss."

WHAT MAKES A METABOLIC RATE

Although basal metabolic rates don't vary all that widely among people, Peter Vash, M.D., points out that certain factors can influence your BMR:

1. Your age. Metabolic rate decreases with age, regardless of sex.
2. Your sex. Men have a slightly higher metabolic rate than women because they have more lean muscle mass; women's BMR is slightly lower to maintain their bodies' greater fat content.
3. Temperature. Your metabolic rate is higher in colder temperatures, lower in warmer temperatures.
4. Activity level. The more you move, the higher your metabolic rate will be.
5. Time of day. Metabolic rate slows toward the end of the day, becoming very slow during sleep. This means you shouldn't eat your heaviest meal at night, when you can't burn calories as well.
6. Food intake. After you eat, your metabolic rate rises for several hours, whether or not you exercise.

EATING DISORDERS: NOT FOR WOMEN ONLY

Mention anorexia, and who comes to mind? Karen Carpenter? Gymnast Christy Henrich? Most people think of a young white woman from a well-to-do family, starving herself to achieve some distorted ideal of thinness. But the first person ever diagnosed with anorexia nervosa was a man, and as doctors have always known, anorexia and other dietary dysfunctions don't discriminate by age, race, class or, more to the point, gender. Approximately 10 percent of the nation's estimated seven million people with eating disorders are male.

What's more, the familiar definitions of anorexia (self-starvation caused by an irrational fear of fat) and bulimia (eating huge meals, then purging by vomiting or using laxatives) are changing. Eating disorders, experts now say, actually encompass a broader range of behaviors, suggesting that more men suffer from distorted body image and dangerous eating habits than previously thought.

Men and women with eating disorders are alike in many ways. "A person who'd seen anorexia nervosa in a woman would have no trouble spotting it in a man," says James B. Wirth, M.D., Ph.D., director of the

Eating and Weight Disorders Clinic at Johns Hopkins Hospital. "It's the same intense preoccupation and discomfort with one's shape and weight."

No one is sure what causes an eating disorder, but patients of both sexes frequently share similar characteristics. Anorexics tend to come from families that stressed high achievement and the importance of physical appearance. Both anorexics and bulimics are likely to suffer from depression (40 percent of the patients Wirth treats require antidepressants) and lose their sex drive.

Low self-esteem is common, too; for many sufferers, losing weight is perceived as a way of gaining attention and approval. Ultimately, people with these unhealthy eating patterns seem to use food to mask feelings of inner turmoil. "Behind every eating disorder is one of the three deadly emotions: anger, fear or guilt," says Gregory L. Jantz, Ph.D., director of the Center for Counseling and Health Resources near Seattle.

If the idea of male anorexia seems oxymoronic, it's probably because the public's perception is that eating disorders are caused by living in a sexist society that holds women to unrealistic physical standards. This feminist argument contends that waiflike supermodels—like the near-skeletal Kate Moss—induce aberrant eating behaviors in women.

But what about the Soloflex guy in the TV ads? Billboards of Arnold Schwarzenegger flexing his biceps? Gossip-page photos of pop star Marky Mark lifting his shirt and dropping trou' to bare his chiseled pecs, washboard tummy and muscle-bound butt? The pressure to be perfect has become omnipresent and gender-blind.

A study of eating disorders among bodybuilders cited media images as a possible factor in producing not only a higher-than-average rate of anorexia but a bizarre new phenomenon known as "reverse anorexia." Harvard Medical School psychiatrist Harrison G. Pope Jr., M.D., the study's lead author, says that 9 of the 108 subjects—whom he describes as large and muscular men—saw themselves as scrawny and weak. The men spoke of wearing heavy sweatshirts at the beach to hide their bodies and turning down social invitations out of embarrassment. Steroid abuse was common.

A study published in 1993 demonstrated that when men feel intense pressure to lose weight, they, too, will go to extremes. Psychologists at Ithaca College examined the dietary habits of 131 football players in a special lightweight league, in which players had to weigh less than 158 pounds. Two-thirds of the subjects said they had fasted in the previous month; 17 percent had at some time induced vomiting to lose weight. One man in five reported that controlling his weight had interfered with his thoughts and/or extracurricular activities.

In 1994, Pope oversaw what may be the first study to compare men with eating disorders against a control group. The yet-to-be-published survey, conducted at Tufts University, concluded, among other things, that men with eating disorders are more likely than their female counterparts to have a history of obesity, and that eating-disordered people in general have a high rate of substance abuse. Contrary to earlier studies, it found no connection between eating disorders and sexual orientation.

Perhaps most intriguing, though, was the merciless attitude many of the study's subjects showed toward working out. When asked how they'd feel about missing a day at the gym, nearly half of those with eating disorders said very or extremely uncomfortable, compared to just 4 percent of normal eaters.

This exercise addiction didn't surprise Pope, who points out that people with eating disorders tend to be pathologically single-minded. Their behavior reminds him of obsessive-compulsive disorder, whose victims can't shake persistent thoughts or stop performing some action.

So what's wrong with being a dedicated gym rat? It's one thing to be committed to fitness, but the mental-health community now recognizes overexercise as a form of bulimia. The problem is particularly critical among men; in fact, most male bulimics don't use the familiar finger-down-the-throat method or a dose of Ex-Lax to purge, preferring to obsessively sweat away their meals (see "Exercise Addiction" in Chapter Ten).

And it's not just the guys camping out at the gym who are fooling themselves into thinking they can achieve better bodies by bulimia. Jogging junkies are at risk, too. According to the *New York Road Runners Club Complete Book of Running*, increasing your mileage to compensate for a fatty-food binge is a sign of running addiction. The late club chairman and coauthor Fred Lebow used to say that he knew a lot of people—single men in particular—with fatal attractions to roadwork. "Running is their date," as Lebow put it.

Compulsive exercisers, who might spend up to six hours a day at the gym, risk damaging more than just their job performance and personal relationships, says psychologist Ron A. Thompson, Ph.D., codirector of the eating disorders program at Bloomington Hospital in Indiana. Stress fractures or fatigued limbs may lead to even more serious problems. "We've had people in our clinic who, if they can't exercise because they're injured or ill, won't allow themselves to eat," he adds.

Not that they were eating right to begin with. Thompson, coauthor of

Helping Athletes with Eating Disorders, has worked with men who claimed to know a lot about nutrition but maintained rigorous workout schedules while living on 200 to 300 calories a day (2,000 to 2,500 is average for an active adult male).

At the other end of the compulsiveness scale is a variation of bulimia that's beginning to receive more attention; some psychiatrists think it's a distinct and equally important phenomenon. Binge-eating disorder is the urge to eat uncontrollably—without purging. The binge eater isn't necessarily obese but usually feels pangs of guilt for his indulgences.

Nick, thirty-eight, a Boston-area salesman, says he's gone through periods when he pigged out on burgers and pizza every night, gorging "until I felt like I'd swallowed a brick." Nick, who stands five-foot-nine, has watched his weight swing from his ideal of 155 pounds to 180 pounds and more. At times he's ballooned to more than 200 pounds. Naturally shy, he has learned through psychological counseling that he uses his weight to avoid romantic and social situations. "If I got to my ideal weight, I'd be all out of excuses for not going out and meeting people," Nick says.

Psychotherapist Donald Branum runs a support group Nick recently joined, one of the first in Boston. Branum feels overeating is a great threat to men. After all, it's more socially acceptable for guys to pig out at mealtime than it is for women, and many of his bingeing male patients seem to identify too closely with larger-than-life male figures, like NFL linemen. "Body size and weight can be seen as power," he says. "But a lot of these men who go home and clean out the fridge every night are dealing with frustration and pain."

Eating disorders can be notoriously difficult to treat; between 10 and 20 percent of all anorexics die as a result. Treatment may involve hospitalization, depending on the severity of the case, but will always require intensive counseling to help the patient deal with underlying psychological issues. Prozac and other antidepressants have been used to treat anorexics and bulimics. When the patient shows obsessive-compulsive symptoms, Thompson says, the task is to shift his or her focus. "We're not going to change the personality of the compulsive person," he says, "but we try to get him to be compulsive about remaining healthy."

Therapists monitor the patient's eating habits but avoid placing too much emphasis on food as a component of the treatment program. "We steer away from the word *diet*," Jantz says. "We don't think food is the issue." Again, depending on the severity of the problem, the duration of a treatment program can vary, from six months to several years. The upside of seeking help, of course, is that it can add decades to the life of a young man who is starving or overeating himself to an early grave.

For therapist referrals and more information on eating and exercise disorders, contact ANRED-the Anorexia Nervosa and Related Eating Disorders Association, P.O. Box 5102, Eugene, OR 97405; 503–344–1144.

Cultivating a healthy body image can mean confronting a subject as complex and emotionally freighted as an eating disorder. Fortunately, feeling better about your body can also be as simple as standing up straight.

POSTURE

Here's one of life's best-kept secrets: good posture provides us with a psychological advantage in our social and professional lives, radiating a healthful and attractive image that's important to our emotional needs and, to some extent, our success in life. Moreover, good posture is the key to long-term freedom from back pain and is crucial to keeping the spine from disintegrating before its time.

Like motherhood, no one is against good posture. Yet if you stand in a crowd and look around, you'll discover a sizable number of people who don't have it. Why? Some people, unfortunately, have anatomical or structural deformities or disease-related problems, but for the majority of us, slumping results primarily from lack of awareness.

The mention of "good posture" for many of us brings to mind the exaggerated upright stiffness of Marines on parade. Theirs may be good posture, but it's also unnatural and impractical for daily civilian life. In truth, an exact definition is elusive. In general, though, it's agreed that the head, upper and lower body and legs need to be in line. Stand sideways in a doorway or next to some other vertical line and have someone check your body's alignment. Your ears, shoulders, hips, knees and ankles should all be even with the vertical edge.

One specialist, Arthur H. White, M.D., medical director of the San Francisco Spine Institute and current president of the North American Spine Society (and the orthopedic surgeon who operated on quarterback Joe Montana's back), offers a better image for active individuals: "I call it the 'readiness posture.' If I were about to serve to you on the tennis court, would you be standing there with your knees locked and your belly hanging out? No. You'd strike the readiness posture, with your head directly over your spine, your pelvis slightly tucked, belly in, knees bent, as if you were at the ready for a mugger. "

Dr. White's readiness posture intuitively brings your spine into correct alignment. A healthy spine comes with four built-in curves: the forward curves of the neck and lower back and the backward curves of the center back and sacrum (the section of rigid vertebrae at the bottom of the spine). This natural curvature enables the spine to better absorb shock than, for instance, having a spine like a two-by-four. Poor posture usually occurs when one of these four curves becomes exaggerated to the point where the spine's structural integrity is threatened and the individual bones, discs and muscles no longer fit properly.

A common example of poor posture in men is the "beer belly" swaybacked look, when the forward curvature of the lower spine becomes exaggerated. This places undue pressure on the rear portion of the discs separating the lumbar vertebrae—the classic cause of lower-back pain. Over the long haul, White explains, the vertebrae grind together until they finally "crumble and corrode like rust." Long-term poor posture can also leave the discs "like pounded abalone after ten or twenty years. You bend forward one day to pick up your shoes, and the disc herniates." While it takes many years of poor posture for this to happen, when they finally blow out there's no real cure, although surgery can help. Often, the resulting back pain will be chronic—and extremely painful.

If you hold your head erect, the top curves of the spine naturally tend to assume the correct shape. Likewise, if your pelvis is tipped up correctly, the lower curves of the spine assume theirs. Holding your head and hips correctly requires considerable effort. But consider this inducement: White comments that by holding good posture instead of bad, "You are burning off one more calorie a minute [during] the time on your feet each day. "

Naturally, if you've allowed your posture to deteriorate, you'll have to condition your muscles to support your body correctly. Until then, standing straight will be tiring. To build up these muscles, White suggests you try "rowing machines, rotator cuff machines, all the back machines that take the arms behind the plane of the body. Use them first and last and do everything else in between."

Abdominal exercises (crunches, ab machines and so forth) strengthen the ab muscles, which in turn assist in straightening and supporting the spine. Losing excess weight also helps, since most men tend to put their extra weight on their belly, which further promotes swayback syndrome. How do you know when you've improved your posture? "The solution I've come up with is to have someone take a side-view picture of you every year and put it up on your wall," White says.

If you've ever seen a kicked dog, you've noticed that he yelps, then slinks off, head hung low, with his tail tucked between his legs. The same thing happens to us when we're defeated or abused. Our head hangs forward, our shoulders slump, our chest caves in. Setting aside questions of what this says about our self-esteem, walking around like a kicked canine is simply bad for us.

"The first thing I do when I meet a new client is look at how he carries himself," says Risa Sheppard, who has been a personal trainer in Los Angeles for the past fifteen years. "I believe that a person who has rounded shoulders and stooped posture feels like he's carrying the weight of the world on his shoulders." She gives clients mental and physical exercises, including visualization of the body becoming taller and straighter, along with daily affirmations intended to mold a more positive, relaxed psyche.

One cheering thought is that with a little effort you can have good posture even when your self-esteem is in the gutter. If there's anything worse than low self-esteem, it's low self-esteem and a bad back. After a while you may be surprised to discover that as you begin to look better, you actually begin to feel better as well. That's reason enough to stand tall.

6 HEALTHY LIVING

At first glance, the concept of "healthy living" seems like an oxymoron. What's the alternative—healthy dying? But when you think about it, there's a significant difference between healthy living and mere existence. Even those with seriously unhealthy habits—like Keith Richards' heroin use or Winston Churchill's penchant for early morning whiskey-and-soda—can manage to live to ripe and productive old ages, although the odds are not in your favor. If healthy living doesn't necessarily buy you a longer life, then what's the point?

Healthy living—which encompasses good nutrition, a nontoxic environment and a positive lifestyle—doesn't just increase the quantity of your life: it also greatly augments the quality. It means that even if you don't live a day longer than you otherwise would have, you're sick less often. You have more energy. You're not giving in to self-destructive habits. You're more excited by life's possibilities. In short, you're living—not just existing.

This chapter will discuss diet and nutrition, the dangers that can lurk in our environment, and "lifestyle issues" like drinking and smoking that greatly affect overall health. An integral part of healthy living is, of course, exercise. That topic will be dealt with separately in Chapter Ten.

Living longer may well be the result of a healthy lifestyle, but its aim is to increase your day-to-day quality of life. A few changes made to your diet, your environment and your habits will yield demonstrable dividends—and not in some pie-in-the-sky future, but when it really counts. Today.

HEALTHY EATING

Understanding Dietary Fat

Everyone agrees that too much dietary fat is bad. But how much is too much? One source of confusion about fat is the dietary experts themselves.

Most of us have heard we should get no more than 30 percent of our total daily calories from fat, the U.S. Department of Agriculture's recommendation. But then there are revisionists like Dean Ornish, M.D., who suggests that people adhere to a diet of only 10 percent fat to drastically reduce their risk of heart disease. Who's right?

While Ornish's program was designed for heart patients—and may thus be somewhat draconian for the purposes of healthy living—no research has proven that 30 percent is a magic figure, either. "The number was picked rather arbitrarily," says David Schardt, associate nutritionist at the Center for Science in the Public Interest (CSPI) in Washington, D.C. "It was chosen because it's less than what Americans currently eat, and it was a round figure that could be remembered. But I think many [experts] agree that Americans might be better off consuming closer to 25 or even 20 percent."

- Be aware, however, that fat does have useful functions. Along with providing a reserve of energy, it aids in the absorption of the fat-soluble vitamins (A, D, E and K) and helps maintain healthy hair and skin. The essential fatty acids omega–3 (found in fish oil) and omega–6 (in safflower and corn oils) are the raw materials for prostaglandins, hormonelike compounds that help regulate body functions.
- Until science comes up with ways to curb our craving for more than the small amount we actually need, there's Mother Nature's way. A Monell Center, Philadelphia, study found that when people cut out the "added" fat (salad dressings, mayonnaise, butter) in their diets, their preference for fat declined as well. But when the dieters used low-fat substitutes for toppings and spreads, they continued to crave the taste of fat. In other words, the simplest way to curb your fat hankering may be to eat less fat and low-fat substitutes.
- While you're at it, pay attention to how much saturated fat (mainly from meat, butter and milk fat) you do swallow; 10 percent of daily calories should be tops. Saturated fats raise blood levels of LDL, or "bad," cholesterol—a leading risk factor for heart disease. One study showed that even when fat intake is reduced from 35 to 30 percent, LDL levels don't drop if the proportion of saturated fat and cholesterol remain high.
- You may have noticed that men tend to store excess fat around their belly, whereas women pack it on their hips, thighs and butts. The difference stems from hormones, and the happy news (for you) is that it's easier to deflate a spare tire than to thin thunder-thighs.

Now the bad news: a big belly poses considerably more risk to your health than do hefty hips. The other blubber tends either to stay put or enter into the general circulation; extra abdominal fat empties directly into the liver. "In the liver, fatty acids interfere with the breakdown of insulin," says C. Wayne Callaway, M.D., an associate clinical professor of medicine at George Washington University. This in turn can raise blood pressure and cholesterol, putting men at greater risk for heart disease, stroke and adult-onset diabetes.

- Overweight people could also blame genetics. According to Swedish researcher Per Bjorntorp, fat may wear down the body's natural stress response (the release of hormones such as adrenaline). He believes the body "gives up," releasing too much of the hormone cortisol instead, which promotes fat storage in the belly. And in a late-breaking study, Brown University's Catherine Stoney, Ph.D., found that people who suppress their anger—a great way to augment stress—burn dietary fat slowest of all.
- A simple way to determine whether your waistline poses a hazard to your health is by measuring your waist-to-hip ratio: Divide your waistline circumference (measured at its narrowest) by that of your hips (measured at their widest). "If the ratio is greater than .95 in a man," Callaway says, "you are probably at high risk for weight-related health problems."

Being too lean may not be a boon, either. Research on male anorexia and bulimia show that in excessively thin men, testosterone levels appear to decrease, while osteoporosis (loss of bone density) increases. For a long life, take the middle road. "The curve for mortality rates is U-shaped," Callaway says. "Death rates go up at either extreme, morbid obesity or excessive thinness."

Power from Protein

Listen closely to athletes, coaches and nutrition consultants, and you'll hear that Americans don't get enough protein. You'll also hear that Americans get too much protein. Someone will claim that protein boosts performance. Then someone else will say emphatically that it doesn't. Confused? Part of the problem is that not much is known about protein's role in our lives.

Of prime importance to proteins are groups of hydrogen, nitrogen, carbon and oxygen atoms called amino acids. Lysine, tryptophan, phenylalanine, leucine, isoleucine, threonine, valine, methionine and histidine are the nine essential amino acids, the ones you must get from food because your body can't make them. You also need cystine and tyrosine, which your body does make. Your body can also manufacture the remaining nine aminos, for a total of twenty. For a protein to do what it's designed to do, you need a good balance of all nine essentials, what's called a complete protein.

While meat has long been branded the prime source of complete protein, the humble egg white actually holds that distinction. Fish, milk, lean beef and poultry follow. Contrary to antiquated arguments that vegetarian diets lack adequate protein, vegetarians can still ensure complete protein intake by combining plant foods that together offer the essential amino acids. But how do you know what adequate is? The average man gets 90 to 100 grams of protein a day, about twice the Recommended Dietary Allowance of 56 grams a day for a 150-pound man (to customize this number, multiply your body weight in pounds by 0.37). So, you could meet two-thirds of your daily protein need with a six-ounce burger.

But you may not be so typical. While you may virtuously eschew that fatty hamburger (many foods high in protein pack loads of fat, too), you may at the same time be giving up needed protein. Add exercise to the formula and your protein shortage may worsen. Even the minimum amount of protein the RDAs specify may not suffice because, as a number of experts believe, physical activity drives up the basic requirements.

Researchers have examined the protein needs of two groups of athletes: bodybuilders and people who participate in endurance events. Surprisingly, studies suggest endurance athletes need the most; they burn more calories, including those from protein, so they need more protein.

"A man who does a minimum of three hours a week of aerobic exercise can need as much as 50 percent more protein than a sedentary person," says William J. Evans, Ph.D., director of the Noll Laboratory for Human Performance Research at Pennsylvania State University. Exercisers who are losing weight need a little extra protein too, he says. "Otherwise, the body tends to eat away at its own muscle mass."

Chris Rosenbloom, Ph.D., a spokesperson for the American Dietetic Association and nutritionist for the 1996 Olympics, says a man who runs fifty miles a week may need double the RDA. The protein requirements for weight trainers are less clear. Though certain studies demonstrate that those men need as much as 20 percent extra protein, others show no increased requirement.

Either way, it's clear that protein is not a magical formula. Extra protein probably won't give you any measurable boost of speed or strength.

At the same time, not getting enough (whether enough it is the RDA or some figure adjusted to your activity level) could definitely slow you down. The under-proteined athlete may find himself petering out prematurely. He may feel moody or cranky, catch more colds and have trouble amassing muscle.

But let's say you eat more protein than you need. Your kidneys would have to flush out the excess, which most experts agree is harmless in healthy people if the amounts are moderately low. "I know of no evidence that eating 50 percent more protein than the RDA is detrimental to health," Wolfe says. However, those in early kidney failure could suffer from the extra demands made by protein. At the least, eating too much protein may give you cramps, diarrhea or an upset stomach.

Rather than fiddle with a calculator and a list of protein-rich foods, many people opt for the convenience of protein powders and amino-acid tablets. A well-balanced protein supplement (containing the essential amino acids) has very little fat, unlike many protein-bearing foods, and can save a lot of time and effort. These supplements are positively a godsend for the athlete who spends hours a day working out and can't stop to cook, eat and digest.

Those opposed to supplements often argue that they're expensive and that cheaper substitutes exist in the grocery store. Such as? "My recommendation to athletes or anyone who feels he can't get enough protein from food is to add nonfat dry milk to other foods," Evans says. "It's twenty times less expensive, gives you some extra calcium and has no fat." Others recommend simply drinking more milk.

If you're seriously into weightlifting, it probably won't hurt—and it may help—to get about 20 percent more than the 0.37 grams of protein per pound of body weight each day (roughly 0.44 grams per pound), Evans says. An "average exerciser" who puts in a few hours a week of aerobic exercise might want to increase his intake to one gram of protein per kilogram of body weight (that's about 0.45 grams per pound), Ward says. An endurance runner in hard training could increase protein to 50 percent more than the 0.37 grams (to 0.56 grams per pound), Evans says.

What we do know is that while protein isn't an elixir for strength and speed, it's a basic building block of muscle, meaning you can't have much strength and speed without it. Protein may not be magic, but it's still an essential part of a healthy diet.

PROTEIN PERFORMERS

FOOD PROTEIN	(GRAMS)	FOOD PROTEIN	(GRAMS)
Poultry, light and		Egg, 1 large	7
dark, no skin, 3 ounces	25	Brussels sprouts, 1 cup	7
Pork, 3 ounces	23–28	Pasta, 1 cup	5–7
Fish, 3 ounces	20–25	Bran cereal, half cup	5
Beef, ground, 3 ozs.	20–23	Rice, oatmeal, 1 cup	4.5
Cottage cheese, 4 ozs.	12–15	Wheat germ, 2 tbs.	4
Tofu, 4 ounces	9	Nuts, seeds, 2 tbs.	2–5
Peas, fresh, 1 cup	9	Bread, 1 slice	2–3
Milk, 1 cup	9		

Though meat is a ready protein source, vegetarians can still easily get plenty of protein with all the essential amino acids. Over the course of the day, the trick is to mix and match foods that supplement one another's amino profiles. (The old thinking was that you had to do this for every meal.) Some classic combinations:

- Cereal grains plus legumes. Examples: bean tacos; chili and corn bread; lentils and rice; red beans and rice; peanut butter on whole-wheat bread.
- Legumes plus seeds and nuts. For instance, hummus (chick-pea and sesame paste); split-pea soup and sesame crackers.
- Eggs or milk products plus vegetable-protein foods. Examples: macaroni and cheese; vegetable omelet; eggplant parmesan; cereal with milk.

The 30-Day High-Performance Menu

As teenagers and men in our twenties, our bodies can rebound from just about any kind of abuse and perform to our highest expectations. As we get older, however, we notice that without the right rest, exercise and food, we just can't move as briskly or think as clearly as before. We need high-power fuel from a high-performance diet to maintain mind and body fitness.

Here's that diet—a 30-day menu developed by Susan Kleiner, Ph.D., R.D., a sports nutritionist in Cleveland, Ohio, and a member of the *Men's Fitness* Advisory Board—geared for an active man who's 6 feet tall and 170 pounds, and who needs 3,000 calories daily to meet energy demands during the week as well as on more active weekends. Sixty-five percent of the calories come from carbohydrates, 15 percent from protein and 20 percent from fat. The month's menus have variety to keep them interesting, as well as dining-out suggestions to make the plan practical.

The program can be personalized by figuring your own energy needs using the chart below. Then, using a calorie guide purchased from a drug-, grocery- or bookstore, add or subtract foods to modify the calorie content of the diet. Add grains and fruits, or delete fats and sugars, first.

MEN'S FITNESS 30-DAY HIGH-PERFORMANCE MENU

WEEK ONE

Day 1: Wednesday

Breakfast: Apple Oatmeal*, 1 bagel, 1 tablespoon fruit jam, 1 cup low-fat milk

Brown-Bag Lunch: 1 cup fruit yogurt, 2 large squares seasoned Ry Krisp, handful cherry tomatoes and cucumber slices, 1 cup fruit juice

Afternoon Snack: 3 ounces (1½ cups) pretzels, 2 tablespoons honey-roasted peanuts, 1 cup vegetable juice

Dinner: 5 slices lean roast beef, 1 roll, 1 teaspoon butter or margarine, 1 cup noodles with olive oil and garlic, small tossed salad, 2 tablespoons no-oil salad dressing, ½ cup frozen yogurt with fruit syrup, 2 (1 ounce total) small Peppermint Patties

Day 2: Thursday

Breakfast: Old Reliable*, 1 bagel, 1 tablespoon fruit jam, ½ cup orange juice

Lunch: Your Best Fast-Food Bet*

Afternoon Snack: 6 Fig Newtons, 1 cup low-fat milk

Dinner: Low-Fat Burrito (1 cup beans, 2 tortillas, 1 tomato, ½ cup salsa, lettuce, 2 ounces shredded mozzarella cheese, 2 tablespoons sour cream), 1 cup sorbet with fresh raspberries, 2 small Peppermint Patties

*See recipes on pages 193–94.

Day 3: Friday

Breakfast: Grilled Grapefruit and a Danish*, 1 cup low-fat milk

Brown Bag Lunch: Peanut butter and jelly sandwich on whole wheat, 1 apple, green and red pepper slices, 1 cup low-fat milk

Afternoon Snack: 1 cup fruit yogurt, ½ cup grapes, 6 graham cracker squares

Dinner: Enjoy a high-carbohydrate restaurant meal.

Day 4: Saturday

Breakfast: Peach Melba*, 1 English muffin, 1 tablespoon fruit jam

Lunch: 1 cup bean soup, 3 slices whole-wheat bread, tossed salad, 1 table-spoon salad dressing, 1 apple, 1 cup low-fat milk

Afternoon Snack: 1 cup fruit yogurt, 2 large squares seasoned Ry Krisp, 1 cup juice

Dinner: Enjoy a night on the town, complete with dessert.

Day 5: Sunday

Breakfast: 1 cup orange juice, 4 slices French toast, 3 tablespoons maple syrup, 1 cup low-fat milk, 1 cup coffee

SPORTS DAY
Drink lots of water.

Packed Lunch on the Road: Swiss cheese sandwich on whole-wheat bread (2 slices cheese), carrot and celery sticks, 1 apple, 2 Nature Valley Granola Bars (1 package), 1 box (8 ounces) sports drink

Packed Afternoon Snack: 1 box sports drink, ½ cup dried apricots, 8 graham cracker squares

Dinner: 1 quarter BBQ chicken without skin, large tossed salad, 2 tablespoons salad dressing, 1 large baked potato, 1 teaspoon butter or margarine, 1 cup cooked broccoli, 2 slices French bread, 1 cup frozen yogurt topped with fresh strawberries, cranberry juice seltzer spritzer (½ cup cranberry juice mixed with soda water)

Day 6: Monday

Breakfast: 1 Aloha Muffin*, ½ cup orange juice, 1 cup low-fat milk

Lunch: 1 cup fruit yogurt, 3 large squares Ry Krisp, green pepper and cucumber slices, 1 cup fruit juice

Afternoon Snack: 3 ounces pretzels, 2 tablespoons dry-roasted peanuts, 12-ounce soft drink

Dinner: Chicken and broccoli stir-fry (4 ounces chicken), 2 cups brown rice, small tossed salad, 1 tablespoon salad dressing, ½ cup fruit sorbet, 1 cup low-fat milk, 4 small oatmeal-raisin cookies

Day 7: Tuesday

Breakfast: Apple Oatmeal*, 1 bagel, 1 tablespoon cream cheese, 1 cup orange juice, 1 cup low-fat milk

Lunch: Low-Fat Burrito (see Day 2), 1 cup rice, tossed salad, 1 tablespoon salad dressing, 1 cup soft-serve ice milk

Afternoon Snack: 1 cup fruit yogurt, 3 tablespoons honey-roasted peanuts, 1 cup vegetable juice

Dinner: Tofu Spaghetti (½ pound crumbled tofu, browned in skillet, 1 cup whole-wheat noodles, spaghetti sauce), 1 slice garlic bread, 1 cup steamed zucchini and mushrooms sprinkled with Parmesan cheese, 1 cup low-fat milk, 1 cup sherbet

WEEK TWO

Day 8: Wednesday

Breakfast: Fast 'n' Easy*, ½ cup orange juice, 1 cup low-fat milk

Brown-Bag Lunch: Turkey and Swiss cheese sandwich on whole-wheat bread (2 slices turkey, 1 slice cheese), carrot and celery sticks, 1 pear, 2 Nature Valley Granola Bars, I cup fruit juice

Afternoon Snack: 3 cups microwave popcorn, 12-ounce soft drink

Dinner: 4 ounces fresh fish, broiled or grilled, large tossed salad, 2 tablespoons light salad dressing, 1 large sweet potato, baked, 1 corn on the cob, 3 slices whole-grain bread, 2 teaspoons butter or margarine, 1 cup low-fat milk, ½ cup frozen yogurt, 4 small oatmeal-raisin cookies

Day 9: Thursday

Breakfast: Grilled grapefruit and a Danish*, 1 cup low-fat milk

Lunch: 3 slices pizza with cheese, large tossed salad, 2 tablespoons light salad dressing, 2 slices garlic bread, 1 cup low-fat milk

Afternoon Snack: 1 apple, 6 graham crackers, 1 cup low-fat milk

Dinner: Low-Fat Burrito (See Day 2), 1 cup sorbet with fresh raspberries, 2 small Peppermint Patties

Day 10: Friday

Breakfast: Old Reliable*, 1 raisin English muffin, toasted, 1 cup orange juice

Brown-Bag Lunch: Peanut butter and jelly sandwich on whole-wheat bread, 1 apple, green and red pepper slices, 1 cup low-fat milk

Afternoon Snack: 1 cup fruit yogurt, 3 ounces pretzels

Dinner: Enjoy a restaurant meal, complete with dessert.

Day 11: Saturday

Breakfast: Peach Melba*, 1 cinnamon-raisin bagel, 1 tablespoon cream cheese

Lunch: Beans and tortillas left over from Thursday dinner, 1 cup low-fat milk, 1 frozen fruit juice bar

Afternoon Snack: 6 Fig Newtons, ½ cup grapes

Dinner: 1½ cups whole-wheat pasta with meat sauce and Parmesan cheese, large tossed salad with shredded mozzarella cheese, 2 tablespoons salad dressing, 2 slices garlic bread, ½ cup frozen vanilla yogurt with peanuts and chocolate sauce

Day 12: Sunday

Breakfast: 6 pancakes, 2 tablespoons maple syrup, 1 cup orange juice, 1 cup low-fat milk

OUT FOR A DAY TRIP
Drink lots of water.

Packed Lunch on the Road: Peanut butter and apple butter (2 tablespoons each) on whole-wheat bread, carrot and celery sticks, 1 apple, 2 Nature Valley Granola Bars, 1 box sports drink

Packed Afternoon Snack: 1 box sports drink, ½ cup dried apricots, 8 graham cracker squares

Dinner: Enjoy a high-carbohydrate restaurant meal.

Day 13: Monday

Breakfast: Breakfast Pizza*, 1 cup V–8 juice, 1 cup low-fat milk

Brown-Bag Lunch: 1 cup fruit yogurt, 3 large squares seasoned Ry Krisp, handful cherry tomatoes and cucumber slices, 1 cup fruit juice

Afternoon Snack: 4 oatmeal cookies, 1 cup milk

Dinner: 4 slices lean roast beef, 1 roll, 1 teaspoon butter or margarine, 1 cup noodles with olive oil and garlic, large tossed salad, 2 tablespoons light salad dressing, ½ cup frozen yogurt with fruit syrup

Day 14: Tuesday

Breakfast: Garden Delight*, 1 cup low-fat milk

Lunch: Your Best Fast-Food Bet*

Afternoon Snack: 1 cup fruit yogurt, 3 ounces pretzels

Dinner: 2½ cups spaghetti with marinara sauce and Parmesan cheese, 2 slices garlic bread, 1 corn on the cob, small tossed salad, non-fat salad dressing, 1 cup low-fat milk, 1 cup fruit sorbet

WEEK THREE

Day 15: Wednesday

Breakfast: Old Reliable*, I cup orange juice

Lunch: 1 cup leftover spaghetti heated in a microwave with Parmesan cheese, 1 apple, 1 pear, 1 cup vegetable juice

Afternoon Snack: 6 Fig Newtons, 1 cup low-fat milk

Dinner: 5 ounces fresh fish, broiled or grilled, 1 teaspoon butter or margarine, large tossed salad, 2 tablespoons salad dressing, 1 large baked potato, 3 slices whole-grain bread, 2 teaspoons butter or margarine, 1 cup low-fat milk, 1 cup fruit sorbet

Day 16: Thursday

Breakfast: McBreakfast*

Lunch: Enjoy an ethnic vegetarian restaurant meal.

Afternoon Snack: Microwave popcorn, ½ cup grapes, 12-ounce soft drink, 3 ounces pretzels

Dinner: 1 cup vegetable soup, 2 pieces chicken, broiled or roasted, 2 rolls, 2 teaspoons butter or margarine, 2 cups rice pilaf, tossed salad, 2 tablespoons light salad dressing, 1 cup frozen yogurt

Day 17: Friday

Breakfast: Banana Dip*, 1 cup orange juice, 1 cup low-fat milk

Lunch: Chicken sandwich on rye using last night's leftovers, 1 cup (2 packages) applesauce snack pack, 1 cup vegetable juice

Afternoon Snack: 2 tablespoons dry-roasted peanuts, 12-ounce soft drink

Dinner: Enjoy a high-carbohydrate, restaurant dinner and popcorn at the movies.

Day 18: Saturday

Breakfast: 1 Aloha Muffin*, 1 cup low-fat milk, 1 cup cranberry juice

Lunch: 1 cup bean soup, 3 slices whole-wheat bread, tossed salad, 1 tablespoon salad dressing, 1 apple, 1 cup low-fat milk

Afternoon Snack: 1 cup fruit yogurt, 1 large square Ry Krisp

Dinner: Enjoy a restaurant meal, complete with dessert.

Day 19: Sunday

Breakfast: 1 cup orange juice, 4 slices French toast, 3 tablespoons maple syrup, 1 cup low-fat milk, 1 cup coffee

OUT FOR A HIKE
Drink lots of water.

Packed Liunch on the Road: Swiss cheese sandwich on whole-wheat bread (2 slices cheese), carrot and celery sticks, 1 apple, 2 Nature Valley Granola Bars, 1 box sports drink

Packed Afternoon Snack: 1 box sports drink, ½ cup dried apricots, 8 graham cracker squares

Dinner: 4 ounces fish, grilled, large tossed salad, 2 tablespoons salad dressing, 1 large baked potato, 1 teaspoon butter or margarine, 1 cup broccoli, steamed, 2 large squares corn bread, 1 cup frozen yogurt topped with fresh strawberries, cranberry juice seltzer spritzer

Day 20: Monday

Breakfast: Apple Oatmeal*, ½ cup orange juice, 1 cup low-fat milk

Lunch: 1 cup fruit yogurt, 3 large squares corn bread left over from last night, 1 cup cold broccoli left over from last night (with 1 tablespoon Italian dressing), 1 pear, 12-ounce soft drink

Afternoon Snack: 2 Nature Valley Granola Bars, 1 cup low-fat milk

Dinner: Chicken and snow peas stir-fry (5 ounces chicken), 2 cups brown rice, small tossed salad, 2 tablespoons salad dressing, 1 roll, 6 Fig Newtons, 1 frozen fruit juice bar

Day 21: Tuesday

Breakfast: Grilled Grapefruit and a Danish*, 1 cup low-fat milk

Lunch: 1 Low-Fat Burrito (see Day 2), 2 cups rice, tossed salad, 1 tablespoon salad dressing, 1 cup soft-serve ice milk

Afternoon Snack: 1 cup fruit yogurt, 3 tablespoons honey-roasted peanuts, 1 cup vegetable juice

Dinner: 2 cups Tofu Spaghetti (see Day 7), 3 slices garlic bread, 1 cup steamed vegetables, 1 cup low-fat milk, 1 cup fruit sorbet

WEEK FOUR

Day 22: Wednesday

Breakfast: Peach Melba*, 1 bagel, 1 tablespoon fruit jam

Brown-Bag Lunch: 1 cup leftover Tofu Spaghetti heated in a microwave, carrot and celery sticks, 1 apple, 1 cup vegetable juice

Afternoon Snack: 4 Fig Newtons, ½ cup raisin-nut mixture

Dinner: 2 cups macaroni, tuna and cheese casserole (regular mac and cheese plus 6 ounces chunk white tuna packed in water and drained), 1 corn on the cob, tossed salad, 1 tablespoon light salad dressing, 2 rolls, 1 cup low-fat milk, [fr 1/2] cup frozen yogurt with fruit syrup, 4 graham cracker squares

Day 23: Thursday

Breakfast: Old Reliable*, 1 cup orange juice

Lunch: Your Best Fast-Food Bet*

Afternoon Snack: 1 cup yogurt, 2 squares Ry Krisp

Dinner: 2½ cups spaghetti with marinara sauce and Parmesan cheese, 2 slices garlic bread, 1 corn on the cob, small tossed salad, nonfat salad dressing, 1 cup low-fat milk, 1 cup fruit sorbet

Day 24: Friday

Breakfast: Fast'n' Easy*, 1 cup low-fat milk

Brown-Bag Lunch: Turkey and Swiss cheese sandwich on whole-wheat bread (2 slices turkey, 1 slice cheese), carrot and celery sticks, 1 pear, 2 Nature Valley Granola Bars, 1 cup fruit juice

Afternoon Snack: 3 ounces pretzels, 1 cup vegetable juice

Dinner: 2 Low-Fat Burritos (see Day 2), 1 cup rice, large tossed salad, no-oil salad dressing, 1 cup low-fat milk, 1 cup sherbet with fresh berries, 4 small Peppermint Patties

Day 25: Saturday

Breakfast: Garden Delight*, 1 cup low-fat milk

Lunch: Large whole-wheat pita stuffed with two slices cheese and lots of fresh veggies, 3 ounces pretzels, 2 frozen fruit juice bars, 1 cup vegetable juice

Afternoon Snack: 1 cup fruit yogurt, 1 bagel, 1 tablespoon peanut butter, 1 tablespoon fruit jam

Dinner: Enjoy a restaurant meal, complete with dessert.

Day 26: Sunday

Breakfast: 6 pancakes, 2 tablespoons maple syrup, 1 cup orange juice, 1 cup low-fat milk

SPORTS DAY
Drink lots of water.

Packed Lunch on the Road: Peanut butter and apple butter (2 tablespoons each) on whole-wheat bread, carrot and celery sticks, 1 apple, 2 Nature Valley Granola Bars, 1 box sports drink

Packed Afternoon Snack: 1 box sports drink, ½ cup dried apricots, 8 graham cracker squares

Dinner: 1 quarter BBQ chicken without skin, large tossed salad, 2 tablespoons no-oil salad dressing, 1 large baked potato, 1 teaspoon butter or margarine, 1 cup steamed broccoli, 2 slices French bread, 1 cup frozen yogurt topped with fresh berries, 2 small Peppermint Patties

Day 27: Monday

Breakfast: McBreakfast*

Brown-Bag Lunch: 1 quarter BBQ chicken left over from last night, green pepper and cucumber slices, 2 large squares seasoned Ry Krisp, 1 cup applesauce snack pack, 1 cup low-fat milk

Afternoon Snack: 1 cup fruit yogurt, 4 Fig Newtons

Dinner: 2 cups spaghetti with marinara sauce and Parmesan cheese, 2 slices garlic bread, 1 corn on the cob, large tossed salad, 2 tablespoons salad dressing, 4 oatmeal-raisin cookies, 1 cup fruit sorbet

Day 28: Tuesday

Breakfast: Breakfast Pizza*, 1 cup V–8 juice

Lunch: Enjoy an ethnic vegetarian restaurant delight.
Afternoon Snack: 3 cups microwave popcorn, 1 cup fruit juice, 1 apple

Dinner: 4 ounces fresh fish, broiled or grilled, small tossed salad, 1 tablespoon light salad dressing, 1 large baked sweet potato, 1 corn on the cob, 3 slices whole-grain bread, 2 teaspoons butter or margarine, 1 cup low-fat milk, 1 cup frozen yogurt with fruit syrup, 4 small oatmeal-raisin cookies, cranberry juice seltzer spritzer

Day 29: Wednesday

Breakfast: Fast 'n' Easy*, 1 cup low-fat milk

Lunch: Half of 10" pizza with ground beef, small tossed salad, 1 tablespoon salad dressing, 1 cup cranberry juice

Afternoon Snack: 1 cup yogurt, 2 large squares seasoned Ry Krisp, 12-ounce soft drink

Dinner: 1 cup vegetable soup, 1 piece broiled or roasted chicken, 1 roll, 1 cup rice pilaf, tossed salad, 2 tablespoons light salad dressing, ½ cup frozen yogurt with fresh berries, 2 small Peppermint Patties

Day 30: Thursday

Breakfast: 1 cup orange juice, 4 slices French toast, 3 tablespoons maple syrup, 1 cup low-fat milk

Lunch: Swiss cheese sandwich on whole-wheat bread (2 slices cheese), carrot and celery sticks, 1 apple, bottled water

Afternoon Snack: 1 cup low-fat yogurt, 1 cup dried apricots, 8 graham cracker squares

Dinner: 4 ounces fish, grilled, large tossed salad, 2 tablespoons salad dressing, 1 large baked potato, 1 teaspoon butter or margarine, 1 cup steamed broccoli, 1 large square corn bread, 1 cup frozen yogurt topped with fresh strawberries, cranberry juice seltzer spritzer

Ten One-Minute Breakfasts

Banana Dip

1 banana
1 tablespoon peanut butter
Toasted wheat germ
Spread peanut butter over banana, dip in wheat germ and enjoy.

Aloha Muffin

1 multigrain English muffin
¼ cup cottage or ricotta cheese
¼ cup crushed pineapple
Toast muffin, spread with cheese and pineapple.

Grilled Grapefruit and Danish

½ grapefruit
2 slices raisin bread
2 ounces ricotta or cottage cheese
Cinnamon
Sprinkle grapefruit with cinnamon, then broil in oven or toaster oven for 2 to 3 minutes or until top bubbles. Spread each slice of bread with 1 ounce of cheese, sprinkle with cinnamon and broil.

Peach Melba

½ cup sliced peaches (fresh, frozen or packed in light syrup)
1 cup low-fat raspberry yogurt
½ cup orange juice
Combine ingredients and blend in blender until smooth.

Apple Oatmeal

1 cup applesauce
Dash pumpkin pie spice
2 servings quick rolled oats, prepared according to directions
Pour applesauce and spice into cooked rolled oats and stir.

Garden Delight

1 ounce (two thin slices) havarti cheese
2 slices fresh tomato
4 slices fresh cucumber
2 slices whole-grain bread
Toast bread lightly. Make 2 open-face sandwiches of tomato, cucumber and cheese. Broil in oven or toaster oven until cheese melts and bubbles.

Old Reliable

1 cup bran cereal
1 cup low-fat milk
½ cup fresh berries

McBreakfast

1 serving fast-food pancakes
2 tablespoons syrup
1 cup orange juice
1 cup low-fat milk

Fast 'n' Easy

2 whole-grain frozen waffles
1 tablespoon peanut butter
1 sliced banana
Toast waffles. Slice banana lengthwise. Spread waffles with peanut butter and top with banana slices.

Breakfast Pizza

1 whole-wheat pita
1 ounce mozzarella cheese
2 tomato slices
Place tomato slices on pita and cover with cheese. Broil or toast until cheese melts and bubbles.

YOUR BEST FAST-FOOD BETS

	CALORIES	% CALS. FROM FAT
McDonald's		
Regular Hamburger	260	18
Regular Cheeseburger	310	40
Quarter Pounder	410	45
Chef's Salad (with full.packet dressing; use a light dressing to lower the fat)	230	52
Burger King		
BK Broiler Chicken Sandwich	379	43
Wendy's		
Grilled Chicken Sandwich	340	34
Chili (regular serving)	240	30
Chili (large serving)	360	30
Plain Baked Potato	250	7
Salad Bar (select low-fat items)	N/A	N/A
Generic		
Burrito	392	31
Pizza (with cheese, one slice)	290	27
Pizza (with pepperoni, one slice)	306	34
Roast Beef Sandwich	347	35
Taco (skip sour cream to lower the fat)	187	50

How to Personalize This Menu

STEP 1. Determine your healthy body weight. Find it on a height-weight table or use this formula to estimate it: Take 106 pounds for the first five feet of your height, and add 6 pounds for every additional inch to get to the midpoint of your healthy weight range.

STEP 2. Estimate your activity level. Based on whether you are currently overweight, normal or underweight, select the activity factor from the chart below that corresponds to your activity level. A moderately active person exercises three to five times a week for 20 to 30 minutes per session.

	SEDENTARY	MODERATE	ACTIVE	VERY ACTIVE	EXTREMELY ACTIVE
Overweight	10	11	12	13	15
Normal	13	14	15	17	20
Underweight	16	17	18	20	22

STEP 3. Calculate your daily energy needs. In this equation, calories equal your activity factor multiplied by your healthy body weight.

STEP 4. Adjust for your weight goal.

If you need to lose weight: Subtract 250 to 500 calories per day.

If you need to maintain your weight: Keep the same caloric level unless you change your activity level.

If you need to gain weight: Add 500 calories per day and increase muscle-resistence training.

Healthy, Healing Foods

When it comes to healthy foods, not all are created equal. Even among the most virtuous food choices, some are definitely better than others. While you shouldn't say "no" to any vegetable, the following ones are the triple-A-rated—the ones that pack the most nutrition and the greatest protection into the smallest packages.

Beans (snap): Snap beans—as well as wax, Italian and other fresh varieties—share most of the attributes of their dried counterparts. But since they're not as dense, they are lower in fiber and certain vitamins and minerals. Still, they are brimming with vitamins A and C, nutrients that are lacking in dried beans. That makes them ideal immunity boosters. Fresh beans also have just enough iron—coupled with the vitamin C that enhances its absorption—to be a help against anemia.

Beets: Look to these red globes for a nice shot of no-fat, no-cholesterol, low-cal potassium to help lower blood pressure and protect against stroke. A cup of beets has 3.4 grams of fiber, about the same as 1.5 cups of cooked oatmeal.

Broccoli: One of the true superstars of the produce bin. A member of the cruciferous family of vegetables; studies have suggested that eating a diet rich in these veggies may decrease cancer risks. Broccoli is also packed with beta-carotene and vitamin C, two powerful cancer battlers. Broccoli is rich in potassium, a mineral that's credited with lowering incidence of high blood pressure and stroke. Its high fiber content also helps lower cholesterol, which—along with the green giant's low sodium and fat levels—lowers the risk of heart disease. Preliminary studies suggest that the vitamin C in such produce as broccoli may even head off heart disease before it starts, by protecting against free radicals, the unstable molecules thought to transform cholesterol into building blocks of artery-clogging plaque. It's also a great source of bone-building calcium, which can reduce your chances of developing osteoporosis.

Brussels sprouts: Another cruciferous powerhouse. These "little cabbages" are almost as impressive in all areas of healing potential as is broccoli. Although they have, when cooked, considerably less calcium than broccoli, the two are on par when raw. And cooked sprouts have as much vitamin C and iron as broccoli and almost twice as much stroke-preventing potassium as broccoli. (One tip: If you're one of those people who think they don't like brussels sprouts, try cooking the little vegetables until just tender. Overcooking accounts for the characteristic strong flavor that many people object to.)

Cabbage: King of the anticancer clan. This wonderful cancer-fighting vegetable comes in so many varieties that you'll never tire of it. And that's good, because studies have suggested that consumption of crucifers in general may reduce the risk of gastrointestinal and respiratory-tract cancers. Other studies indicate that the vitamin C in such vegetables as cabbage protects against stomach and esophageal cancers. There's also lots of evidence that fiber (high in this vegetable) helps reduce the risk of colon cancer, and may slow cancer's spread once it has developed in the body.

Choose from regular green and red varieties, plus savoy, bok choy and napa (Chinese) cabbage.

Carrots: They're a rich source of vitamin A and, perhaps more important, beta-carotene. This vegetable form of vitamin A is credited with activity against various cancers, including those of the larynx, esophagus, lung, colon, stomach and cervix. Just half a cup of cooked carrots has almost four times the recommended daily allowance for vitamin A. And although vitamin A is toxic in large doses, the beta-carotene form found in carrots and other vegetables is not. Researchers from the U.S. Department of Agriculture say just two carrots a day can reduce cholesterol by as much as 20 percent, which can help lessen the threat of heart disease.

Cauliflower: A tasty half cup of this cruciferous vegetable has just fifteen calories. And for those few calories, you get lots of potassium and just a little sodium—the perfect formula for blood-pressure and stroke control. What's more, the same half cup contains about 50 percent of your daily quota of vitamin C, a nutrient that helps build immunity, fight fatigue, and aid iron in countering anemia.

Garlic: Scientists are seriously examining the potential of this odoriferous bulb, so prominent in cuisines worldwide, to protect against heart disease. Studies have shown that garlic raises levels of beneficial cholesterol in the body while also lowering total cholesterol levels. Garlic also "thins" the blood, reducing the chances of clotting. Blood clots are one of the most common causes of heart attack and stroke. And this herb lowers blood pressure and blood-sugar levels. A preliminary study from China suggests that allium-family vegetables, which include garlic and onions, may reduce the risk of stomach cancer. The theory is that these vegetables have anti-bacterial and antifungal properties that may inhibit tumor growth.

Onions: Along with leeks, scallions, shallots and other members of the pungent allium family, onions are excellent health boosters. They appear to share some of garlic's cholesterol-beating punch, and it's thought that onions may help offset the artery-clogging effects of a high-fat diet, which explains why Mediterranean diets are so heart-smart. And white onions have been found to raise protective HDL cholesterol, to help forestall heart disease. Certain substances in onions seem to inhibit the formation of blood clots, a principal trigger of most heart attacks. In addition, onions, scallions, garlic and similar bulbous vegetables may guard against the development of stomach cancer. A compound in onions may even help relieve asthma attacks.

Potatoes: They're a fabulous source of potassium, making them top priority for those with high blood pressure. They are also high in vitamins C and B$_6$, which help fight fatigue and infections. A large baked potato has nearly half your daily requirement of vitamin C, plus lots of beneficial minerals, including iron and magnesium. And they contain virtually no fat. All of which means healing potential on many fronts, particularly heart disease and stroke. Even better, potatoes contain certain compounds called proteinase inhibitors, which may be potent cancer fighters.

Red Peppers: A good source of vitamin C, with one cup supplying over 150 percent of the RDA for that important vitamin. (Hot chili peppers have twice that amount.) All that vitamin C also comes with a healthy portion of fiber.

Squash (winter): This variety has even more healing potential than its warm-weather counterparts, thanks to the amazing amount of vitamin A some specimens contain. A half cup of baked butternut or hubbard squash contains much more than a full day's supply of this anticancer crusader. A helping of both vitamin C and fiber secures their position as cancer fighters. All varieties are good sources of potassium (with very little sodium), for help on the blood-pressure and stroke fronts. And like summer varieties, winter squash has a bit of calcium—plus some iron—thrown in for extra measure.

Turnips: For some reason, turnips don't get as much respect these days as they deserve. As cancer-fighting crucifers, they're good sources of fiber and vitamin C. And they're extremely low in calories, for a healthy heart and a trimmer profile.

Food and Mood

There was a time when the food-mood connection seemed as easy as "Have a brownie, you'll feel better." Nowadays, it's no secret that there's more to it than simply the morale boost that comes from eating something sinfully tasty. What we eat can play a significant role in our energy level and mood, depending not just on what but also on when, where and how much we eat. The more we learn, the less simple the link appears.

In the eighties, a popular theory was that complex carbohydrates, like bread or cereal, relax us, even make us sleepy. Now it's being argued that sugar—once blamed for making us "hyperactive"—does the same because it, too, is a carbohydrate, albeit a simple one. Fat, meanwhile, is blamed for making us sluggish, whereas protein peps us up, making us more alert. According to food-mood researchers Richard and Judith Wurtman of the Massachusetts Institute of Technology, the physical reactions go like this:

- *Protein for energy.* When we eat something that's predominantly protein, a batch of amino acids is released. Among them is tyrosine, the principal ingredient of dopamine and norepinephrine, the pleasure chemicals in the brain. Eating protein stimulates production of dopamine and norepinephrine, giving a quick pick-up.
- *Carbohydrates beat stress.* The relaxing amino acid tryptophan is also present in protein foods, but when all the amino acids are fighting their way into the brain, tryptophan gets shoved aside. When we eat a carbohydrate, however, tryptophan has a clear road into the brain, where it is used to manufacture serotonin, the body's natural calming chemical. Insulin does the street-sweeping, clearing the bloodstream of all amino acids except tryptophan. Mixing protein foods—cottage cheese or poached eggs, say—with carbohydrates may give you a slightly bigger boost.
- *The post-lunch lag.* Now what about that slump we sometimes feel after lunch? For one thing, our natural biorhythms sink in the afternoon, and this alone can make energy dip. If you end up feeling too full and relaxed—perhaps even sluggish—look to the fat content. Fat digests more slowly than protein or carbohydrate, leaving you dragging for hours.

  In other cases, you may be sluggish because you haven't eaten enough throughout the day, leaving your blood sugar low (the same situation you face upon waking in the morning). "People get moody, irritable, sleepy or whatever when they haven't eaten enough calories," says registered dietitian Nancy Clark, director of nutrition science at SportsMedicine Brookline in the Boston area. Her advice: "If you eat breakfast, lunch and an afternoon snack, you'll be even-keeled." Clark emphasizes making complex carbohydrates—bread, rice or cereal—the foundation of every meal, giving you sources of readily available, sustainable energy.
- *Sugar spikes.* Sugar offers readily available energy, but as a simple carbohydrate it burns up significantly faster than its complex cohorts. Many experts point out that sugar leads to a sudden rise in blood sugar, then an equally sudden drop, as insulin shepherds the stuff out of the body.

Clark clarifies, however, that unless you're one of the few truly sugar-sensitive people, it won't have you bouncing off the walls with the so-called sugar buzz. Think of when one ordinarily consumes sugar: with coffee or sodas, leading to a caffeine high, or on holidays like Halloween and Christmas, when stimulation already abounds. What sugar will do, adds Madelyn Fernstrom, Ph.D., of the University of Pittsburgh School of Medicine, is quickly boost your alertness.

- *Other stimulants.* Coffee, tea, sodas and other caffeinated drinks can perform the same trick. Caffeine stimulates the central nervous system, but, as with food, you have to consider a number of variables when anticipating how it might affect you—your tolerance to the stimulant, your expectations of what it can do for you, whether you're on deadline and so forth.

  As Fernstrom points out, "People expect to be stimulated by caffeine, but it can also be a sedative." A warm caffeinated drink on a warm evening, after a warm dinner enjoyed with a warm companion, could prove just as soothing and relaxing as a warm glass of milk before bed.

- *Comfort foods.* Why should milk be soothing? Past arguments to the contrary, milk doesn't have enough tryptophan to do this. A more likely, albeit partial, explanation could be milk's fat content. Even more influential may be our expectations: You want it to soothe, therefore it does. That's a very important aspect of the food-mood connection. For many of us, the comfort and pleasure we derive from certain foods is sparked by warm, fuzzy memories associated with that food, be it pizza, ice cream, french fries or Cracker Jack.

  However, there's also a tangible physiological reason why we get caught with our hand in the cookie jar, says Adam Drewnowski, Ph.D., director of the University of Michigan's human nutrition program. In rats, chocolate elevates endorphins, the brain's natural opiates, and stimulates pleasure. Although the exact mechanism isn't known, Drewnowski theorizes that something in the mix of sugar and fat is responsible. He and his colleagues are also investigating the natural analgesic effects of chocolate that could be sparked by the release of endorphins; they expect results later this year.

In fact, as complex as the relationship is between how we feel and what we eat, you can probably expect a lot of findings to be forthcoming. Until then, perhaps the best way to eat, drink and be merry, in addition to eating a well-balanced diet, is to listen to your body. It knows what it's talking about.

VITAMINS AND MINERALS FOR MEN

Twenty years ago, physicians and nutritionists agreed that a well-balanced diet provided all the vitamins and minerals necessary for optimal health. Three beliefs followed from this view: Supplements were a waste of money, supplement sellers were hucksters, and the few scientists who touted them, notably Nobel laureate Linus Pauling, were nuts.

How things have changed. Today, thousands of medical professionals take large doses of supplements and advise their patients to do the same. Part of the reason: Most Americans don't eat a balanced diet.

While the National Cancer Institute urges us to strive for five servings each day of fruits and vegetables, which are rich in key nutrients, only about 9 percent of the population do so. In fact, a recent dietary analysis of 12,000 Americans showed that 41 percent ate no fruit at all, and only 25 percent ate even one fruit or vegetable rich in the antioxidant vitamins A or C daily.

As you know, antioxidants are hot stuff. They've been proven to help prevent every major form of cancer. "They're rapidly becoming the cutting edge of medicine, and as a result, supplementation with the entire range of vitamins and minerals has become increasingly accepted," says Sheldon Saul Hendler, M.D., Ph.D., an assistant clinical professor of medicine at the University of California, San Diego, and author of *The Doctors' Vitamin and Mineral Encyclopedia.*

The current recommended dietary allowances (RDAs) for vitamins and minerals are extremely controversial. They were established in 1943 by the National Academy of Sciences (NAS) as "the intake of essential nutrients . . . adequate to meet the known needs of practically every healthy person." NAS RDAs are expressed as a range. The FDA took the highest amount for each nutrient and created the USRDAs, making "RDA" a household term.

Growing numbers of scientists contend that RDAs should be raised to a level that Shari Lieberman, Ph.D., a clinical nutritionist in New York City and co-author of *The Real Vitamin and Mineral Book*, calls the "optimal daily allowance," or ODA. This is the level the latest studies show helps prevent cancer, heart disease and other health problems.

"The RDAs have never been set in stone," says Paul Thomas, director of the NAS Food and Nutrition Board, the group that actually sets the RDAs. "RDAs represent a consensus of the nutrition community, and the consensus has changed." Thomas expects to release revised RDAs sometime this year or next.

So how much should they be raised? No one knows for certain. "Extremely large doses of some supplements—vitamin D, for example—can cause problems," says Gladys Block, Ph.D., a nutritional epidemiologist at the University of California at Berkeley. But, by and large, supplements are safe, even at doses substantially above the RDA. (See the chart on pages 204–210.)

Adding to the confusion among consumers is the overwhelming array of products available. As a result, many people buy more supplements than necessary. *Men's Fitness* asked nutrition experts around the country to explain how to take supplements without getting taken. Here's what they said:

- Supplements don't replace food and can't undo damage caused by a chronically poor diet. "Before you buy supplements," Block says, "fill your shopping cart with fresh fruits and vegetables, and eat them." Get your five a day, and then take a supplement.
- Start with an "insurance formula." Packed with some of every vitamin and mineral, they're convenient and economical. They're also better for you than supplements made of individual nutrients. "Nature packages [vitamins and minerals] together in foods, and it's best to take them that way in supplements," Lieberman says. For instance, vitamin E works better when combined with vitamin C, and calcium works better with vitamin D. "Some minerals compete with one another," she adds. "Iron interferes with the body's ability to absorb zinc. Zinc interferes with copper absorption. Taking an insurance formula that contains some of all the essential minerals largely compensates for any competition among them."

  Of course, bigger, heavier men need more nutrients than smaller, lighter guys. Many supplement labels anticipate this with directions that say something like: "Take one to three tablets daily." If you're lighter than average, stick to the low side. If you're huskier, take more.
- Supplement your insurance formula; it may not provide all the nutrients you need. The RDA of some minerals—say, magnesium and calcium—won't fit into one little pill. Moreover, if you have a family history of cancer or heart disease, you may want larger doses of antioxidants. If you're a serious athlete or have a chronic medical condition (asthma, diabetes, arthritis, kidney disease, etc.), consult a registered dietitian to determine your specific needs. Ask your trainer or physician for a referral or call the American Dietetic Association (800–366–1655).
- Forget brand names. "Only about a half-dozen drug companies—for example, Hoffman-La Roche—actually make vitamins," Hendler explains.

"They supply all the hundreds of companies that sell them. What you're paying for is packaging and advertising."

- Ignore the word *natural*. Chemically, there's no difference between the vitamin C in an orange and the C synthesized in a lab. Some "natural" vitamins come from plants, like vitamin C from rose hips. But frequently, packagers mix a tiny amount of a natural vitamin with the synthetic, calling it natural.

  Three exceptions: E, folic acid and calcium. Natural vitamin E (d-alpha-tocopherol) is absorbed more easily than the synthetic version (dl-alpha-tocopherol). The words "with d-alpha" on a label may mean that a tiny amount of the natural vitamin is mixed with lots of the synthetic. Meanwhile, synthetic folic acid is more easily absorbed, and natural calcium, whose sources include bone meal and dolomite, may have lead contamination. Go with calcium carbonate, a less expensive synthetic.

- Ignore the hype. Some supplement labels promise they can do everything except raise the dead. Vitamins and minerals do play important roles in virtually every body system and process. But by themselves, supplements don't eliminate fatigue, alleviate stress or boost your libido.

  Likewise, forget claims of "newly discovered" vitamins. There aren't any, though several nutrients, like coenzyme Q–10, have recently caused significant excitement among researchers.

- Don't pay extra for vitamins that claim to be sugar-free or starch-free. Unless you're seriously allergic, a little starch or sugar won't hurt you.

- Don't pay more for "chelated" (KEY-lated) minerals. Chelation combines minerals with other substances, often amino acids. Although proponents claim it promotes absorption, ordinary minerals are absorbed just fine.

- Unless a health professional advises otherwise, steer clear of time-released supplements. These typically cost more but may not provide a steady stream of nutrients. It's usually cheaper to take a few pills throughout the day.

- Look for a dissolution statement on the label. To do any good, supplements must dissolve completely in the digestive tract. Forty-five minutes is the voluntary industry standard.

- Don't buy any supplements within six to nine months of the expiration date. They've probably been on the shelf several years and may already be past their prime. If there's no date at all, move on.

- If you're taking doses of vitamin A above the RDA, switch to beta carotene. The body converts it into vitamin A, so for all practical purposes they're the same thing. Plus, long-term use of A at daily doses above 50,000 IU may cause problems, whereas beta carotene is nontoxic

even at high doses. Beware of labels that say "vitamin A with beta carotene": If the label doesn't specify, you can't be sure how much of either you're getting.
- Look for biotin, the most expensive vitamin. Many packagers skimp on it. Buy the cheapest insurance formula containing at least 25 micrograms.
- Unless your physician advises otherwise, don't exceed the RDA for iron. Most people don't need more, and at high doses, iron can cause problems. Also, a recent study suggests that high blood levels of iron may increase risk of heart disease, yet some supplements contain several times the RDA.
- Check for selenium. Research suggests this mineral helps prevent esophageal and stomach cancer.

One last tip before you go shopping: $10 a month should do it. If you pay any more, you're probably wasting cash you could spend on things like . . . more fruits and vegetables.

Note: While no one knows the "best" dose for all vitamins and minerals, the RDAs are increasingly looking like minimum daily requirements. Based on recent research, clinical nutritionist Shari Lieberman, Ph.D., recommends "optimal daily allowances" (ODAs). They're presented on the following pages in consultation with Gladys Block, Ph.D., and Sheldon Saul Hendler, M.D., Ph.D.

A MAN'S GUIDE TO VITAMINS AND MINERALS: OPTIMAL DAILY ALLOWANCES

	USES	FOOD SOURCES	RDA	ODA	TOXICITY
Vitamin A (or Beta Carotene)	Helps maintain good vision, enhances immunity, prevents cancer, repairs tissue. Possibly helpful in treating skin problems and gastrointestinal ulcers.	Green and yellow fruits and vegetables, fishliver oils, animal livers.	4,000 to 5,000 IU	10,000 to 75,000 IU	Possible after long-term daily ingestion of 50,000 IU of Vitamin A, but beta carotene is nontoxic.

	USES	FOOD SOURCES	RDA	ODA	TOXICITY
Vitamin B$_1$ (Thiamine)	Helps maintain healthy hair, skin, eyes, nerves, digestive tract. Involved in energy production. Helps deal with physical and emotional stress.	Whole grains, green leafy vegetables, beans, nuts, fish, poultry, liver.	1.2 to 14 mg	25 to 300 mg	None known.
Vitamin B$_2$ (Riboflavin)	Same as B$_1$. May help prevent cataracts and, with B$_6$, treat carpal tunnel syndrome. Strenuous exercise increases need.	Same as B$_1$.	1.2 to 14 mg	25 to 300 mg	None known.
Vitamin B$_3$ (Niacin)	Same as B$_1$. Also lowers cholesterol.	Same as B$_1$.	1.2 to 14 mg	25 to 300 mg	Reversible liver damage can occur at doses of 2,000 mg per day. ODA dose may cause temporary itching and reddening known as "niacin flush."
Vitamin B$_6$ (Pyridoxine)	Same as B$_1$. May help asthma and carpal tunnel syndrome.	Same as B$_1$.	1.2 to 14 mg	25 to 300 mg	Reversible damage to the nervous system is possible at doses above 2,000 mg.
Vitamin B$_{12}$ (Cobalamine)	Necessary for fat and carbohydrate metabolism. Helps the nervous system function properly. May help minimize anxiety and depression.	Milk, seafood, tofu, cheese, eggs, liver, herring, mackeral.	2 micrograms (mcg)	25 to 300 mcg	None known.

	USES	FOOD SOURCES	RDA	ODA	TOXICITY
Vitamin C (Ascorbic Acid)	Protects against cancer and heart disease. Effective cold treatment at 2,000 mg a day. Enhances immunity. Protects against pollution. May help reduce cholesterol and blood pressure. Stress increases need.	Citrus fruits, green vegetables.	60 mg	500 to 5,000 mg	Diarrhea is possible at high doses. If you have a history of kidney stones, consult a doctor about appropriate dose.
Vitamin D	Required for calcium and phosphorus absorption. Prevents and treats osteoporosis (which affects men as well as women). Enhances immunity. May help reduce blood pressure.	Fortified milk and dairy products, eggs, fatty saltwater fish (salmon, mackeral, etc.), fish-liver oils.	400 IU	400 to 600 IU	Doses above 1,000 IU a day may be fatal.
Vitamin E	Antioxidant. Cancer and heart disease prevention. Important for circulation and tissue repair.	Whole grains, vegetable oils, green leafy vegetables, nuts, legumes.	8 to 10 IU	200 to 800 IU	Nausea, diarrhea, headache, flatulence, fainting and heart palpitations are possible at daily doses greater than 1,200 IU.
Vitamin K	Important in blood clotting. May play a role in bone health.	Green leafy vegetables.	65 to 80 mcg	65 to 80 mcg	Death of red blood cells (helolytic anemia) is possible at doses above the RDA/ODA.

	USES	FOOD SOURCES	RDA	ODA	TOXICITY
Biotin	Necessary for the metabolism of protein, carbohydrates and fat. Deficiencies may play a role in high cholesterol and skin and nervous system problems.	Whole grains, salt-water fish, eggs, milk, soybeans, poultry, meats.	None	25 to 300 mcg	None known.
Calcium	Necessary for healthy bones and teeth, nerve and muscle function. May help reduce blood pressure. Dairy foods, leafy vegetables, salmon, seafood, sardines.		800 mg	1,000 to 1,500 mg	None known.
Chromium	Required for glucose metabolism. May help prevent diabetes and high cholesterol.	Whole grains, beer, cheese, meats, brewer's yeast.	None	200 to 600 mcg	No known toxicity as a nutritional supplement.
Choline and Inositol	Involved in the metabolism of fat and cholesterol and in the synthesis of an important neurotransmitter in the brain.	Fruits, milk, egg yolks, whole grains, vegetables, organ meats.	None	25 to 300 mg	Nausea and depression are possible at very large doses.

	USES	FOOD SOURCES	RDA	ODA	TOXICITY
Copper	Necessary for blood formation, bone development, nerve function, sense of taste and energy production.	Widely distributed in foods. Copper pipes enrich many home water supplies.	None	0.5 to 2 mg. Most people ingest the ODA from water and food.	Excessive amounts can produce nausea, vomiting, abdominal pain, diarrhea, headache, dizziness and a metalic taste in the mouth. Long-term use of excessive amounts can be fatal.
Folic Acid	Necessary for healthy cell reproduction. Involved in protein metabolism. May help minimize anxiety and depression. Stress may increase need.	Bran, whole wheat, green leafy vegetables, chicken, beef, lamb, pork.	180 to 200 mcg	400 to 1,2000 mcg	None known.
Iodine	Necessary for thyroid gland function. Deficiency causes goiter.	Iodized salt, seafood, saltwater fish, kelp.	150 mcg	50 to 150 mcg	Safe up to 1,000 mcg.
Iron	Necessary for blood formation, energy production and immune-system functioning.	Green leafy vegetables, whole grain or enriched breads and cereals, eggs, meat, poultry, fish, liver.	10 to 15 mg	15 to 30 mg	Adverse affects are rare with daily doses below 75 mg. New research suggests that high iron levels may increase risk of heart disease.

	USES	FOOD SOURCES	RDA	ODA	TOXICITY
Magnesium	Necessary for healthy bones, nerves, muscles and blood vessels. Used in energy production. May help reduce blood pressure.	Dairy foods, fish, seafood, meats.	280 to 350 mg	500 to 750 mg	Rare except in people with failing kidneys. Doses above 3,000 mg are laxative.
Manganese	Necessary for bone growth, reproduction, blood-sugar regulation, protein and fat metabolism, energy production and healthy immune and nervous systems.	Nuts, seeds, whole grains, avocado, seaweed.	None	15 to 30 mg	Rare when ingested. Possible if inhaled.
Pantothenic Acid	Necessary for metabolism, hormone synthesis, red blood cell production and healthy adrenal glands. May help traet arthritis, anxiety and depression.	Beans, fresh vegetables, whole wheat, milk, beef, pork, eggs, saltwater fish.	None	25 to 300 mg	None known.
Phosphorus	Necessary for energy production, healthy bones and metabolism.	Available in most foods.	800 mg	Optimal amounts available from food.	Large amounts increase calcium excretion to the detriment of bones and teeth.
Potassium	Necessary for nerve transmission, muscle contraction, hormone secretion and energy storage. May help reduce blood pressure.	Whole grains, vegetables, beans, fruit, fish, dairy, poultry, meat.	None	99 to 300 mg	No problems at doses below 18,000 mg.

	USES	FOOD SOURCES	RDA	ODA	TOXICITY
Selenium	Cancer and heart-disease prevention.	Amounts in foods depend on soil conditions.	55 to 70 mcg	50 to 400 mcg	High doses poison animals. No toxic effects in humans at doses up to 750 mcg.
Zinc	Necessary for male reproductive health, wound healing, senses of taste and smell, and liver health.	Seafood, whole grains, beans, poultry, meats.	12 to 15 mg	22 to 50 mg	Amounts of 300 mg a day may raise cholesterol. Vomiting possible at 2,000 mg.

COFFEE, TEA AND THEE

Coffee is terribly confusing. Judging by the coast-to-coast proliferation of Starbucks and other coffee bars, America's longtime love affair with the dark, rich fluid seems hotter than ever. We glug a third of the world's coffee crop a year—ten to fifteen pounds of beans per person.

But frequent news reports of coffee's purported health hazards are enough to give even decaf drinkers a case of jitters. It's been blamed for everything from high blood pressure to cancer to birth defects. Recently, a study in the *Journal of the American Medical Association* called coffee not just habit-forming (we already knew that), but comparably addictive to crack or heroin—java junkies, indeed.

The truth? "There is no persuasive evidence that consuming moderate amounts of caffeine—a cup or two of coffee a day—is harmful," says Nancy Clark, director of Nutrition Services at SportsMedicine Brookline, near Boston, and a fellow of the American College of Sports Medicine.

Caffeine, a powerful central nervous system stimulant, is the world's most widely used psychoactive drug. And though tea, colas, chocolate and some pain relievers and cold remedies contain it, most Americans get theirs from coffee. The average daily dose in the US is about 280 milligrams, the equivalent of two five-ounce cups of brewed java, two to three cups of instant, six cups of tea or six 12-ounce Cokes. Among coffee's benefits:

- *Increased speed and stamina.* Aside from perking you up, caffeine really can give you an athletic edge. On nine different days, British researchers had 18 male runners race 1,500 meters after drinking one to two cups of either regular or decaffeinated coffee. When caffeinated, the runners ran 4.2 seconds faster. In a similar study, researchers had endurance athletes run and cycle to exhaustion, then retested them an hour after they drank about five cups of coffee. Their stamina improved 44 percent in the running test, 5 percent in the cycling test. The international Olympic Committee bans caffeine levels higher than 12 micrograms per milliliter of urine—about what you'd get from five cups of coffee.

  "The early studies on caffeine and athletic performance suggested that it helped only people who were not well-conditioned," says Ellen Coleman, a nutrition consultant at The Sport Clinic in Riverside, California. "However, the latest research shows that caffeine . . . helps every athlete excel." But only if you exceed your tolerance. A non-coffee drinker might benefit from a cup or two. A one-cup-a-day drinker might have to knock back three or four, along with plenty of plain water. As a diuretic, coffee increases urination and thus your risk of dehydration, which hurts athletic performance.
- *Cold relief.* Caffeine opens up bronchial passages, which can help relieve chest congestion. "If you'd rather not take a decongestant, have a cup or two of coffee," says James Duke, Ph.D., an expert on plant-based drugs at the U.S. Department of Agriculture's Research Station in Beltsville, Maryland. "It produces a similar effect."
- *Asthma prevention and treatment.* This bronchodilating effect also helps prevent asthma attacks. A survey of 70,000 Italian households showed that as coffee consumption increased, asthma incidence decreased. A standard asthma medication is theophylline, a close relative of caffeine. Joe Graedon, co-author of *The People's Pharmacy* books and a syndicated newspaper column and the host of a national radio program, recalls, "We got a thank-you note from a woman who forgot to pack her asthma medication for her honeymoon in Hawaii. She started wheezing and got panicky, then recalled a column of ours that recommended caffeine as an emergency substitute. She had a few cups of coffee and was fine."
- *Pain relief.* Several studies have shown that a combination of aspirin and a small amount of caffeine (perhaps 60 milligrams) relieves pain more quickly and effectively than aspirin alone. Scientists aren't sure why: it

could be that caffeine provides an emotional lift that helps dampen pain sensations, or it may have true analgesic properties. Next time you have a headache or any injury that makes you reach for aspirin, wash it down with a cup of coffee. Or take Anacin, a combination of aspirin and caffeine.

- *Jet lag prevention.* Coffee helps shift the body's natural time cycle (circadian rhythm) after abrupt time-zone changes. Researchers at New York Hospital-Cornell Medical Center in New York housed five men in rooms without windows, clocks, radios or TVs for sixteen days, producing the equivalent of jet lag by abruptly changing their wake-up and bed times. When the men were awakened in time to drink about 1.5 cups of coffee at their "destination's" breakfast hour, jet lag was minimized.

We seldom consider how much of a drug caffeine is. And like all drugs, it has its drawbacks:

- *Addiction.* Use caffeine regularly, and you develop a tolerance. Deprived of caffeine, you may experience withdrawal symptoms, including lethargy, depression and headaches.
- *Jitters.* As every coffee drinker knows, when you drink more than you're used to, you get jumpy and impatient and may have trouble falling asleep. Some people swear coffee doesn't make them wired, but it's a rare coffee drinker who switches to decaf without feeling calmer and more patient.
- *Fat.* Black coffee is virtually fat-free, but any milk other than skim adds fat. Two percent fat milk adds only a smidgen, but foamy espresso drinks are another story. A large Starbucks Cafe Mocha made with whole milk has 409 calories and 31 grams of fat, 180 more calories and twice the fat of a half-cup of super premium ice cream.
- *Stomach distress.* Coffee increases secretion of acid in the stomach, so drinking a lot more of it than you're used to may upset your stomach. If you have an ulcer or a chronic digestive disorder, drink caffeinated coffee sparingly, if at all.
- *Pesticide residues.* Of the 170 pesticides used on coffee crops worldwide, 76 are prohibited in the U.S. because they're considered hazardous to health. Yet an FDA survey showed that 30 to 50 percent of imported coffee beans contain illegal pesticide residues. If you're concerned, try organically grown coffee. Two mail order sources: Equal Exchange, 191 Tosca Dr., Stoughton, MA 02072 (call 617–344–7227 or fax 617–344–7240); and Frontier Coffee, c/o Frontier Cooperative Herbs, Box 299, Norway, IA 52318 (800–669–3275).

Coffee has been accused of increasing heart disease and cancer risk. Here's what's left once you filter out the sensationalism of these reports:

- *Heart disease.* A "weak association" between heart attacks and a daily coffee intake of four or more cups has turned up in several studies. But the typical American consumes only one or two cups, so coffee drinking can't be a major risk factor. If you have an elevated risk for heart disease—a personal or family history, smoking, obesity, high blood pressure or a Type-A lifestyle—keep it to a cup or two a day, tops. "Moderate coffee drinking poses no major risk for heart disease," says Varro Tyler, Ph.D., professor of pharmacognosy (natural-product pharmacy) at Purdue University. "But I had some cardiac arrythmias a few years ago, so I stopped drinking it."
- *High blood pressure.* Caffeine increases heart rate, leading to speculation that it might boost blood pressure enough to increase risk of heart attack and stroke. Here, too, however, the evidence is iffy. Caffeine produces a sharp spike in the blood pressure of the uninitiated, but in coffee-tolerant people, blood pressure remains in the normal range. And though several studies have shown small decreases in blood pressure among people who switch to decaf, other studies have not. If you have high blood pressure, you're probably best off switching to decaf. But if your blood pressure is normal, a modest coffee habit won't give you hypertension.
- *Cholesterol.* Though many studies have shown that coffee raises cholesterol levels slightly, the ones showing the strongest link have come from Europe, where people often boil coffee. Most Americans filter theirs, minimizing the effect, which is small to begin with. If your blood cholesterol level is well above 200 milligrams per deciliter, ask your physician if you should cut down on the java.
- *Cancer.* Coffee has been tied to cancers of the bladder, pancreas, prostate, breasts and ovaries. All of these reports have subsequently been disputed, and several thoroughly debunked. Coffee's contribution to human cancer, if any, remains unclear. The roasting process does introduce many carcinogens into coffee beans, but research to date has generated about as much scientific nervousness as a cup of Sanka.

"My best advice is to know yourself, and drink coffee consciously," says Roland Griffiths, Ph.D., professor in the departments of psychiatry and neuroscience at the Johns Hopkins University School of Medicine and co-author of major studies on caffeine dependence and withdrawal. "You should understand that by drinking it, you're using a powerful drug. Pay attention to how it affects you, and respect your own limits."

Tea

When Isao Kubo was a child growing up in Japan, his grandmother would tell him to drink a cup of green tea every time he ate something sweet. Green tea, she said, would help prevent cavities. "I thought it was an old wives' tale until I proved it myself as a scientist," says Kubo, a professor of natural-products chemistry at the University of California, Berkeley. "Now I follow her advice."

Kubo is one of an increasing number of scientists who believe that tea—including the green, black and yogi varieties—may offer a host of health benefits. His research, for example, indicates that two compounds in tea battle the bacteria responsible for tooth decay. The first group, known as tannins, prevent plaque by inhibiting bacterial production of a substance that binds acid to teeth. The second group are flavor compounds called linarols that have been shown to kill decay-inducing bacteria in test tubes.

Next to water, tea is the world's most popular drink. It is made from the leaves of the *Camellia sinensis* evergreen plant and comes in three general varieties: black, green and oolong. Herbal teas don't really count since they aren't made from real tea leaves.

Black tea, used to make teas like Lipton, makes up nearly 80 percent of world tea consumption. Green tea accounts for about 20 percent, and oolong, popular in China, only about 2 percent.

It's green tea that is most steeped in research. Tests on laboratory animals show it may be effective in reducing tumors of the lungs, liver, skin and digestive tract. In one study, Fung-Lung Chung, Ph.D., a chemist and associate chief of the division of chemical carcinogenesis at the American Health Foundation in Valhalla, New York, exposed mice to the carcinogens found in cigarette smoke. Up to 45 percent fewer lung tumors occurred in mice given green tea than in those who drank water. "The results may explain why Japanese smokers have a lung cancer rate approximately half that of American smokers," says Chung.

Allan Conney, Ph.D., director of the Laboratory for Cancer Research at Rutgers University in Piscataway, New Jersey, had even more encouraging results. He subjected mice to ultraviolet light and found that up to 87 percent fewer skin cancers developed in mice who drank green tea instead of water.

And two studies by Hirota Fujiki Ph.D., a chemist at the National Cancer Research Institute in Tokyo, showed that mice fed green tea extracts were less likely to develop liver and intestinal cancers. Fujiki estimates that to reap any protective benefits from green tea, a human would have to drink 10 cups daily.

Most American researchers, however, don't recommend drinking green tea in unusually large quantities. "These studies are not conclusive," says Rutgers's Conney. "Certainly, no one should go out and start drinking excessive amounts of green tea. It's still very much an open question." The argument is that because studies have been carried out only in animals, it is still unclear if green tea has any cancer-preventing benefits for humans.

Some scientists even see danger in drinking tea. "It's an open-and-shut case against tea," says Julia Morton, an economic botanist at the University of Miami. Morton says that tannins—the same ingredient Kubo credits with fighting plaque—cause esophageal cancer and points to several epidemiological studies as evidence.

For instance, a century ago the Dutch were big tea drinkers, and esophageal cancer was rife in Holland, she says. When coffee supplanted tea as the national drink, this type of cancer became rare. In Japan, the esophageal cancer rate is very high, compared to the low rates in the parts of China where oolong tea, which is low in tannins, dominate.

Interestingly, esophageal cancer is rare in England, famous for its citizens' heavy tea-drinking habit. The reason, says Morton, is that most Britons drink their tea with milk, which binds to tannins, making them harmless. "I don't advise anyone to drink tea without milk in it," Morton says.

Herbal teas, which have been prescribed for centuries for their healing qualities, are low in tannins. Nevertheless, Morton is skeptical of them, too, contending that their health benefits are "obsolete and marginal." She adds that some herbal teas may even be harmful if overused: "[Many herbs] are not necessarily suitable for daily beverage use." For example, tea made from juniper berries has the potential to cause kidney damage.

While most experts believe that herbal teas pose little danger, they find the notion that herbals offer specific health advantages misleading. According to a Food and Drug Administration (FDA) spokeswoman, no data have ever been submitted to the FDA to substantiate any health claims for herbal teas. As a result, most manufacturers promote them with vague adjectives like "soothing" or "relaxing."

One company that does make health claims about its tea is the Yogi Tea Company in Los Angeles. It offers, for example, a line of "ancient healing formulas," including one called Male Vitality that is supposed to "heighten strength, increase vigor and improve endurance" in men. Their "teas" are a blend of cinnamon, black pepper, cloves, cardamom and ginger and based upon the 5,000-year-old Indian philosophy of *ayurveda*.

Waheguru S. Khalsa, a Los Angeles chiropractor, explains that the philosophy involves "the science of using herbs to help somebody whose body is out of balance get back in equilibrium." Khalsa concedes that there has been little Western research in this area but says that is merely a reflection of our cultural bias.

Despite the lack of scientific support for their health benefits, herbal and other teas are big business. In 1991, Americans spent nearly $120 million on them. One reason for their popularity may be the public's concern over caffeine.

But Arthur Bassett, Ph.D., a professor of pharmacology at the University of Miami School of Medicine, says that concern may be overstated. Some reports have linked caffeine to heart disease, but an equal number have contradicted those findings, he says. While caffeine can produce small increases in blood pressure, Bassett explains that most tea and coffee drinkers quickly develop "caffeine tolerance."

In reasonable amounts, caffeine may even be desirable for some people, he says: "It certainly picks you up and makes your mind more alert. For people who want a stimulant, tea is generally a good choice. It has less caffeine than coffee and most carbonated beverages." Although tea has about twice as much caffeine as coffee by weight, you have to brew four times more coffee than tea leaves to yield one cup. Thus tea, with about 30 to 46 milligrams per cup, has about half the caffeine of an equal-size cup of coffee.

Bassett says that while the scientific debate over tea can be a steamy one, it shouldn't keep you from sipping the leafy brew: "People should just remember that, like any drug, too much tea can probably cause some problems. But in moderation, it's probably reasonable to enjoy it."

ENVIRONMENTAL HEALTH

In 1981, American scientists embarked on the largest and most publicized microbe hunt in history in an effort to learn the cause of a new "gay cancer." But despite all the attention and money expended in the battle against AIDS, the virus that causes it is only one of several deadly microorganisms threatening us with a virulence unseen in this country since the early 1900s.

Unthinkable as it may have been even five years ago, airline passengers are spreading tuberculosis to fellow travelers, and otherwise healthy people are succumbing to bacterial infections that used to be child's play for antibiotics. We've seen people die after eating tainted hamburgers in fast-food restaurants, hundreds of vacationers get sick aboard a cruise ship, a man in rural California die from pneumonic plague and a half-million residents of one city become ill from a waterborne bug. Overseas, deadly epidemics like cholera, plague and diphtheria have returned. But others once considered vanquished are returning to the United States in changed and sometimes incurable forms. It appears that hygienic America is suddenly being besieged on all fronts by invisible enemies.

In fact, diseases, epidemics and plagues are as old as history, but when people remained relatively confined to their own corners of the world, germs had less of a chance to spread. Today, things are different. "We live in a global village," says Laurie Garrett, author of *The Coming Plague: Newly Emerging Diseases in a World Out of Balance,* an exhaustive documentation of how biological factors, in addition to politics, medical mismanagement and social changes, have created the potential for a worldwide health disaster.

"Globalization is great culturally," Garrett says, "but the downside is that we're also making microbes global. They hitchhike on people, on shipments of foods, animals, plants and so on." In the era of jet travel, it has taken less than a day for some viruses to appear on one continent, then jump to another.

A second factor is the changing global landscape. In the tropics, for example, previously untouched forests have been cleared for farmland, bringing villagers in contact with formerly remote areas and microbes that never before confronted humans on any large scale. The farmers, in turn, bring these exotic viruses and bacteria with them to teeming megacities where public-health measures may be nonexistent.

All this began at a time when Americans had become complacent, believing that scourges such as influenza, measles and gonorrhea were under control. Indeed, in 1969, the U.S. surgeon general declared the battle against infectious diseases won. Researchers and medical schools began focusing on chronic and degenerative conditions such as cancer, aging and heart disease. Pharmaceutical companies made antibacterial research a low priority.

"The return of old diseases and the emergence of new ones are both related to the misconception that infectious illnesses had gone away, " explains Stephen Ostroff, M.D., associate director for epidemiologic science at the National Center for Infectious Diseases in Atlanta. In fact, smallpox was the only one ever really conquered. Others keep returning in waves.

The situation isn't helped any by the fact that our arsenal of antibiotics, which were highly effective disease fighters just a few years ago, is becoming increasingly impotent. Bacteria have built-in survival mechanisms; given half a chance, they not only survive, but mutate and reproduce, spawning more virulent and drug-resistant versions of themselves.

One major cause of this resistance is the inappropriate use of antibiotics. For example, doctors know that the drugs are effective only against bacterial diseases, not viral infections such as influenza and colds. Yet many a flu-plagued patient has sauntered out of his doctor's office with a prescription for tetracycline or amoxicillin. This type of overuse allows the bacteria that normally exist in a person's body to "read" the drug, mutate and pass on to other bacteria the enzymes that allow for drug resistance.

Patients are also guilty. "Perhaps 50 percent of the resistance problem comes from patients playing doctor once they have antibiotics in their hands," says Stuart Levy, M.D., director of the Center for Adaptation Genetics and Drug Resistance at Tufts University Medical School and author of *The Antibiotic Paradox: How Miracle Drugs Are Destroying the Miracle.* "In particular, when patients stop taking them as soon as their symptoms subside, stronger and drug-resistant bacteria are allowed to survive and reproduce."

Rheumatic fever, ear infections and pneumonia caused by Streptococcus bacteria have appeared in virulent new forms. Pneumococcal bacteria, responsible for pneumonia, middle-ear, upper-respiratory and sinus infections, are increasingly antibiotic-resistant. Group A streptococci, the incorrectly nicknamed flesh-eating bacteria, are responsible for a rise in toxic shock and can invade chickenpox lesions and other small skin breaks. The chances of a person becoming infected with these bacteria is small, but because new strains have appeared, their potential to inflict harm is uncertain.

The resistance problem is greatest in hospitals, where potentially deadly Staphylococcus aureus (staph) bacteria, invulnerable to a dozen or so previously effective antibiotics, may soon become resistant to vancomycin, the only drug that now can kill it. Some strains of enterococcus, which cause serious gastrointestinal, urinary-tract and wound infections, are already resistant to vancomycin—and are potentially fatal. Tuberculosis, the leading fatal infectious disease worldwide, is spreading among immigrants, the homeless and HIV-infected people in the U.S., and many cases are multidrug-resistant.

In the contest between mutating bacteria and the race to find new drugs to kill them, many experts are pessimistic about which side will win. Techniques that pharmaceutical companies used successfully in the past no longer work. Finding new methods will be a slow, expensive process with greater potential for toxicity and liability.

Even if they have changed, most bacterial infections at least have familiar names. But what about threats that only recently entered our vocabulary? Emerging diseases—those that have either increased within the past two decades or threaten to do so soon—include the following:

- Acquired Immune Deficiency Syndrome (AIDS), caused by HIV, the human immunodeficiency virus, has probably afflicted humans for at least two decades. "We learned from HIV that any once-obscure, isolated microorganism now has the opportunity to reach increasing numbers of people," says Stephen S. Morse, Ph.D., assistant professor of virology at Rockefeller University in New York City and author of *Emerging Viruses.*
- Lyme disease, first described in 1975, has exploded nationwide out of its original Connecticut home as suburbs expand into formerly wooded areas, increasing people's exposure to ticks that transmit the bacterium.
- Hantavirus pulmonary syndrome, also called Four Corners disease, is a new and frequently fatal form of an old rodent-borne viral illness that first appeared more than two years ago in the Southwest and now has been reported in more than twenty states.
- Legionnaires' disease is a serious respiratory illness caused by a tougher strain of an old bacterium. "The organism was around before the first outbreak, in 1976, but mass water- and air-treatment centers made transmission possible," Ostroff says.
- Cryptosporidiumm, a waterborne parasite that can live in chlorinated water, sickened approximately 400,000 Milwaukee residents in 1993. More than 100 people died.
- Staphylococcus aureus, toxic shock syndrome, which rose to fame during the early '80s when it struck large numbers of women who used superabsorbent tampons, largely disappeared as a problem. But it's increasing again, and about half of recent cases have no connection with tampons.
- Salmonella has become more and more resistant to antibiotics and is increasingly found in the food supply. The U.S. Department of Agriculture estimates 40 percent of the poultry sold here contains the microorganism. E. Coli also causes food poisoning. Widespread illness and the deaths of four children in the Pacific Northwest in 1993 were caused by a new strain, E. coli 0157:H7, in undercooked hamburger.

Until very recently, the public health response has been frighteningly inadequate. In 1994, the Centers for Disease Control and Prevention (CDC) described the nation's early-warning system for infectious diseases as "crumbling into disrepair" and in desperate need of a massive infusion of federal money. But things are beginning to turn around, with the American

Medical Association, the CDC, the World Health Organization and other groups expanding their attacks on the growing threats.

"Having international disease 'listening posts' is not terribly expensive when compared with defense spending or dealing with diseases after the fact," suggests Robert E. Shope, M.D., professor of epidemiology at Yale University School of Medicine. "If a new influenza strain emerges, it could infect millions, as did the 1918–19 pandemic that killed 20 million people worldwide. International monitoring could alert us in time to prepare a vaccine."

Hopefully, such preparedness would extend to some of the more exotic, gruesome diseases we hear about. Lassa fever, the Ebola and Marburg viruses and the like, made into household names by Richard Preston's book *The Hot Zone* and in the movie *Outbreak*, are not threats to America at this time, but the emergence of an airborne viral microbe could become a global nightmare.

Still, most experts believe that, for now, we should be most concerned with things we can control. What's needed more than paranoia or panic are common sense, personal responsibility and community action, they warn. "There's a fine balance between caution and hypochondria," says Edward McSweegan, Ph.D., of the National Institute of Health's Division of Microbiology and Infectious Diseases. "Be aware of local risks and take appropriate precautions. For example, if you live in the Northeast, protect yourself against tick bites. Be cautious about exposure to rodents if you're in the Southwest." Finally, he adds, don't let fear of disease keep you from leading a normal life: "Chronic worry isn't good for your health."

Home, Hazardous Home

As autumn falls, appreciation soars for the great indoors—and the central heating that comes with it. Yet your home may not be a safe haven, especially if routine maintenance ranks somewhere below death and taxes on your priority list. In that case, shutting out the cold could mean sealing in viruses, bacteria, mold, mildew, insects and toxic chemicals for the winter— a kind of Biosphere gone bad.

Even seemingly minor problems can pose health risks. Fumes from mothballs and new carpeting do you wrong just as easily as, of all things, a leaky pipe: By causing dampness in walls, that pipe encourages mold growth which, in turn, triggers allergies in susceptible individuals. If the moisture causes paint to peel, and the paint is old, you could be augmenting your exposure to brain-damaging lead. (Young children are at particularly high risk.) Moisture under the kitchen sink could cause metal containers stored there to rust and emit toxic chemicals or fumes. And it could attract cockroaches—you know, those things which haul around Salmonella, Streptococcus and Staphylococcus bacteria that can make you sick.

The point? Creating a home sterile enough to perform surgery in isn't realistic (or sane), but improving your home environment with simple cleaning and maintenance is. The following is a collection of homebody horrors to sweep out from under the rug.

Like them or not, bacteria and viruses are everyone's invisible room-mates. Leave problems unchecked, and you roll out the welcome mat for guests like influenza, Salmonella, hepatitis, E. coli and Streptococcus. Some of the best defenses are simple ones. Frequent hand-washing, for example, discourages the spread of germs from household surfaces to your body (and vice versa). In cleaning up your act, also consider the following:

Problem: Some viruses live on household surfaces for twenty-four hours or more.

Solution: Fussy as it sounds, you can reduce the spread of viruses if you disinfect doorknobs, light switches, faucets, toilet handles, railings, telephone handsets, remote-control devices and any other commonly touched items weekly.

Problem: Refrigerator science projects yield sickening results. "Juices from raw meat and poultry may contain bacteria, including Salmonella and others, which cause food poisoning," says home economist Susan Conley, manager of the U.S. Department of Agriculture's Meat and Poultry Hotline (800–535–4555). "If these juices drip onto other foods [or touch them via unwiped spills], those foods could become contaminated."

Solution: "Refrigerate raw meat and poultry in containers or on trays so juices don't drip," says Conley. Wipe up spills using hot, soapy water. Refrigeration slows bacterial growth but doesn't kill the little buggers, so make sure you thoroughly cook food to kill them, and toss any affected item that can't be cooked.

Problem: Plastic boards may be less effective at keeping food-poisoning contaminants at bay than old-fashioned wood ones. A study by the University of Wisconsin Food Research Institute recovered fewer bacteria from intentionally contaminated wooden boards than from plastic.

Solution: Wash your (preferably wood, not plastic) cutting board with hot, soapy water after and between its encounters with raw meat or poultry.

Problem: Your water cooler may be swimming with bacteria. According to the Tufts University Diet and Nutrition Letter, researchers sampled water from water coolers on the Northeastern University campus and found 2,000 potentially harmful organisms per liter—four times the government-allowed limit. Although that level's not life-threateningly high, it's enough to cause gastroenteritis, an inflammation of the membrane lining the stomach and intestines.

Solution: Clean your cooler's reservoir monthly. Run a half-gallon of bleach through the system, then flush it with four or more gallons of tap water. Also, wipe dirt, soot and debris off water bottles before using.

Problem: Your mother doesn't approve of your housecleaning habits, but household pests do. Food debris and water attract ants, roaches, rodents and other scavengers, while piles of newspapers and magazines invite rats and mice.

Solution: Keep a clean, uncluttered domicile. Regular vacuuming helps control fleas in your carpet—especially if you put pyrethrum flea powder or a flea collar in your vacuum bag to help the pests expire. Outdoors, turn empty flower pots, buckets and other receptacles upside down, and get rid of old tires. Standing water makes a great love nest for procreating mosquitoes.

Unfortunately, even cleanliness leads to hazards. A quick survey of the typical home reveals enough cleaners, waxes, solvents, pesticides, detergents, finishes and fungicides to create an alternative universe. And with homes being more energy-efficient (read: more airtight, with less air exchange between indoors and out) than ever, the resulting chemical soup can be annoying at best, poisonous at worst. Here's a brief sampling of what might ail you:

Problem: Formaldehyde exists in everything from plywood and particle board to permanent-press fabrics, adhesives and carbonless copy paper. "At the levels at which most people are exposed to it, formaldehyde is only an irritant," says David Mannino, M.D., a pulmonologist with the U.S. Centers for Disease Control and Prevention in Atlanta. Symptoms include throat irritation, respiratory problems and headaches. Industrial exposures may cause long-term effects.

Solution: Whenever feasible, avoid formaldehyde-containing products. Wash permanent-press clothes repeatedly before wearing them; this removes offending finishes. If symptoms arise when you work with plywood, particle board or any other formaldehyde products, ventilate the area aggressively and continue doing so as long as symptoms persist.

Problem: "It's not uncommon to smell solvents when you bring home your dry cleaning," Mannino says. Though most exposure is relatively harmless, "in high enough concentrations, those solvents can cause symptoms," including dizziness and fatigue.

Solution: Remove the plastic bag and air out dry cleaning before stowing it in your closet. (Dispose of the bag safely so that babies or young children can't get hold of it.)

Problem: In addition to having formaldehyde-containing adhesives and backing, new carpeting may reek with moth- and stainproofing. And? Well, in one study, mice that were exposed to air blown over new-carpet samples died within twenty-four hours. No human deaths are recorded, but many complaints of headaches and respiratory ills have been. The suspected culprit is a carpet-backing chemical, 4-phenylcyclohexene (4-PC), although evidence is inconclusive.

Solution: Sorry, but until evidence is more conclusive, options are few. Besides living on hardwood flooring or ceramic tile, your only real alternative is to avoid exposure to new carpeting after installation. "I advise patients to wait a month or two before moving in after any remodeling project," says Oak Park, Illinois, allergist Anne Szpindor-Watson, M.D. If that's impossible, even a few days' evacuation while the carpet breathes will help.

Problem: According to the *University of California at Berkeley Wellness Letter*, infants reportedly have died and whole households have become ill after heavy exposure to clothing and blankets stored in naphthalene mothballs. Eating even one mothball can be fatal to an infant. Paradichlorobenzene mothballs are less toxic but more carcinogenic in the long term.

Solution: Nix the mothballs and store clean clothes (stains attract bugs) in tape-sealed, airtight plastic bags or containers. (Added bonus: You won't smell like everyone's great aunt.)

Problem: For every cockroach you see, fifty or more may be hiding undetected. Not only can roach allergies cause rhinitis (runny nose) and asthma, but the insects can also spread disease.

Solution: Keep food areas free of dirty dishes, crumbs and water. Caulk crevices where roaches may enter the house. Skip the pesticides; Most roaches are immune. Sprinkling boric acid in roach-traffic zones is effective but not safe around children and pets.

Problem: Carbon monoxide (CO) is present wherever combustion takes place—near gas furnaces, gas ranges, wood stoves, kerosene heaters and auto exhaust. Without warning, it can cause headaches, drowsiness and (a sure sign of overexposure) death.

Solution: Again, maximize ventilation. Home inspector Tom Corbett, owner of Tomacor Inc. in Chicago, warns against carbon monoxide buildup in attached garages and from windows that open onto streets and alleys. He also says, "Have a licensed service person check your furnace for CO backdrafting to make sure it isn't blowing CO throughout your house."

Of course, there are countless other substances to avoid—not just the obvious ones like asbestos, lead dust and radon gas. Poorly-ventilated refinishing projects send up toxic clouds; wantonly sprayed pesticides find their way into foods; even fumes from art supplies, cleaning solutions and paint solvents can do your health wrong.

"Just about every product can be used in a dangerous way," says Michael Hodgson, M.D., an associate professor working in the department of occupational and environmental medicine at the University of Connecticut in Farmington. "That doesn't necessarily mean you shouldn't use these products, only that you should put some thought into how you use them." (But: "With 35 hazardous agents in it, tobacco smoke is far and away the worst indoor pollutant and probably the most avoidable," David Mannino adds.)

If you are plagued with allergies, chemical irritants and indoor allergens can team up to make dwelling in your domicile a real gasp. According to Anne Szpindor-Watson, allergic individuals should be doubly vigilant in avoiding the home-maintenance pitfalls we've already covered. "Whenever [mucous membranes] become inflamed and exposed [as the result of illness or irritation], they are likely to react to things they normally don't react to," she says.

And there's plenty for allergic people to react to in the average home. Some ubiquitous sneeze-makers include the following:

Problem: Dust mites dwell everywhere but are partial to high humidity, low elevations and wherever human dander—flakes of skin and scalp—collects. These include carpeting, upholstery, mattresses, bedding, pillows and piles of dirty clothing. Regular vacuuming and cold-water washing don't faze them.

Solution: The American Academy of Allergy and Immunology suggests removing wall-to-wall carpeting and upholstered furniture. Encase mattresses and pillows in airtight coverings. Wash bedding weekly in hot (130 degrees Fahrenheit) water. Remove clutter. Keep humidity below 50 percent.

Problem: Bathrooms, kitchens and basements are prime real estate for humidity-loving mold. Also check windowsills, leaky outdoor walls and any area that has been flooded. Forced-air heating and humidifiers can circulate mold throughout the house.

Solution: Use exhaust fans in baths and kitchens to control humidity. Dehumidify basements. Remove visible mold from walls with bleach or trisodium phosphate (TSP). Follow the manufacturer's instructions, cleaning humidifiers regularly. Find and fix leaky plumbing, roofs, walls and windows.

"There is really no limit to the number of allergies one can develop," says Szpindor-Watson. Past immunity is no safeguard, either, she observes.

"If you're allergic to one thing now, you're likely to develop more allergies in the future." The best strategy is to reduce exposure before problems begin. "The fewer things you're exposed to," she says, "the less chance you have of developing a reaction."

By now severe paranoia and bewilderment may be setting in. If it's any consolation, even your best efforts will probably never result in environmental nirvana. Home inspector Corbett, who ferrets out environmental problems for a living, notes, "Some people want to fine-tune everything to perfection. Realistically, you can't do that, though you can address a lot of problems."

Just enough, perhaps, so you can fire up the recently-serviced central heat, pull up the well-laundered flannel sheets, lie back on the moderately-upholstered sofa and breathe deeply.

A HEALTHY LIFESTYLE

Addressing Addictions

Today, addiction of all kinds seems to be epidemic. People aren't just having problems with alcohol and drugs, but with food, smoking, gambling, shopping, chocolate, exercise, coffee, work and sex. Indeed, almost everything these days has been labeled an addiction. But what is the nature of addiction, and how do we explain its hold over certain individuals? When and how does a simple experiment or indulgence spiral into a full-blown addiction?

Though addiction is better understood these days, its root cause remains a mystery. One theory is that some addicts have abnormally low levels of some of the body's naturally occurring neurochemicals, such as endorphins. These neurochemicals affect mood and behavior, and when the balance is tipped, an addicted person may try to compensate by ingesting a substance that produces a similar, or a far more intense, feeling. In this light, addiction seems to stem from an effort to self-medicate. A user's first attempts to medicate himself with drugs or other substances usually lies within his control. Gradually, however, he loses control, and choice becomes compulsion.

How do compulsive shopping, gambling, and other non-chemical addictions fit the self-medication model of addiction? Some experts believe that every addiction is a search for wholeness or inner peace, and compulsive behavior is yet another misguided attempt to fill an individual void. If this is true, then any effort to conquer an addiction must be accompanied by an exploration of what has created this feeling of incompleteness in the first place. Are these "true addictions?" However you choose to classify them, the pain they cause is real enough.

Contrary to popular mythology, no genetic basis for addiction has been firmly established. Scientists have yet to turn up an "alcoholism gene," for instance. But some studies do suggest a genetic predisposition to addiction. For example, children of alcoholics have been shown to be more prone to developing drinking problems. But Alcoholics Anonymous and other self-help groups with a similar approach argue that the substance *itself* creates the need. The important thing is absolute avoidance—a goal achieved through the group support of people with the same addictions, along with recognition of self-destructive behavior patterns, and assistance in overcoming them.

In fact, Alcoholics Anonymous (as well as many medical experts) consider addiction to be a disease. The disease concept of alcoholism is an old one, the idea being that the individual is powerless over his or her drinking due to a biological vulnerability. This theory is now applied very broadly, not just to alcoholism, but to every conceivable form of addictive or compulsive behavior.

Some experts support the view that addiction is influenced by external factors—that family environment plays a part, as do cultural norms, peer pressure and other factors. Another view is that the proliferation of addictive behavior reflects social problems—for instance, the rising divorce rate. And still another group suggests that our over-reliance on drugs and medical technology to cure everything from bad breath to bad moods has made us too ready to try to "fix" every twinge and unpleasant feeling we experience.

What is known is that, in combating addictions, knowledge and will alone are rarely enough. Smoking-related illnesses, for example, kill tens of thousands of people a year in the U.S., yet most nicotine addicts can't kick the habit—despite numerous attempts and the knowledge that this behavior is potentially deadly. Legions of alcoholics have traded away family and career rather than quit drinking. The key isn't recognizing that addictions exist; it's recognizing that they might exist in one's own life.

Fortunately, many treatment options provide hope for those who realize that they have lost control of their lives. Some are able to stop their addictive behavior either on their own, or with the encouragement of family and friends. Many turn to support groups such as Alcoholics Anonymous, or seek professional help from a therapist or physician. For others, enrolling in an outpatient treatment program, or entering an inpatient facility, is the only way to make a clean break from addiction.

Innovative techniques to curb addictions are also available. Hypnosis and autogenics (a self-hypnosis technique) have been used successfully by some overeaters. Those who wish to stop smoking have had good results using hypnosis and acupuncture. And acupuncture, visualization and even massage have all been used to treat alcohol and drug addiction, with varying degrees of success.

But kicking the habit might only be the first step. For lasting recovery, addicts need to think about rebuilding their lives, and finding the meaning and motivation to move ahead. It's open to debate as to whether many of today's so-called addictions are actually diseases, but they certainly qualify in one respect. You have to recover before you can move on.

Alcohol on Trial

Heavy drinking—more than six drinks a day for a man, according to most experts—can cause cirrhosis (scarring) of the liver, heart disease, accidents, birth defects, ulcers, psychiatric problems and cancer of the esophagus, colon and rectum. But dozens of studies in recent years have shown that moderate drinking, no more than three drinks a day, provides some health benefits.

The most obvious is temporary stress reduction. That's because when the ethanol in a drink hits your brain, levels of dopamine, serotonin and endorphins—chemicals linked to feeling good—rise. Your worries seem to ease, you feel more confident, and you may even be able to express yourself more clearly.

Recent research has also shown that moderate alcohol intake protects against coronary artery disease. In fact, moderate drinkers may have a 40 percent lower risk than either teetotalers or people who drink more heavily. Researchers aren't sure why this is so. Some say an antioxidant found in the grapes used to make red wine helps prevent atherosclerosis. Others say that alcohol itself from any source, not just red wine, raises levels of the "good" high density lipoprotein (HDL) cholesterol, which helps prevent the buildup of arterial plaque. Still another theory is that alcohol triggers an enzyme that breaks down blood clots.

In addition, moderate alcohol consumption can protect against strokes and some types of food poisoning, such as salmonella. It may help you fall asleep more quickly and alleviate long-term depression. And at least one study has shown that alcohol may actually help you think better. An Indiana University study of middle-aged male twins found that those who regularly had one or two drinks a day displayed slightly stronger cognitive skills than non- or heavy drinkers, perhaps because alcohol improves circulation to the brain.

But even moderate drinking has its risks. One clear danger is that of behaving inappropriately. "Alcohol deinhibits people," explains Collins Lewis, M.D., an associate professor of psychiatry at Washington University School of Medicine in St. Louis. Alcohol is heavily implicated in domestic violence and child abuse. Conservative estimates are that one of every four American homes has been struck by an alcohol-related family problem.

Alcohol also impairs judgment and coordination. The dangers of drinking and driving have been well publicized. But fewer people know that alcohol and sports also don't mix. Booze is often a factor in recreational accidents, particularly skiing, skating, swimming and boating, and in athletic injuries. "Both exercise and alcohol break down muscle fibers," says Max A. Schneider, M.D., medical director of Chemical Dependency Services at St. Joseph Hospital in Orange, California. "Doing them together puts too much stress on your body. "

While you have to drink heavily to get cirrhosis of the liver, even three drinks a day can contribute to a fatty liver, the earliest stage of the disease. "The liver is like a chemical factory that burns fat for energy," says Charles Lieber, M.D., director of the Alcohol Research and Treatment Center at the Bronx Veteran Affairs Medical Center. "When alcohol is present, that burning gets interrupted, fat piles up, and the liver's functioning is disrupted."

Your gut may get fatty, too. A 12-ounce beer has about 150 calories; a glass of wine or an ounce of hard liquor, around 100. Mix liquor with fruit juice, chocolate or cream, or start having three drinks a day, and you take in an extra 500 to 1,500 calories daily, which may end up on your gut. That classic "beer belly" increases your risk of heart disease, because abdominal fat enters the bloodstream more easily than fat from other parts of the body.

As you drink, you may also be tempted to eat more fattening foods. "When your blood alcohol is elevated, it's hard to concentrate on eating right," says Charles Halsted, M.D., professor of internal medicine at the University of California, Davis. And alcohol not only provides little, if any, vitamins, minerals or protein, it also actually impairs their absorption.

Chalk up another big zero for romance. The alcohol industry pummels us with advertisements displaying virile men, sexy women and suggestions of great things to come, but even a couple of drinks can impair your libido, erections and orgasms. Chronic heavy drinking decreases testosterone and has a feminizing effect—a man can actually develop breasts and lose his pubic hair. And if you snuggle down to snooze instead, your sleep may be disturbed.

Perhaps the greatest danger is addiction. Ten percent of alcohol users are "problem" drinkers; 3 percent are alcoholics, according to the National Council on Alcohol and Drug Dependence. Researchers aren't sure why alcohol is addictive, but they do know that certain people, including those with a family history and those who displayed antisocial behavior as children or adults, are predisposed to alcoholism.

They also believe that if you drink steadily, your brain stops producing the chemicals that normally make you feel relaxed. You become dependent on alcohol for that effect and lose the emotional skills needed to cope with difficult feelings or situations. "I call it 'emotional muscle,'" says Marc F. Kern, Ph.D., executive director of Life Management Skills, a Los Angeles clinic that helps people learn to drink moderately. "You unlearn sophisticated skills in dealing with anger, anxiety or even falling asleep. You have to use alcohol to tolerate that discomfort."

At the same time, your tolerance for alcohol will increase. "The more you drink, the more you can drink," Kern says. "After a while, the same amount doesn't make you feel relaxed. It just makes you feel normal, which means you need even more alcohol to actually relax."

The threshold at which a moderate drinker becomes a problem drinker is unclear. "The best way to look at it isn't in terms of how much you drink, but what happens when you drink," Lewis says. "One person can have six drinks a day and not have problems with it—although he may be uncomfortable physiologically when he stops. Someone else could have two drinks a day and suffer bad effects. It depends on the individual."

Some people should never drink. That category includes people with heart disease and those who take sedatives, sleeping pills, antianxiety or antidepressant medications, even under a doctor's care.

Second, if you don't drink now, don't start for the sake of the supposed benefits. "You can get the same benefits by eating well and exercising," says Ernest P. Noble, Ph.D., director of the Alcohol Research Center at UCLA. And if you are drinking now and training hard, consider abstaining. "Alcohol affects your reflexes, your sleep and your nutritional balance. If you're concerned with peak performance, you're better off without it," Noble says.

If you still want to drink, the key is moderation. Three drinks a day for men is the max. If you think that sounds easy, be sure you know what a drink really is: between 1 and 1.5 ounces of hard liquor (one jiggerful), 4 or 5 ounces of wine or one 12-ounce beer.

Make sure you eat before drinking, and don't have more than one drink an hour. Alternate alcoholic drinks with juice or water. If you're dying for a beer after a workout, be sure to drink water, too. Alcohol, like exercise, dehydrates the body.

Don't keep drinking to stay exhilarated—spikes of giddiness or good cheer only occur as your blood alcohol is rising. If you drink to maintain that high, you'll probably drink too much. And make at least a day or two a week (three is better) alcohol-free to allow your liver to rest, cut down on the empty calories and, as Kern says, "see what it's like to be awake and conscious."

Most of all, be straight about how much you're drinking. As Noble points out, "People are clever at taking data and using it to their advantage."

HOW MUCH IS TOO MUCH?

Worried that you may be drinking too much? One easy guideline is the commonly used CAGE Index. Ask yourself the following four questions. If you answer yes to two or more, you're flirting with danger.

1. Have you ever felt you should Cut back on your alcohol intake?
2. Have you ever felt Annoyed by people telling you to drink less?
3. Have you ever felt Guilty about your drinking?
4. Do you ever need a drink as an Eye-opener in the morning?

Other warnings: loss of control (if you have one drink, you can't stop), blacking out, becoming aggressive or depressed under the influence and drinking your buddies under the table. If you're still not sure, take thirty days off from drinking. "Alcohol leaves your body in five days," says Life Management Skills' Marc F. Kern, Ph.D. "If you still yearn for it, you're psychologically ensnared."

Cigarettes: Minimizing the Risk.

Okay. You smoke.

You know you shouldn't, but you ignore the warnings. Statistics like a 73-year lifespan for you verses 81 years for non-smokers (and 400,000 smoking-related deaths annually) bounce off your armor. So does mounting harrassment from friends, family, colleagues, the EPA, AMA, FDA and the American electorate. Short of quitting, what's a guy to do?

For starters, you can make smoking your only bad habit in a generally healthy lifestyle. You can exercise often and eat wisely. Doing so won't prevent much smoke-related damage, but it may stave off other problems.

Antioxidants and vitamin supplementation may be a key second step. Free radicals, which accelerate the rate of aging and the progression of age-related problems, are formed by, among other things, cigarette smoke. Antioxidants, including vitamins C and E and beta-carotene, may counteract some of the molecular damage caused by free radicals. These vitamins employ an "Uzi approach," says J. Jean Hine, Ph.D., of the University of Arkansas for Medical Sciences. They contain the nutrient variety that smokers need. Studies suggest that key nutrients such as B-complex vitamins are as much as 42 percent lower in smokers, despite the fact that smokers probably need them more.

Since it would be virtually impossible to get the amounts of vitamin C and beta-carotene, which has been shown to give the most effective protection against lung cancer in your diet, smokers should consider supplementation. However, since there is little definitive research and since doctors are reluctant to recommend anything, fearing it gives the smoker a false sense of security, you're pretty much going to have to experiment. (A very high, but safe, dosage would be 1,200 I.U., vitamin E; 2,000–3,000 mg, vitamin C; and 50,000 I.U., beta-carotene.)

Humans evolved on a diet of wild plants and fish, which are both rich in antioxidants. Consuming the ingredients that helped form our genetic patterns and defenses is a good move. Fish, in fact, is high in omega–3 fatty acids, which are thought to be partially responsible for low lung-cancer rates among Japan's large smoking population.

Another such ingredient is purslane. Usually considered an annoying garden weed, it is abundant in vitamin E, beta-carotene and omega–3 fatty acids. For centuries, the Chinese have used purslane for a variety of ailments, including tumors. The biggest problem with purslane is its availability. Short of finding a field in which it grows or a Chinese herbalist who can supply it, your best bet is ordering seeds from a catalogue and growing the plant yourself.

But if the idea of a purslane salad doesn't excite you, try the more mundane green tea and garlic. Both have compounds which appear to neutralize cancer-causing chemicals. Again, no definitive dosages have been established, but most boosters recommend one to three cloves of garlic and/or one to four cups of tea a day.

Above all, of course, you should consider kicking the habit. What works best? Accupuncture, hypnotherapy, meditation, aversion therapy, self-help groups and nicotene patches can all work—but be prepared to try several methods before you hit on the one that works best for you. The key element in successfully beating the habit can be the love of friends and family who want to see you around for as long as possible. Quitting cigarettes might be the hardest thing you ever do, but it's the most important step you can take toward a healthy lifestyle.

Getting a Good Night's Sleep

During an important client meeting, your head does that weird bobbing thing. You peer out through one bleary eye and notice there's quite a bit of head bobbing going on around the table. It's like a sleep-deprived take on *Dawn of the Dead*. What's going on here?

By many accounts, we're becoming a nation of somnambulists. Fully one-third of Americans today suffer from chronic or periodic sleep disorders, according to the National Commission on Sleep Disorders Research (NCSDR). In fact, some doctors say a silent epidemic of sleep deprivation is sweeping the country, with effects ranging from mild forgetfulness to sexual dysfunction to heart attacks.

"We're taught that the way to keep up with increasing demands is to get less sleep—in short, that sleep is unimportant," says Mark Mahowald, M.D., director of the Minnesota Regional Sleep Disorders Center in Minneapolis. Big mistake: Sleep is vital to both mind and body. But as researchers learn just how essential sleep is and why, our society is incurring a burgeoning sleep debt.

By some estimates, we're snoozing up to 20 percent less than our grandparents did at our age. You can blame most of our sleep-related ills on industrialization. Our forebears had few alternatives but to sleep once the sun went down. Watching fires flicker was big during the Stone Age, but that grew old fast. ("Fifty-seven campfires and nothin' on!") As recently as twenty years ago, you couldn't see much more than a test pattern on the TV screen after 2 A.M.; now you can channel surf all night long. To make matters worse, as sleep time has diminished, annual work hours have increased 158 hours, nearly a full month, since 1969 alone.

How does sleeplessness steal funds from your health account? Let us count the ways.

The big debit is immunity. Healthy old people often cite healthy sleep habits as one of the keys to their longevity. Science is beginning to confirm that link. In one study, researchers found that depriving rats of sleep wiped out their immune systems, resulting in lethal bacterial infections. Another study found that when healthy humans are deprived of sleep for three days, their immune systems go on red alert; levels of monocytes, granulocytes and other natural "killer" cells rise as though sleep deprivation was itself some type of invading organism. In still another study, researchers found that when cytokines, the immune system's "messengers," are injected into animal brains, the animals fall asleep.

Sleep is also essential for higher levels of mental functioning, though simpler ones seem to be unaffected. James Horne, a psychophysiologist at Loughborough University in England, found that people who were deprived of sleep for thirty-two hours could handle rote tasks—like organizing files, sending out documents or answering phone calls—but couldn't do tasks that demanded spontaneity or creativity, such as developing a business plan or responding to an emergency.

Fatal accidents—including those on the scale of Chernobyl, Three Mile Island and Exxon Valdez—are often linked to sleep deprivation. One-third of all heavy-trucking accidents in which the driver is killed are due to fatigue, according to the National Transportation Safety Board. And the U.S. Department of Transportation estimates that 200,000 car accidents each year may be caused by sleepiness; 87 percent of such crashes are fatal.

Science is even beginning to correlate sleep patterns with cardiovascular disease. For example, University of Iowa researcher Virend Somers, M.D., found in a 1994 study that heart attacks are most likely to occur just after waking. The reason appears to be that the entire sympathetic nervous system, which governs the pulse-quickening shifts your body undergoes in response to a fight-or-flight threat, is twice as active during sleep as when you're awake.

Add the exertion of waking up, and if you're a man predisposed to cardiac trouble, you've got the ingredients for heightened risk. The rapid eye movement (REM) portion of sleep is characterized by the highest increase in heart rate, blood pressure and blood clotting. Because sleep-deprived people have longer REM cycles when they finally do crash, their susceptibility to heart problems is further compounded.

Also in physical danger are people—usually men—with obstructive sleep apnea, a syndrome associated with heavy snoring, obesity, alcohol intake and smoking. Apneics drift in and out of sleep as they gasp to breathe through an obstructed air passage. In such cases the heart may work harder to compensate for lowered blood-oxygen levels, putting the victim at greater risk for heart attack and stroke. In fact, 38,000 cardiovascular deaths are attributed annually to sleep apnea.

But for most of us, sleep deprivation surfaces in our emotional states. It can trigger irritability, restlessness, anxiety, hostility or depression. People who chronically undersleep feel out of control as they watch their family and work lives deteriorate. Sex lives also take a tumble. "Given a choice between having sex or sleeping, sleep-deprived men will choose sleep," says Patrick Strollo, M.D., a pulmonary sleep specialist at the University of Pittsburgh Medical Center in Pennsylvania. "That doesn't make them the most satisfying bed partners."

The first step toward a good night's sleep is to listen to what your body tells you and respond to it, just as you respond to the messages it gives you about your food intake or workout regimen. Generally speaking, you need between seven and nine hours of sleep a night, although a small percentage of people can get away with six and some of us don't feel right with less than nine.

When you awaken in the morning, you should feel well-rested, if not refreshed. Throughout the day, you should feel alert and functional. If you fall asleep within three or four minutes of hitting the sack at night, you may need more sleep than you're getting; well-rested people generally take between fifteen and twenty minutes to fall asleep.

And don't begrudge yourself the sleep you need, even if it's a bit over the average. In a study of twenty-four healthy men who typically slept seven or eight hours a night, Timothy Roehrs, Ph.D., director of research at the Sleep Disorders Center at Henry Ford Hospital in Detroit, found that extending the subjects' sleep to ten hours per night for six nights reduced daytime sleepiness, increased alertness and improved performance on mental tests. While you may not be able to sleep for ten hours a night, even one extra hour may help your mood and performance considerably.

7

SEXUALITY

An erection, too, defies gravity, flirts with it precariously. . . . Men's bodies, at this juncture, feel only partly theirs; a demon of sorts has been attached to their lower torso, whose performance is erratic and whose errands seem, at times, ridiculous. It is like having a (much) smaller brother toward whom you feel both fond and impatient; if he is you, it is you in a curiously simplified and ignoble form.

—JOHN UPDIKE

I s it any wonder that the dearly departed King of Rock & Roll used to refer to his penis as Little Elvis? That nickname—and the many others like it—speaks volumes about how a man views his sexuality. Our whole vocabulary for referring to our sex organs ("That thing has a mind of its own") hints of a certain detachment (in the non-Bobbitt sense) we have from our sexual selves. After all, when was the last time you heard a woman give a pet name to her vagina?

Where women may see their genitals and their sexuality as fundamental parts of themselves, men view their penises Janus-faced and cross-eyed. The penis is ruled alternately by both the good and bad angels of our nature: it leads, and we follow. Women have the reproductive cycle, inextricably linked to the phases of the moon and the rhythm of the universe. For men, the penis is an erratic divining rod to the eternal mysteries of life, to the places that we can never fully understand.

For a man to fathom his own sexuality is challenge enough. It is a much more ambitious goal to try to understand what sex means for women. That's an endeavor worth a lifetime of study—and a topic too ambitious for these pages. But for starters, perhaps we can learn something about male sexuality by exploring a particularly mysterious aspect of women's sexuality: the female orgasm.

A LAYMAN'S GUIDE TO A WOMAN'S ORGASM

Was it good for you? Did you like it? (Probably, you did.) But what about her? Her movements, pulsations and moans are mysteries to you. Which shudders signify pleasure and which ones discomfort, frustration or dissatisfaction?

Appearances to the contrary, male and female orgasms feel very similar. Says Kenneth Reamy, M.D., professor of gynecology and psychiatry at West Virginia University Health Sciences Center, "Written descriptions of orgasms by men and women are indistinguishable." Here's what is different: Many women take longer to become aroused and climax than men do, but they also rate higher in the variety of orgasms they experience. Like most men, some women have one intense explosion, after which a second orgasm may be unlikely. Others will climax, then experience a slight drop and subsequent rise in arousal, often followed by another orgasm. Still others may have one "big" orgasm, followed by a succession of smaller ones—kind of a ripple effect.

Multiple orgasms are a huge source of fascination for men. While many women do have the capacity for them, they shouldn't be the goal of lovemaking; any pressure by either party is self-defeating. According to Lonnie Barbach, Ph.D., a sex therapist, psychologist and author, "A single, terrific climax is perfectly satisfying for most women." Barbach describes a female client who claimed to have 100 orgasms in 15 minutes using a vibrator but says that person's experience isn't necessarily better than that of the woman who has one intense orgasm.

Are orgasms essential to women's enjoyment of sex? Generally speaking, yes. The twist is, they don't necessarily expect them to happen during intercourse. In fact, about half of American women don't climax consistently or easily that way. Some 25 percent say they've never even had a coital orgasm. That doesn't mean they don't get a kick out of vaginal sex; most sex therapists agree that women find intercourse pleasurable whether they climax during the act or not.

But the orgasm should fit into a woman's sex life somewhere, and that's where the clitoris comes in. Use a finger, your tongue, or . . . well, use your imagination, but remember this: According to *The Kinsey Institute New Report on Sex*, 75 percent of women require some kind of clitoral stimulation in order to climax. Before and/or during intercourse, it's the key to female orgasm. (Though intercourse alone generally doesn't provide direct stimulation of the clitoris, there are coital positions and techniques that lend themselves to increased clitoral contact; more on these later.)

Some women climax noisily—panting, moaning, yelling; others are virtually silent. Some women thrash around; others barely move at all. But physiologically the process is the same: As orgasm nears, breathing becomes more rapid, muscles tense, and the vaginal opening narrows, gripping the penis more tightly (a sensation the man may or may not feel). With orgasm, a series of muscular contractions, lasting several seconds, occurs in the vaginal, uterine and anal areas.

"There's a whole range of female orgasmic response," says Carol Ellison, Ph.D., a clinical psychologist who, with psychologist Bernie Zilbergeld, Ph.D., has studied female sexuality. "Sometimes a woman's muscular contractions and her whole orgasm are very powerful and intense. Other times, orgasm is just a gentle wave of release."

If you think your partner isn't having orgasms, talk to her about it (though not while you're making love). The best approach, Barbach says, is the caring and direct one. For instance: "What do you like and not like about our sex life? Is there something I can do to make our sex life better?"

If she masturbates, that's good for her. And for you. David Hurlbert, a marital and sex therapist at the Adult and Adolescent Counseling Center in Belton, Texas, found that women who masturbated on a regular basis had orgasms through a variety of sexual acts with partners (intercourse, oral sex, manual stimulation), while the vast majority of women who didn't masturbate could only climax with their partners during oral-vaginal sex. In addition, if she knows how to explore her own terrain, she can more easily guide you toward her pleasure.

Vibrators have become increasingly popular among couples as well. Besides adding variety to your sexual sessions, these devices provide an almost surefire way to give your partner an orgasm—especially useful if she's in the mood and you're not.

Apart from the thrill of an occasional quickie, the key to pleasurable sex for a woman, Barbach says, lies in three words: "foreplay, foreplay, foreplay." Let your partner's responses guide you. It's usually best to talk about lovemaking preferences, turn-ons and other sexual "positives" in bed, but save discussions about sexual difficulties and turn-offs for later.

Keeping in mind that each woman has her individual sexual preferences, here are a couple of general tips.

- Go easy on the clitoris; it's highly sensitive. Start out gently, with fingers or tongue touching only lightly and sporadically and gradually building up to direct pressure as she becomes more aroused. "As a woman approaches orgasm," Barbach says, "it's useful for her partner to keep on doing whatever he's doing and maintain a steady rhythm. This isn't the time to vary the pace, pressure or activity." More rapid breathing, increased muscle tension throughout her body and a tendency to focus on herself rather than you are all signs that she's about to climax.

- If you both want her to have orgasms during intercourse, here's how you can raise your odds: 1) Relax; make clear that it's no big deal either way. Trying too hard can backfire. 2) Get into positions that allow you or her to touch her clitoris during intercourse; rear-entry and woman-on-top positions are your best bets. In fact, if she's on top, the pressure of her clitoris against your pelvic bone might do the trick. 3) Try the coital alignment technique (CAT), a new twist on the old missionary position in which you rest your body against hers, positioning yourself far forward between her legs so the shaft of your penis presses against her clitoral area. With this technique, instead of thrusting, the two of you move your pelvises together in short, rocking motions. (CAT is discussed in more detail in the following section.)

The one surefire way to demystify the female orgasm is to simply talk. "The best teacher for you is the woman you're with," Ellison says. "And if she doesn't really know what she wants sexually—some women don't—the two of you can experiment together. "

TERRA INCOGNITA:
THE FEMALE SEXUAL ANATOMY

Clitoris: Located where the labia minora join on top (the forward part) of the vaginal opening. For most women, it's by far the most sexually sensitive part of the genitals. It's also the only human organ whose sole function is sexual sensation. Like the penis, the clitoris contains specialized nerve endings so it gets erect when a woman is aroused.

Graefenberg spot: The "G-spot" according to some sex researchers, is a dime-sized area on the vagina's front wall that's very sensitive to sexual stimulation. While there is still no conclusive evidence that it exists, some women report that the area is stimulated by penile thrusting, which can trigger orgasm.

Labia majora: Literal translation: "large lips." These are the larger folds of flesh around the vaginal opening.

Labia minora: "Small lips," located inside the labia majora. These are sexually sensitive and swell with blood when a woman is excited.

Mons veneris (or mons): The cushiony, hair-covered mound of flesh over a woman's pubic bone.

Vagina: About four to five inches long (it lengthens when a woman is aroused), it's more like a drawstring purse than a canal or tunnel; vaginal walls touch each other and mold themselves around whatever goes inside.
Vulva: The outer, visible part of the genitals, including the vaginal opening.

COITAL ALIGNMENT TECHNIQUE

The Kama Sutra, an ancient hindu love catalog of sorts, never once mentioned it. China's Taoist masters never mentioned it, either. Miriam Stoppard's *The Magic of Sex* has more than one hundred photos, none of which illustrate it. Alex Comfort's *The Joy of Sex*, twenty-four years old and still going, has helped millions of people achieve happier sex lives without ever once referring to it.

"It" is the Coital Alignment Technique, or CAT, a new variation on the old missionary position. As outlined in *The Perfect Fit*, written by sex therapist and researcher Edward Eichel, the promise of CAT is that we can "achieve mutual fulfillment and monogamous passion through the new intercourse."

Here's how CAT works: The man enters the woman in the standard missionary position, resting his weight on his elbows. Now he makes what Eichel calls "a small but significant adjustment": He shifts his pelvis a couple of inches higher, into an "override" position. Then he takes his weight off his elbows and rests the full length of his upper body flat over his partner's, distributing it evenly. She, in turn, wraps her legs around his thighs and rests her feet on his calves, keeping her pelvis flat.

In that position, thrusting is virtually nonexistent. Instead, the partners gently rock their pelvises: She presses upward with enough force to lift him two inches or so while he resists a little; then he presses downward while she resists. With this basic pattern, the couple can either climax quickly or make a weekend of it.

What makes CAT work, in theory, is that the base of the penis is in constant contact with the clitoris—a boon for both woman and man, says Eichel, who asserts that men have an erogenous zone at the base of the penis. For the man, the position offers the control of the top position without the responsibility of having to do all the work. For the woman, the position offers a slow, steady rhythm and lots of clitoral stimulation. Eichel says both partners will experience orgasm in a much more mutually satisfying way and, quite often, score the Loch Ness Monster of sex: the rarely seen but often-discussed simultaneous climax.

If there's a drawback to CAT, it's that the technique takes time to learn. And the single man who's not in a committed relationship will have to file the information away for a time down the road when he's more settled. But Eichel, a fan of marriage and monogamy, says the complications of the technique are no vice. "There's a natural design to it," he says. "You're learning something as natural as swimming. You don't complain that you have to learn to swim."

But what about men who practice CAT? Wouldn't they miss the sort of deep thrusting that, after all, is our most natural post-pubertal physical reflex? No, Eichel says. Intense thrusting dulls sensitivity, moving the body's focus away from the pelvis and into such muscular areas as the lower back and abdomen. CAT does just the opposite, increasing sensation in the groin while relaxing the major muscle groups. More important, he says, is that it makes men and women equal partners in the sex act. "The man is not 'doing it' to the woman," he says. "She's just as active, and it's just as dependent on her motion. She has to do her part or it doesn't work."

Fair enough, but how about this: Shouldn't there be some variety? Doesn't having sex in the same position every time, even if it's a great position, get old? Eichel, who has been married since 1975, says that in his experience and that of his patients, it doesn't. "Foreplay will always vary according to individual tastes," he says, "and each time [CAT] happens, there can be variation in the intensity. It kind of has a life of its own."

"Sex has always been a mystery," Eichel concludes, "and [with CAT] it stops being one. The mystery is in love, not in the sex act."

1. Assume the standard missionary position with your partner.
2. Slide forward, with your pelvis above hers and the base of your penis in direct contact with her clitoris. Rest your entire torso on hers.
3. Maintaining full-body contact, your partner presses upward, lifting you about two inches as you gently resist. Then you press down about two inches as she gently resists. Continue that rocking motion with neither partner shifting weight or going for deeper thrusts.
4. If you lose your erection, shift back to the standard missionary position and thrust until you're back at attention. Then start again at step 1.

MULTIPLE ORGASMS—FOR MEN

Imagine being able to achieve five orgasms in a row without losing your erection. Sound impossible? According to William Hartman, Ph.D., and Marilyn Fithian, D.A., with a little practice any man can. *Any Man Can* is, in fact, the title of the book that earned Hartman and Fithian the distinction of being the first sexologists to present scientific proof of the existence of multiorgasmic men. Their work was based on laboratory data recorded at the Center for Marital and Sexual Studies (CMSS) in Long Beach, California, during an eighteen-year clinical study of the arousal and response patterns of men and women during masturbation and coitus.

In the course of their study, the pair logged 10,000 hours of physiological research and monitored the orgasms of 751 volunteers. Of the 282 men studied, 33 proved multiorgasmic. "Our most prolifically orgasmic subject was an athletic young man we call John," Hartman recalls. "He holds the record: 16 orgasms in a 50-minute period. We tested John once a week for 25 weeks, and he consistently gave us the same results, both in volume and intensity."

If you never considered yourself multiply orgasmic, you're not alone. According to Hartman, most naturally multiorgasmic men—an estimated 10 to 15 percent of the male population—remain unaware of their sexual potential.

"The problem is that men fail to make a distinction between orgasm and ejaculation," Hartman explains. You can experience orgasm without ejaculating. In fact, the key to multiple orgasms is controlling the release of ejaculate. In the multiple-orgasm phenomenon, a man experiences repeated climactic feelings by using one of several techniques to inhibit complete ejaculation. Little or no ejaculatory fluid accompanies the early orgasms, and more accompanies the later orgasms.

In the CMSS lab, multiple orgasms were impossible to fake. Hartman and Fithian used highly sensitive instruments to monitor and record eight separate sets of data. The most important was the subject's cardiovascular rate, which showed a direct correlation with the level of arousal.

Using this cardiovascular-response data, the researchers could identify two distinct types of multiple orgasm. "The first," Hartman says, "which is generally experienced by some women, consists of a series of discrete orgasms. The heart rate starts at a baseline of 70 beats per minute and peaks at approximately 120, then returns to a resting state before peaking again. The second type, the continuous orgasm, is the kind almost all multiply orgasmic men experience. Here, the heart rate peaks at around 150 beats per minute and drops down to only 130 before going right back up again."

When beginning his study, Hartman had not expected to find a multiple-orgasm response in males. By his own admission he'd never even considered the phenomenon. "A student from the university came to my office one day and said, 'I want to teach men to be multiorgasmic,'" Hartman recalls. "I was very skeptical, so I invited him to be tested in the lab. The results were exciting—the data showed he had three or four continual orgasms."

Based on his work with several such male subjects, Hartman designed a training program through which, he maintains, almost any man can teach himself to become multiply orgasmic within six months.

"The secret to achieving multiple orgasms," Hartman says, "lies in learning to control ejaculation via the pubic, or pubococcygeus (PC), muscle," which runs from the pubic bone in front to the coccyx, or tailbone, in back. Also known as the voluntary urinary sphincter muscle, the PC muscle starts and stops the flow of urine. Once strengthened, it can provide the same sort of control over ejaculation. "Just prior to the moment of ejaculatory inevitability [more on that later], you clench the PC tight and hold it until the urge to ejaculate passes—roughly fifteen seconds."

According to Hartman, men in good physical condition are the quickest learners. "Orgasms come more easily when you're in good shape," he notes. "You'll climax at a lower heart rate and rate the orgasm as more intense than will less fit men. They have to struggle to reach orgasm, and when it's over they don't have the energy to continue."

Hartman's program focuses on two separate concerns: learning to identify the moment of ejaculatory inevitability, and educating and strengthening the PC muscle. The former is of critical importance: Squeeze the PC muscle prematurely and you won't reach orgasm. Squeeze too late, and you'll be unable to postpone ejaculation—and once you've ejaculated, continual orgasms are no longer possible.

Identifying the moment of ejaculatory inevitability requires at least a cursory understanding of the mechanics of ejaculation. During sexual arousal, sperm from the testicles and seminal fluid from the prostate gland accumulate at separate points near the ejaculatory duct. When the level of arousal peaks and ejaculation becomes inevitable, the seminal fluid is suddenly released from the seminal vesicles, washing the sperm into the urethral bulb. From there, the mixture is then propelled down the urethra and out the penis. The moment of ejaculatory inevitability is the split-second before the release of the seminal fluid.

Unfortunately, you'll feel no tingle or twinge to signal the impending release of seminal fluid. However, certain pleasurable sensations can be used as signposts, and to discover these Hartman suggests masturbating while you experiment with the squeeze technique to inhibit ejaculation. He explains, "Each time you get close to the point of ejaculatory inevitability, you squeeze the penis just below the tip to halt the release of ejaculate."

Once you've experienced your first set of multiple orgasms, Hartman advises that you continue to use the squeeze technique, either alone or with a lover, to train your body to sustain increasingly longer orgasmic periods. "This is something you can begin immediately and continue doing because it will take a couple of months of 'muscle education' before you can control with the PC muscle what you controlled with your hand at the outset," the sexologist says. "Your goal is to be able to masturbate and climax for at least fifteen or twenty minutes this way. "

Another technique for delaying ejaculation, one that's particularly suitable when you're with a partner, is to gently pull the testicles away from your body just before the moment of ejaculatory inevitability. During ejaculation the testicles are drawn tightly up against the perineum, and you won't be able to ejaculate unless they're fully elevated. However, as with the squeeze technique, you will still be able to experience orgasm with them descended.

The second part of Hartman's program aims at developing the PC muscle, which is most easily trained by adopting a regimen of exercises known as Kegels. Named after the late gynecologist Arnold Kegel, M.D., who developed the program to aid pregnant women who were suffering from incontinence, Kegels are designed to provide conscious control over an otherwise involuntary physiological event.

Once ejaculation has begun, muscles within the penis involuntarily contract at 0.8-second intervals, propelling the semen down the urinary tract. If, just prior to ejaculation, you clench the PC muscle and hold it tight for ten to fifteen seconds, you suppress the urge to ejaculate and experience only orgasm.

To familiarize yourself with the workings of the muscle, Hartman suggests that you practice stopping and starting the urine flow while facing the toilet. "This way you identify the muscle and get used to squeezing it," he explains. The next step is to begin a regular program of Kegels. "It's best to do them before you get out of bed in the morning because when you're standing or sitting, the weight of your internal organs presses down on the muscle," Hartman notes. "Then, you can repeat the exercises throughout the day, no matter what position you're in."

The first phase of exercises focuses on flexing, or flicking, the PC muscle—that is, raising and lowering the penis by tightening and relaxing the muscle. "You should begin with maybe ten flicks in the morning and increase the number by five each day until you get up to forty or fifty, " Hartman recommends. "Then you can add clenching-and-holding exercises to the routine. Begin with two or three reps, tightening and holding each for three or four seconds. Gradually increase the time to fifteen seconds and add two more reps. Doing five of these five days a week is plenty." But Hartman cautions against over-zealousness. "It's like any other exercise program," he warns. "If you go too far too fast, you'll end up sore."

Are these people for real? Or are multiple male orgasms nothing more than a hoax? Hartman and Fithian, who've presented their findings to countless international gatherings of scientists, maintain that their data bear them out. The vast majority of their colleagues agree. If you're one of those who'd like to try this technique, and you'd like further information, you can write to Drs. Hartman and Fithian at the Center for Marital and Sexual Studies, 5251 Los Altos Plaza, Long Beach, CA 90815.

CEREBRAL SEX

You love the woman in your life. She's a terrific companion and a wonderful lover. But sometimes when you're making love, you imagine that you're with Kim Basinger or Michelle Pfeiffer or the new waitress at your favorite lunch spot. Moreover, your thoughts turn to sex several times a day—all right, dozens of times. You're mesmerized by the curves on every woman you see.

Your sexual fantasies usually don't worry you—even Jimmy Carter admitted to having lusted in his heart—but occasionally they seem, well, excessive. Sometimes you wonder: Am I obsessed with sex? Are my fantasies putting my relationship in jeopardy?

No on both counts. Sex fantasies are incredibly common for most men. In one study discussed in *The Kinsey Institute New Report on Sex*, men were asked how frequently they thought about sex. The average teenager, to no one's surprise, reported having a sexual thought every five minutes; the average fortysomething guy admitted to having one once every half-hour.

To be sure, not all sexual thoughts are technically fantasies, but most are. This means that, assuming 18 waking hours per day, the average guy from age 16 to 49 has somewhere between 36 and 216 sexual thoughts and/or fantasies daily. Having frequent fantasies doesn't mean you're obsessive. In truth, entertaining an even hundred or so a day puts you smack dab in the middle of the normal range.

If you're a recent convert to fitness, you're probably fantasizing more than ever. Researchers at the University of California, San Diego, studied ninety-five healthy but sedentary men averaging forty-five years old. Some were asked to participate in strenuous aerobics, others to take nonaerobic walks. After nine months, the walkers reported no change in sexual behavior, whereas the aerobics group boasted major increases in frequency of kissing, caressing, intercourse and orgasm at home. This makes perfect sense: Fitness celebrates the body, and men who become fit celebrate in more ways than one. In turn, positive reinforcement ensures that those who engage in sex more frequently also fantasize about it more often.

Still, many people feel guilty about their sexual fantasies. "They're very concerned that their fantasies are 'abnormal' or 'immoral' or 'mental cheating' on their relationship," explains Suzana Cado, Ph.D., a psychotherapist based in Landover, Maryland. Cado surveyed 178 adults (77 men and 101 women, ages 18 to 83, with 30 as the average age for the men, 25 for the women) and discovered that 84 percent admitted having other-lover fantasies during intercourse. (The true figure is probably higher because some people who have sex fantasies don't 'fess up.) Yet more than one-quarter of that 84 percent expressed guilt about their trysts with these imaginary lovers.

Why? "These fantasies may raise questions about their commitment to their real-life relationship," Cado speculates. A man in an unhappy relationship who has recurrent fantasies about one particular other woman might interpret his daydreaming as an indication that it's time to seek out some change. But for those in basically happy relationships, sex experts say, fantasies of other people do not imply any loss of interest in the primary relationship. "Many people have fantasies about what they'd do if they won the lottery," says San Francisco sex therapist Louanne Cole, Ph.D. "That doesn't mean they hate their [current] lives."

What about "bizarre" fantasies you'd never want to act out in real life? They're fine, too, experts agree. The range of images people find arousing is usually broader than the range of activities they enjoy. But if your fantasies begin to horrify you or start to interfere with your life—your job, your relationship, your family—you should see a therapist.

Despite the benefits, many a man who accepts his own fantasies might resent learning that his lover has dreamt of Mel Gibson and not him. "That's understandable," Klein says. "In our culture, men are taught that it's okay for them to have free-floating sexual desire, but in women, that same indiscriminate sexual desire is seen as unladylike. Women are supposed to desire sex only with a particular partner, their man."

If the thought of your lover having fantasies about William Baldwin upsets you, Klein suggests trying to rechannel your feelings into the arousal between you. "What men want from women is sexual responsiveness," he explains. "Women who fantasize get more turned on, and usually become more responsive, so women's sexual fantasies have a payoff for men."

So give yourself and your partner permission to have fantasies. Just try not to get lost in them when you're crossing busy streets, dealing with your boss or operating farm machinery. After all, there's a time and place for everything.

BEYOND CONDOMS

We've figured out how to send men to the moon, develop babies in test tubes, even build artificial hearts, and still, guys have just two birth control options of their own: condoms and vasectomies. That scenario promises to change in the near future, giving men real choices where few existed before. There aren't any magic solutions in store, but present methods are improving, with breakthroughs on the horizon. Here, a few words intended to raise your hopes about future prospects.

As you probably know condoms are the only (relatively) reliable, reversible birth-control method available to men right now. They help protect against sexually transmitted diseases—notably HIV—which makes them current as well. Yet, frankly, men find wearing a condom as much fun as bathing in a wet suit.

Thankfully, condoms are improving. According to Adam Glickman, co-founder of four Condomania stores nationwide, today's state-of-the-art condoms are a far cry from the old drugstore models. Condomania stocks over 300 types, including extra-small, extra-large, extra-thin and extra-strength. Says Glickman, "In the future, plastic condoms are going to make latex obsolete. They'll be twenty times thinner, have fewer defects, and they'll be heat-conductive." In the meantime, Glickman offers this advice: "Put a drop of water-based lubricant in the tip before putting the condom on. It increases sensitivity by as much as 50 percent."

The much-maligned rhythm method has theoretical efficacy rates as high as 99 percent, with a rate closer to 80 percent (depending on which variety of the rhythm method is used and how careful the participants are). Women can monitor their body temperatures and other physical signals such as their cervical mucus to determine when they're fertile, so couples can either abstain or use barrier methods during fertile periods. Withdrawing before orgasm is (let's face it) not the intuitive choice, so failure rates for coitus interruptus are high. Moreover, enough sperm may be present in pre-ejaculatory fluid to cause a pregnancy.

Then there's vasectomy. It's simple, effective and safe. The only real drawback is its permanence. "I can put anyone back together after a vasectomy, but I can't promise a pregnancy," says andrologist Cappy Rothman,

M.D., a clinical instructor at UCLA. "This is a form of sterilization, not contraception," meaning that vasectomy should be treated as a decision for the long haul. In fact, Rothman advises vasectomy patients to use a sperm bank: "It's a lot easier and more reliable than trying to reverse the surgery."

A new, no-scalpel method may allay the fear associated with vasectomy. The physician clamps the vas deferens (the tube that transports sperm from the testicles) near the surface of the skin, injects a local anesthetic and punctures the skin with a small instrument that severs the vas. The procedure takes less than fifteen minutes, is performed in the doctor's office and is safer than traditional vasectomy. (For information and a list of performing surgeons, send a SASE to Association for Voluntary Surgical Contraception, 79 Madison Avenue, New York, NY 10016).

Researchers at the Population Council are working on a contraceptive implant for men that's similar to Norplant, a device for women that works for five years, to suppress sperm production. The implant will consist of two capsules. One contains a drug called LHRH 13, which will interrupt the function of LHRH, a hormone that regulates production of two others responsible for sperm production. The second capsule will contain MENT, a synthetic androgen to replace male hormones affected by LHRH 13. Rosemarie Thau, Ph.D., director of contraceptive development for the Population Council, says the implants won't be available before the turn of the century.

The World Health Organization is sponsoring a worldwide study of testosterone enanthate (TE) injections. By raising testosterone levels, the injections signal the body to curtail sperm production. According to C. Alvin Paulsen, M.D., professor emeritus of medicine at the University of Washington and head of the Seattle arm of the study, more than 60 percent of TE test subjects achieved *azoospermia*—lack of sperm—within six months of commencing weekly TE injections. Short-term side effects were limited to weight gain, irritability, increased libido and acne and didn't occur in all subjects. Researchers expect introductory trials to begin by the year 2000.

The real stumbling block, says Paulsen, is marketability. "Obviously, weekly injections represents a concept, not a product," he explains. Thus, researchers are working on shots that last months, instead of days. Unfortunately, TE is also years away from the marketplace.

The likelihood of a male Pill is slim since, for men, oral drugs aren't as effective as injections or implants. On the other hand, after literally centuries of inactivity on male contraceptives, new ideas are out there. But even if methods get better and safer and cheaper and easier, will men use them?

Skeptics abound. "I think most men think the current situation is fine," says Lisa Kaeser, a policy analyst with the Alan Guttmacher Institute, a nonprofit research, policy-analysis and public-education organization. "Of course, there are enlightened men who want to share the responsibility, but a lot of men would have problems putting hormones in their systems every month, as women do now. I think a lot of men would rather not think about it."

Birth control isn't fun, but it's a Mardi Gras compared to the cosmic costs of unwanted pregnancy, when a man's choices are minimal at best. And judging by the latest advances, those choices won't be as limited in years to come.

SEXUALLY TRANSMITTED DISEASES

Unless you've been involved in an absolutely monogamous relationship for several years, beware. Today's sexually active man needs to guard against a host of virulent afflictions—and guard is an active verb here: Many give little warning that they've taken up residence in your body, one attribute that's allowed them to quietly reach epidemic proportions in the past decade. They used to be called venereal diseases, or VD. Today they're known as sexually transmitted diseases (shortened to STDs). In their case, ignorance isn't bliss; it's misery.

According to the Centers for Disease Control in Atlanta, about six million men and women in the United States contract either gonorrhea, syphilis or chlamydia yearly. An estimated 30 million Americans are infected with genital herpes, an incurable, often painful disease that claims 500,000 new victims every year and appears to double the risk of HIV infection, at least among heterosexuals, according to two separate studies. The number of new cases of venereal warts, caused by the human papilloma virus (HPV for short), has mushroomed by 500 percent in the past decade. Despite some encouraging recent changes in our sexual behavior, experts believe that STDs will remain at record levels for years to come.

We have good reason to be concerned: What makes STDs particularly insidious is that most prove difficult to detect. Consequently, they're more likely to be transmitted, and victims are more apt to delay treatment until the disease reaches an advanced state. If allowed to progress unchecked, certain STDs can cause permanent damage, including blindness, cancer, heart disease and death.

For example, the telltale symptoms of gonorrhea in a man, which include a burning sensation during urination and a nasty discharge from the penis, normally surface within seven to ten days. In a woman, however, the infection can remain localized in the vagina and go unnoticed for a long time; in the meantime, she's highly contagious to unprotected sexual partners.

Initial syphilis symptoms might not appear for up to twelve weeks after infection, and since they disappear spontaneously, many victims are left with a false sense of security. The first sign of syphilis is a painless, shallow ulcer, called a chancre, which appears at the site where the bacteria entered the body, such as on the lips or genitals. The lesion normally heals within two weeks, but the infection has only begun. If it's not knocked down with antibiotics, the second stage is a total-body rash, sometimes appearing even on the palms or soles, accompanied by flulike symptoms. These also disappear. Untreated, the disease quietly progresses into its late stages, during which it attacks internal organs, bones and the brain, ultimately causing blindness and death.

The task of controlling the spread of these communicable diseases falls to a nationwide system of county-funded health agencies. All physicians are required by law to report the names of people they treat for syphilis and gonorrhea—and various other diseases as mandated by individual states—to their local health agency. Investigators then interview each patient and make sure that each of his or her sexual contacts is warned of the possibility of infection. Without their efforts, STDs would spread like wildfire.

Over the past decade, however, these agencies have had to cope with shrinking budgets and epidemic levels of AIDS-related ailments. As a result, they've been unable to keep enough investigators in the field, thus making it increasingly difficult for them to keep traditional STDs in check.

To complicate matters, some county STDs programs saw their caseloads quadruple when chlamydia was added to the list of STDs physicians are required to report. Chlamydia, which has most of the same symptoms as gonorrhea, is not a new disease. It was previously placed in the catch-all category of nonspecific urethritis or vaginitis. However, when diagnostic lab tests for the disease were developed, it was given a listing of its own.

Genital herpes and genital warts are two other types of STD that are reaching epidemic proportions; together they afflict an estimated one in every four adults in America and claim 1.5 million new victims annually. These STDs first gained notoriety during the seventies. Twenty years later, researchers are just now learning to control them.

Although it's one of the most agonizing genital afflictions, herpes, caused by the herpes simplex II virus, by itself rarely causes serious health complications in adults. When an outbreak occurs, small red bumps, which quickly develop into painful, open blisters, appear on or near the genitals. The body's immune system immediately begins to fight off the infection, and after a few days or weeks the sores crust over and begin to heal. The virus then retreats down into the nerve tissues, where it lies dormant until the next active episode, resurfacing up to twelve times each year, depending upon the individual.

Herpes is transmitted through skin contact with an active site, even if an ulcer hasn't yet appeared. Researchers have discovered that a person with herpes simplex I, which causes "cold sores" around the mouth, can infect his or her partner's genitals if they engage in oral sex during an outbreak. And no part of the body is immune to the virus; while it easily penetrates the thin mucous membranes in the genital and anal areas, herpes also can anchor itself on the upper thighs or abdomen.

Unlike chlamydia, syphilis and gonorrhea—which are infectious at any time—herpes is contagious only just before, during and just after an outbreak, although there's some question as to how long that window of opportunity remains open. Generally, couples are told to refrain from sex as soon as the telltale tingling symptoms signal an imminent outbreak and to abstain until at least four days after the sores have completely healed.

But in a recent study led by infectious-diseases specialist Gregory Mertz of the University of New Mexico in Albuquerque, 10 percent of the healthy partners of genital-herpes sufferers were infected within a year, even though they'd been advised to avoid sex during outbreaks. Most of those infections occurred when no ulcers were evident. Condoms were a big deterrent to transmission: Of the twenty-one couples who routinely used them, twenty made it through the year without the healthy partner becoming infected.

At present, the most effective treatment for herpes is an antiviral drug called acyclovir, marketed under the trade name Zovirax. If taken during a patient's first outbreak, acyclovir often reduces the severity of the episode. In chronic cases, in which recurrences happen as frequently as once a month, daily doses of the drug sometimes eliminate outbreaks altogether.

Genital warts are even more stubborn. Once the human papillomavirus becomes rooted in the soft, moist skin of the penis, vagina or anus, the warts may resist a succession of alternative treatments, even to the point of reappearing after being removed.

Some genital warts can be successfully treated with the drug podophyllin in conjunction with a topical application of trichloracetic acid (TCA), according to David Hardy, M.D., assistant professor of medicine at

UCLA and an infectious-diseases specialist. "This works as an irritant and causes an inflammatory reaction," Hardy explains. "It often requires multiple therapies and is most effective on small warts. However, it is potentially carcinogenic."

If podophyllin proves ineffective, other treatments may help. The physician may perform cryotherapy, which entails freezing the wart with liquid nitrogen or chilled metal probes. Electrocautery and laser therapy can burn warts off. Another option is to inject the drug interferon, an immune-system stimulant, directly into the wart. Although effective, interferon therapy is almost prohibitively expensive.

The most dangerous aspect of genital herpes and genital warts is that they increase the risk of contracting the AIDS virus and certain types of cancer. Five strains of HPV have been associated with cancer of the penis and cervix, while an open herpes sore, like the ulcer that accompanies a syphilis infection, provides an excellent avenue through which the AIDS virus can enter the bloodstream. "The tragedy is that we haven't discovered a vaccine for a single one of these diseases," Fannon laments. "I keep hearing there's not enough money for research, but given the number of victims, that's hard to understand."

While we may not yet be able to vaccinate against STDs, we can do much to prevent transmission by using condoms in conjunction with a spermicidal cream or gel. Studies have shown that contraceptives containing the spermicide nonoxynol–9 can kill the microbes that cause herpes, chlamydia, syphilis and gonorrhea. Latex condoms offer further protection by providing a physical barrier through which neither bacteria nor viruses can pass. In the case of herpes, though, the condom protects only the shaft of the penis and so leaves your testicles and thighs vulnerable.

In putting on a condom, as in lifting weights, form is everything if you want to avoid an exercise in futility. To be effective for both partners, the rubber must be used correctly. This means that you 1) put it on before engaging in oral, genital or even manual contact, 2) carefully roll it down over your erect penis so as not to tear it with fingernails, teeth or whatever, and 3) hold on to it when you withdraw after achieving climax so that you take your ejaculate—and your protection—with you when you leave. Finally, since condoms deteriorate with age, keep a fresh batch on hand, and, of course, never use the same one twice.

Other than that, the main thing to remember is that you need to be on guard in all nonmonogamous sexual relationships. A condom is your first line of defense. Always seek treatment at the first sign of trouble. That burning sensation in your penis may be due to something as harmless as a mild case of nonspecific urethritis that will clear up in a couple of days. On the other hand, it may be caused by an insidious infection that, if left untreated, will cripple you for life. The only way to know for certain is to see a doctor.

AIDS

Myth number one about AIDS: It's a new plague—a scourge that struck out of nowhere in the eighties, scorching the hedonism of the sexual revolution into cinders overnight.

In fact, frozen blood and tissue samples screened for HIV in 1988 fixed the date of the first probable American AIDS death much earlier. A sexually active fifteen-year-old black male, known in the medical files as Robert R., succumbed in St. Louis in 1969 after a sixteen-month illness. So the explosion of new cases that began in the late seventies and early eighties with ominous reports of a strange wasting disease among gay men in New York, Los Angeles and San Francisco was really only the flare-up of an epidemic that apparently had been smoldering unseen for decades.

Now the media and various organizations regularly claim to offer "the facts about AIDS," but often the information is obscured by waves of hysteria that periodically crash around us. Some say that HIV heralds the extinction of the human race, while others embrace another extreme, insisting that the virus is innocuous. A minuscule but vocal minority of scientists, led by Peter Duesberg, a Nobel Prize-winning microbiologist at the University of California at Berkeley, contend that HIV is not, in fact, the cause of AIDS; most reputable researchers emphatically disagree. Others maintain the virus threatens only the traditional risk groups. Such was Michael Fumento's contention in his 1990 book with the self-explanatory title *The Myth of Heterosexual AIDS*.

Throughout these pronouncements, AIDS has continued its relentless spread, with more than 500,000 cases reported in the U.S. so far. If Rock Hudson's 1985 death catapulted awareness of the disease from the gay community into mass-media currency, Magic Johnson's claim in 1991 that he'd been infected by HIV through heterosexual intercourse suggested that the virus doesn't discriminate by sex or sexual preference. Heterosexual AIDS, whatever its prevalence, is no myth.

For the most part, medicine's war against AIDS has been marked by frustrations and obstacles that show few signs of abating. Back in the early eighties, scientists were hoping that a vaccine to protect uninfected people would be available within four or five years. That effort has been far less productive than anyone expected. Even the most optimistic projections say that a first-generation vaccine, available perhaps by the year 2000, would be only about 50 percent effective, certainly not enough to stop the plague in its tracks.

Progress has been somewhat steadier in the development of drugs to treat people who are already infected, but these medications are primarily geared toward controlling the opportunistic infections and organisms associated with late-stage AIDS. HIV itself has so far triumphed over every much-hyped new therapy. One recent sensation, a three-drug cocktail devised by a thirty-one-year-old medical student at Massachusetts General Hospital, was played up in the media as a major breakthrough. Hopes were dashed when an investigative team discovered flaws in his research. Even AZT, the best-documented anti-AIDS medication, took a serious hit when an Anglo-French clinical study suggested that asymptomatic users of the drug were no more likely to ward off eventual illness or death than those who went without it.

Bad enough news for a disease that is painful, disfiguring, overwhelmingly fatal and still, despite all the microscopes focused on it, elusive. AIDS, scientists discovered early on, isn't like other infections. For example, the cellular actions of something like a staph infection or gonorrhea can be charted and usually halted. While the overwhelming evidence is that HIV does indeed cause AIDS, scientists also know it's not HIV that makes you sick. Rather, the virus serves as the doorway to a host of opportunistic invaders otherwise healthy people would have no trouble defeating.

It's not HIV that gives you a typical (and often fatal) AIDS-related pneumonia, but a fungus, *Pneumocystis catinii,* that exploits the vulnerability HIV creates. Another microbe, cytomegalovirus, lives in most humans as a harmless parasite. Unleashed by HIV, it can cause fever, uncontrollable diarrhea, liver failure and blindness. Kaposi's sarcoma, a rare cancer marked by purplish lesions, previously was seen only in elderly Mediterranean men; it is now commonly diagnosed in young AIDS patients.

Also atypical is the long delay between initial infection and the first tangible symptom of illness. Most studies suggest a median lapse of ten years. But some HIV-positive people have remained symptom-free for as long as fifteen years and counting—encouraging if you're HIV-positive, but a conundrum for epidemiologists, since statistics dawdle a maddening decade or more behind the virus.

Just as the disease's spread through the body is complicated, so too is the pattern of its spread through society. In the developed world, men have been the chief targets, with homosexual sex and IV drug use accounting for most infections. But in Africa and the Caribbean, males and females are about equally affected, and heterosexual intercourse is the chief route of transmission.

Such variations don't faze epidemiologists. "Nearly all public-health issues are different in Africa," says D. Peter Drotman, M.D., assistant director for public health in the Centers for Disease Control and Prevention's Division of HIV/AIDS. "It's not as much of a paradox as it seems." Diseases affect public health differently in different cultures, responding to different physical conditions, different medical-care systems and different behaviors.

Which distills to a harsh conclusion: AIDS is here; it's staying; get used to it. Barring a miracle, which nobody in the field is expecting, sobering AIDS statistics are going to form a hard-to-swallow part of our national diet for the foreseeable future. Official projections from the CDC are for a gradual increase to 50,000 or 60,000 new cases per year. And don't count on a cure: Nothing in the pipeline promises one.

Are we defenseless? Emphatically not. Remember, a great deal is known about HIV infection, enough that you can somewhat accurately assess—and substantially lessen—your risk. Start by biting on the harsher facts. Just being American puts you in statistical jeopardy, at least in comparison with people in other industrialized nations. The U.S. has accumulated 1,200 cases of AIDS per 1 million population, three times the rate in Spain and ten times that in the United Kingdom.

While nobody can say for sure where the epidemic will head in the future, the most recent figures make it clear that nobody can blithely assume that AIDS is some other group's worry. In absolute numbers, homosexual and bisexual men remain the most afflicted group; they still account for more than half of all new AIDS cases. And people—male and female, hetero-, homo- and bisexual—with a history of intravenous drug use account for many of the new cases.

Unfortunately, it appears that a second wave of AIDS infection is underway, according to epidemiologists and statisticians. This second wave seems to strike ethnic minorities disproportionately: while new HIV cases rose 11 percent among white males in 1994, the increase for black men was twice that number. Male Hispanics saw a 60 percent increase in HIV cases that same year. Some data indicates that condom use is down among gay men—and infection rates sharply up. Andrew Moss, an epidemiologist at the University of California, San Francisco, projects that for a group of 100 HIV-negative men age 17 when first examined in 1993, 23 will test positive by age 28, and 51 will be positive by age 44. "That [infection rate] is as bad as 1981," he notes.

So, straight or gay, you're vulnerable if you're sexually active. Once an individual is infected, HIV can be found in virtually all body fluids. But the amounts in saliva, breast milk, sweat and tears are so tiny that the risk of infection from these sources seems negligible. Kissing, shallow or deep, seems safe—there is no evidence at all that anyone has ever been infected this way. And AIDS plainly can't be spread through a sneeze, touching, using the same toilet seat or any other casual contact, one fact that Americans finally seem to understand.

But blood, semen and vaginal fluids are dangerous; evidence is overwhelming that they're the major culprits in the spread of the disease among humans. Contaminated blood, of course, is the main vehicle for HIV infection through IV drug use and accidental needle sticks among health workers; it's also a potential danger if it gets onto other, less widely-feared implements, like tattooing needles or ear-piercing equipment.

When it comes to sexual transmission of HIV, semen and vaginal fluids are plainly the major culprits. In hetero sex, women, some experts contend, may be more vulnerable, both because semen carries a larger load of the virus and because of anatomy. Barbara Starrett, M.D., a New York physician with a large AIDS practice, both gay and straight, explains it. "Consider men's plumbing," she says. "A penis is generally well-protected, with good skin around it. The urethral opening is small. Whether it's placed in a vagina or an anus, its potential for [becoming infected with] HIV is much smaller than [that of] the anal or vaginal canal."

Don't breathe a sigh of relief yet. "The insertive male is at less risk," Starrett adds, "but not at nonrisk." While estimates of the relative danger to men and women vary, studies clearly have shown that women can and do pass the infection to men during "normal" sex.

Starrett's take-home advice is practical. "There are ways of getting pleasure without putting anybody at risk," she says. "Men have to learn how to be more sensitive and caring, how to do more holding and kissing, whether they're with men or women. Machismo," she pointedly concludes, "is deadly."

POTENCY PROBLEMS

Ever since man first stood upright, his loins have been depicted as constantly bubbling cauldrons of desire quelled only by the more finicky appetites of the opposite sex. Women, it has been said, get headaches; men get erections.

Of course, the image of the perpetually hard penis has been undergoing more than a little deflation lately. Men's movement author Sam Keen talks frankly about the cycles of desire all men experience, and sex experts increasingly caution that what ultimately derails many men's perfectly normal sex lives is an obsession with unreachable standards of priapic perfection.

But sometimes loss of sexual interest becomes chronic. According to one survey, an estimated 15 percent of American men suffer from what's known as hypoactive sexual desire—a prolonged lack of erotic feeling or activity. Janet L. Wolfe, Ph.D., author of *What to Do When He Has a Headache,* estimates that in 50 to 60 percent of relationships in which lack of sex has become a problem, it's the man who has turned off. Clinically, hypoactive sexual desire means having sexual urges, fantasies and/or activity less than twice a month. Most therapists, however, tend to consider any prolonged and noticeable drop in libido a problem.

"Of all the sexual disorders, this is the one men are least likely to admit to since it's the most devastating," says Eva Margolies, director of New York City's Center for Sexual Recovery and author of *Undressing the American Male.* "It can cause a man to question his virility, and it can plow a deep wedge in a relationship."

In most cases, men with otherwise healthy sex lives may temporarily lose their libido for reasons that can include fatigue, difficulties at work, marital conflict, the birth of a child, medical reasons or, simply, stress. Studies have shown that stress can interfere not just with desire but with actual testosterone production. Many professionals caution against quickly labeling someone who may simply be going through a phase that is temporary and normal.

More chronic sexual aversion may stem from unhealed childhood psychological wounds, including incest. For such men, sex can be a terrifying prospect that best seems avoided. For others in this group, the cause can often be traced to painful, unresolved feelings about their relationship with their mother, says Helen Singer Kaplan, M.D., Ph.D., director of the Human Sexuality Program at the New York Hospital-Cornell Medical Center and author of *Sexual Desire Disorders: 16 Years Later.*

For some men, being sexual is a part of courtship only. "Once the commitment begins," says Kaplan, "they could be dating Cindy Crawford with a trust fund and they'll lose interest." Many such men find that undergoing therapy can help them resolve their problems with commitment.

For others, the cause of low libido is physiological. For example, drugs prescribed to treat high blood pressure (Inderal, Oretic) and anxiety and depression (Prozac, Zoloft) can inhibit arousal, as can depression itself.

Testosterone levels may drop with age, and low levels can be raised by injections or by wearing a patch. However, because these may further diminish the body's natural output of testosterone, any man considering hormone therapy should first determine whether his hypoactive sexual desire is psychological. "Many men have periods when they just aren't having sex and it doesn't mean anything," says Hannah Fox, a psychotherapist in New York City and New Jersey. "If we're too quick to jump to conclusions and put a label on it, it can make someone feel doomed." If you accept sexual down time as a brief intrusion in your cycle of desire and take it as a cue to reduce stress, chances are good that the phase will soon become a distant memory.

GETTING IT BACK

The most important thing to remember if you notice a dip in your desire is not to panic. A diminished sexual craving may work itself out when the stress causing it has been eliminated. But if the problem persists, here are some pointers to keep in mind:

- Get a medical evaluation, including a testosterone-level test, to make sure the problem isn't physiological.
- Talk with your partner to see if you can trace the problem to its cause. When exactly did it begin, and what was going on at the time? Express your feelings honestly and elicit hers. You may be able to find new ways to turn each other on.
- Practice sensate focus, a twenty-minute exercise during which couples touch each other's bodies without sex being the goal. It's a means of becoming more comfortable with physical intimacy while avoiding stress and anxiety.
- Become at ease using fantasy as part of your sex life. Sexually inhibited men are often ashamed of their fantasies and therefore cut them off. Or they may use them to become aroused during masturbation but avoid them during intimate contact.

If the problem continues for more than two or three months, see a therapist who specializes in treating sexual problems (your doctor can recommend one). Unlike premature ejaculation, which tends to remain stable even if untreated, desire disorders may get worse over time since they result in a vicious cycle: The lack of interest causes depression, which only increases the lack of interest.

ARE YOUR SPERM HEALTHY?

In an episode of *Seinfeld,* the character Kramer responds with delirious pride to the discovery that he may have impregnated a woman: "My boys can swim!" he yells.

Arguably, no single event makes a man feel more potent than the discovery that one of his tiny but tenacious "boys" has sailed safely through a woman's viaducts and scored a direct hit, bonding with that persnickety egg.

But the boys don't always succeed the first time out. Reproductive specialists say one out of six couples in the U.S. has trouble conceiving and estimate that the man is lacking spermatic firepower in 35 percent of those cases; some put the number at half. That situation can develop for any number of reasons, many of them reversible. What's pertinent here is what you can do to ensure that your swim team is as strong as it can be.

Most of you have heard that it's better to wear boxer shorts if you're keen on fathering a child. Tight underwear heats up the scrotum, home base to your very own sperm-production factory. And it ideally needs to be a full five degrees cooler than the rest of the body, because sperm are produced more efficiently at slightly lower temperatures.

But what about bike shorts and jockstraps? Your exercise gear is a problem only if you already have a lower-than-ideal sperm count, says Cappy Rothman, M.D., a male-infertility specialist in Los Angeles. "But if your wife can't get pregnant, you might want to reassess the amount of biking you do," he adds.

Another way to get a destructively hot crotch is to lounge around in hot tubs and saunas on a regular basis. Even a fever will temporarily lower sperm production. Since it takes three months to produce new sperm, be aware that your exposure to excessive heat might affect the sperm you produce three months from now.

A hot head, like hot pants, may also impact sperm quality. "Stress is one of the more important factors in male infertility," says Rothman. "I tell my patients not to run their lives as if they were driving a dynamite truck through a forest fire."

If your way of working off stress is a long run, however, you might do your reproductive system more harm than good; excessive exercise can cause you to secrete stress hormones. Rothman explains that marathon runners may have higher levels of adrenal steroids, a stress hormone that lowers the amount of testosterone in their bodies. "This testosterone deficiency in turn decreases sperm production," he says.

A recent study of endurance runners, published in *Fertility and Sterility*, concluded that men who ran more than 65 miles a week had a reduced number of sperm and a higher number of immature sperm. But not all experts agree that distance workouts are counterproductive for would-be fathers. R. Dale McClure, M.D., head of infertility and micro-surgery at Virginia Mason Medical Center in Seattle, did his own study of endurance athletes. "While these men may have had lower counts," he says, "their initial counts were so good that it didn't make a dramatic change."

"We used to think if a man drank too much, took drugs or was exposed to toxins, it might reduce the number of sperm he had but wouldn't damage the hearty few remaining," says Richard B. Johnston, M.D., medical director for the March of Dimes in White Plains, New York, and an adjunct professor of pediatrics at Yale Medical School in New Haven, Connecticut. "It was a survival-of-the-fittest idea—only the strong sperm would make it to the egg. Well, this macho-sperm theory turns out not to be true."

While there are no hard and fast facts on the effects of cigarettes and alcohol on sperm, data suggest that smokers and drinkers are at a higher risk of having a baby with birth defects or low birth weight than those who abstain. "If a man has a compromised sperm count and smokes, he should stop," Rothman says.

Some prescription drugs don't make ideal bed partners for men whose goal is conception. Both McClure and Rothman name two antibi-otics: Azulfidine, used to treat ulcerative colitis, and nitrofurantoin, known commonly as Macrodantin, used for urinary tract infections. McClure adds to the list ketoconazole, prescribed for severe fungal infections (athlete's foot doesn't count).

Most recreational drugs also fall into the don't-know zone. "We have a certain amount of data and a whole lot more suspicion," says Johnston. (Cocaine is a known no-no.) "If you don't want to take any chances, don't take anything that you don't absolutely have to. Stop drinking, smoking, doing drugs and taking any unnecessary medications at least three months before you start working on getting pregnant."

If you're interested in fostering sperm that can go like the Energizer rabbit once they're out of the starting block, you should let them out for training on a regular basis. "If you abstain for too long, say more than five days," explains McClure, "you may have more sperm in your ejaculate. But their motility, because they're older sperm, may decrease."

Old sperm, like sedentary people, are slow-moving. Regular ejacula-tions keep a younger and highly mobile force at the ready. Ejaculate too frequently, though, and you'll deplete those troops. "We recommend that a man who wants to become a father abstain for two to three days before his wife ovulates," says Rothman. "That way you get prime sperm at the prime time."

To ensure that your sperm are healthy and vigorous, you should also take a closer look at your work environment. In 1977, the National Institute for Occupational Safety and Health (NIOSH) in Cincinnati, Ohio, was called in to investigate a strange phenomenon: All the wives of a group of men who worked with a pesticide known as dibromochloropropane (DBCP) were unable to get pregnant. Researchers soon discovered that DBCP significantly reduced or obliterated these workers' sperm counts.

"It was a turning point," says Steven M. Schrader, Ph.D., chief of the functional-toxicology section at NIOSH, "because it was the first study showing that chemicals men work with could affect their sperm production." Since then, a number of hazardous substances have been identified, including lead, paint, radiation, mercury and boron. Most men can recover from exposure to these toxins, producing normal sperm within a year. But McClure points out that in some instances, if the exposure was significant, recovery may take even longer. NIOSH can answer any questions you may have about the safety of your work environment (call 800-35-NIOSH).

Rothman is a proponent of what he calls fertility insurance: "Men working in vocations that could be detrimental to their health, like [being] near radiation or working with chemicals, should consider putting sperm in a sperm bank to ensure their fertility. "

If you're anxious to pass on your twenty-three chromosomes, consider the genes those chromosomes carry, which might include codes for more than just your great teeth and statuesque posture. Medical science has been able to identify people who are carriers of certain genetic diseases, and you might want to participate in a new kind of counseling offered at most medical centers. In the course of genetic counseling, you'll discuss your family's medical history to see if you're at risk for one of a number of hereditary diseases. If so, you can opt for genetic testing, which either evaluates particular proteins in your blood or examines your genes themselves.

Genetic counseling may also be an option if you're older and start a family for the first time. As Rothman explains, "There's more evidence that a male's age could affect his fertility potential and the health of a child." You can contact your local March of Dimes office for more information on genetic diseases. The National Society of Genetic Counselors can't answer questions about specific genetic disorders, but it can locate a counselor near you. Write to them at 233 Canterbury Drive, Wallingford, PA 19086.

Obviously, your fatherly contribution doesn't begin with that orgasm. There's a lot of power in your choices before you even sow the seed. Semen, says Rothman, "is a mirror of a man's state of health. Anything that interferes with his health will interfere with his sperm's health." Respect your sperm, and chances are you'll have a baby who will grow up to be as big and strong as you are.

COMBATING MISCONCEPTIONS

Each year about two million American couples learn they can't have a baby, and it's because of him. As a result, they spend a total of $2 billion a year trying to conceive through artificial means. Now, in a development that lends new meaning to the term *matchmaking*, physicians are able to pluck a single sperm out of the pack and deposit it through a tiny slit directly into the egg's core. The method is a giant step ahead of techniques in which multiple sperm and eggs are thrown together in the hope that they could be coaxed into mating.

ICSI (pronounced "icksy," it stands for intracytoplasmic sperm injection) was first successfully performed by a team of scientists at Brussels Free University in 1992. Since then, there's been an ICSI boom in Belgium; at last count, well over one hundred children had been born as a result of this procedure, a large number when one considers its newness and delicacy. Fertility clinics across the United States are now scrambling to catch up. The technology involved is so cutting-edge that, at last count, only about one hundred pregnancies have been achieved.

ICSI is a refinement of the now-routine, two-decade-old method known as in-vitro fertilization, once considered the last hope for men with very low sperm counts or whose sperm are weak swimmers or misshapen. (By most standards, a "low" sperm count means fewer than 20 million sperm per milliliter of semen; 60 million to 80 million is average.)

In vitro fertilization entails placing semen in a petri dish with eggs extracted from the man's partner. Shortening the distance the sperm must travel to meet up with an egg increases the chance that fertilization will take place. When this first stage succeeds, the resulting embryo is implanted in the woman's uterus. About 17 percent of preliminary tries result in the birth of a child, with success varying by the age of the woman and the clinic where the procedure is performed. Some couples succeed only after repeated fertilization attempts; many never do.

The success rate of in vitro fertilization was enhanced by the addition of a high-tech fertilization procedure known as micromanipulation, in which extremely delicate tools are used to ensure that a sperm and egg connect. In a process called SUZI (subzonal insemination), a superfine needle is used to slip several sperm beneath the egg's protective coat, a process that can take from one-and-a-half to four hours.

Unfortunately, SUZI results in embryos just 25 percent of the time. ICSI takes the technique a step further by leaving even less to chance: A single sperm is injected directly into the egg's core. At first, scientists were amazed, because the conventional wisdom held that breaching the surface of the egg would damage it. But the results have been startling; at some clinics ICSI procedures have produced twice, even three times as many fertilized eggs as SUZI.

Despite the success, some doctors caution that ICSI is not a panacea. Although it results in more fertilizations than other in vitro techniques, the number of actual pregnancies achieved through ICSI remains, in one doctor's words, "not yet spectacular." Even in Belgium, only 28 percent of all fertilizations achieved through ICSI result in ongoing pregnancies or delivered babies. Some of the failures occur when a fertilized egg fails to implant itself to the uterine wall. That deficit, experts say, may be correctable in the near future.

ICSI is expensive, however. In vitro fertilization alone costs between $5,000 and $15,000 (including another $2,000 for fertility drugs), and ICSI adds to the bill; some clinics charge as much as $12,000 to perform the whole process. At this early stage cost still puts ICSI out of reach for many American couples. Belgium has socialized medicine, so infertility treatment is practically free there. But here, some health plans don't even reimburse patients for simple in vitro procedures (Massachusetts now requires insurers to pay, and other states may join this trend).

Observers warn that care should be taken in selecting candidates, since little is known about ICSI's long-term effects. Some worry that manipulating Mother Nature's matchmaking techniques could result in babies born with chromosomal problems. Thus far, most ICSI babies born here and abroad have been healthy. But with few animal studies to draw on, researchers have adopted a wait-and-see attitude.

Finally, some doctors worry that the medical community in the U.S. will be blinded by the flash of modern science and recommend ICSI to patients who could benefit from cheaper, less sophisticated means. After all, male-factor infertility has many causes, and the cures are often relatively simple. But for some couples, this high-tech solution may be the only answer.

PERFORMANCE ANXIETY

It's one o'clock in the morning—do you know where your manhood is? You've been out with this woman since eight o'clock, and everything had seemed so right. From the easygoing hand-holding outside the cafe to the full-mouthed kiss in the parking lot to the fondling in her apartment and the almost instantaneous erection, you were there.

But now it's late and you're running out of ideas. Although each of you is naked and willing, one of you is unable. You're thinking maybe it was the wine, yes the wine, because you don't know why else you would just hang there, limp.

As likely as not, what's happening with your erection—or the inexplicable, terrifying lack thereof—is performance anxiety, a problem that has lots of potential solutions but no surefire ones. Performance anxiety starts with an inordinate focus on the erection and often ends with unbelievable and unsatisfying excuses.

Performance anxiety can halt an erection in its tracks, although most instances have nothing to do with impotence. (Impotence is the inability to get and maintain an erection long enough to complete intercourse in at least 25 percent of attempts.) But there's more to it than that.

Why should men's penises fail them so? Too many demands and unrealistic expectations, which is why the problem might better be called expectation anxiety. Susan Rockwell Campbell, Ph.D., a couples counselor in Columbia, Maryland, relates an example: "I have men who come in saying they have problems with premature ejaculation. 'I can't have intercourse for more than fifteen or twenty minutes [without ejaculating],' they say, and I'm thinking, 'Well, why would you want to?'"

In other words, they wait for their partners to have an orgasm before they have one, and if they can't hold out, they consider themselves failures. Some pressure comes from within, some undoubtedly from their partners. Either way, anxiety ends up hovering about the bedroom during a time that's supposed to be nothing if not blissful and carefree.

Or it may be extreme self-consciousness during sexual activity or a guilty conscience that leads to bad sex, breakups, even divorce. "I see so many couples with this problem," Rockwell says. "I know a lot of couples who are not having intercourse at all anymore, and it started as performance anxiety."

"Having a good partner"—someone to whom you can admit you're anxious—"goes a long way toward correcting the problem," says urologist Kenneth Goldberg, M.D., founder of the Male Health Center in Dallas. "Besides, you don't have to have vaginal intercourse to get pleasure. I see fifty or sixty men a month who have erection problems, and most of them, in an ideal world, wouldn't need to come in," Goldberg says, if they broadened their definition of "normal."

One solution is to take the emphasis off of the sex act itself. William

Masters and Virginia Johnson, the star sex-expert couple, minted the sensate focus method, in which partners "pleasure" each other without working toward the goal of intercourse and orgasm. The idea, to transform foreplay into during play and afterplay, so that play—not performance—will be the emphasis.

Worried men should also remember that women, too, suffer from expectation anxiety. Although women have begun to ask for, even "demand," orgasms, their status in the bedroom hasn't necessarily changed for the better. As Campbell says, "Where men often seem to be hung up on the size of their penis, with women I see far more concern with body image or breast size. They feel their bodies aren't 'perfect' enough. Often, too, a woman will blame herself for her husband's or partner's problem, saying, 'Obviously, I'm not appealing' or something like that."

Which is why it's important to heed how hauntingly familiar one feminine voice on the topic, from *The New Our Bodies, Ourselves,* is: "I feel vaguely guilty if sex isn't great all the time, as though if I'm a real woman I should have an incredible orgasm every time instead of accepting that sometimes there will be little ones and sometimes big ones."

And sometimes there will be missing ones, but if you can believe it, there will be times when even those will be pretty great, too.

PENIS SIZE

It's enough to give a guy a complex. According to the Kinsey Institute, a lot of American men think the average erect penis is 10 inches long, while many women peg it at 4 inches. One wonders how many crossed expectations this misunderstanding causes. But the fact is, both those figures are wrong. The average man's penis measures between 5 and 7 inches when it's erect, something that 30 percent of men questioned in the Institute's recent survey didn't know.

Some people just don't realize when they're ahead of the game.

Concerns about the size, shape and appearance of their genitals are common among men—and not necessarily something to worry about. The vast majority—some 80 to 90 percent, according to experts—fall within the "normal" range. Even an organ as abbreviated as two inches when erect should function just fine, according to Kinsey research. Even so, penis size and shape is the second most popular topic of concern (after impotence) among men who write the Institute for help.

"Men in general think that their penises are either too small or too large," agrees psychiatrist Ron Podell, M.D., director of the Center for Mood Disorders in Los Angeles. Podell, whose patients include men who have physical and psychological problems with sexual performance, believes that there's a direct link between such thoughts and a man's general self-esteem. "It's a question of to what extent a man feels comfortable with his body image and with himself as an attractive person," he observes. The prominence of the penis makes it "a very convenient place for a man to focus a lot of his insecurity about his maleness and attractiveness," says Podell. "So it becomes a focus of negative comparison."

A man's perception of his size usually is based on how he perceives his penis measures up to others, not on its actual dimensions. Consequently, the knowledge that his endowment isn't below average may not in itself allay a man's fears. "It's all a relative thing," Podell explains: "'His is bigger than mine, so mine must be smaller than average.'" The disquiet, however, usually is caused by an inaccurate picture of his own penis size in comparison to what he sees on others.

Boys start checking each other out around ages eleven and twelve, when their own bodily changes cause them to notice the sprouting pubic hair and genital growth taking place among their peers. Such comparisons are "part of a normal adult mental experience when you're going through puberty and adolescence," says Podell, who points out that youngsters usually start taking gym class and communal showers during this developmental period and therefore see a lot more of their peers in the nude. Throughout their lives, men continue to see other men's genitals in locker rooms and restrooms—and to compare.

Here's the rub: What they're comparing isn't erect penises. And that's the only measurement that counts from both the functional and physiological standpoints. On the broadest level, a man compares his penis to others to determine its potential function as a sexual instrument, which speaks to what he does with it in the bedroom when it's in peak operating condition, not what he does with it in the locker room. (Of course, some mistakenly measure their manhood, sexual potency, desirability and the like by their penis size, too.) And from a purely physiological perspective, you just can't get an accurate measurement of a penis that's not erect.

"You have to differentiate between flaccid and erect," explains urologist Bruce J. Joseph, M.D., of Santa Monica, California. A limp penis is no indication of what it will look like in full bloom. Furthermore, it's impossible to determine the actual length of a flaccid penis, says Joseph. "It can change with temperature, time of day, type of clothing or level of excitement."

In general, the smaller the organ when limp, the more it expands proportionately when stimulated. "A longer penis may not increase that much in size when it's erect," Joseph notes, "but the average erect penis is 5 to 7 inches long regardless of whether it's 2 inches or 5 inches when it isn't erect." (And "average" may be a lot closer to 5 inches than 7. A 1995 study at San Francisco General Hospital looked at 80 men and found the average length of their erect penises to be 5.1 inches, with a circumference of 4.9. When flaccid, those numbers dropped to 3.5 inches long and 3.9 inches around. Just 2 percent of those studied were classified as "subnormal," meaning that their erect penis was 2.8 inches or less in length and/or 3.5 inches or less in girth.)

Just as the length of a flaccid penis doesn't indicate its true size potential, neither does the view from which men observe their own genitals. That perspective—looking down on themselves—makes a penis appear foreshortened, or compact. What's more, the length is measured from the pubic bone—under the layer of fat covering it—to the tip, not from the skin covering the abdomen, which is what many men see when they look down, especially if they're carrying excess fat.

Insecurity about penis size is exacerbated by another misconception that plagues the male: the belief that women need about 10 inches of erect penis in order to be sexually satisfied. But Kinsey research indicates that most women don't prefer a larger-than-average penis, which may be a consequence of the fact that only 20 percent of women achieve orgasms through intercourse alone. Due to the position of the clitoris, many women require some stimulation in addition to penile penetration in order to reach a climax, no how matter how large—or small—their partner's genitals are. So a large penis isn't a priority in itself.

"It's not so much a question of size, but how a man and woman fit together," says psychotherapist Joy Davidson, Ph.D., writer and clinical consultant for the Sharper Image/Playboy Enterprises home video *The Secrets of Making Love to the Same Person Forever*. "It has to do with the placement of the clitoris, the lovemaking position or just how physically compatible a couple's bodies are—if they are different heights, different shapes." Penises are long and short, thick and thin; vaginas come in an equal array of shapes and sizes. Multiplying the possibilities, the odds against your finding a partner with whom you "fit" perfectly are something like 16 to 1, experts say.

"With one man but not with another, a woman might have an orgasm while she's being vaginally penetrated without any additional clitoral stimulation," Davidson continues. Even so, a less-than-perfect physical pairing usually will not put a woman off, she maintains. In locker-room conversation, women may intimate that they're impressed with the way a guy fills his trousers, but that's not their bottom line when it comes to choosing partners. "As long as the size is within normal range, it's not an issue," Davidson observes. "In general, women say that what's important is how caring, sensitive and creative a lover is, how emotional and intense a man is in bed."

If a man has decided he's not big enough, he's likely gotten that idea all by himself. "Most women are very sensitive to how fragile men are about this issue, so I don't think a lot of men get feedback from women that says their penis is too small," Podell observes. "A woman might tell her girlfriends before she would tell her boyfriend."

One message that some men do get directly from women is that they are too big. "Women will complain that a man's penis scares them or even hurts," Podell says. "It's not that these men aren't proud of having such a trophy, [but if they've received complaints about being too big] they may feel uncomfortable about it." And if a man is feeling anxious or insecure about himself, such negative feedback can cause just as many problems as the perception that his endowment is lacking. In other words, bigger isn't always better.

PENILE ENLARGEMENT

There is a saying: "Too much is always better than not enough." Most of us, at some time in our lives, have worried that our penises might be on the "not enough" side. Most of us have also concluded that, day in and day out, our members perform their duties in an honorable, yeomanlike fashion. Some men, however, see "not enough" as their misfortune and fate, something that compels them to steer clear of circumstances where penis size might become an issue.

To such men, penis-enlargement operations may represent hope itself, much like now-controversial breast augmentations have to many women in the recent past. Indeed, operations to enlarge the penis may soon prove to be as routine as nose jobs, face lifts or calf implants—procedures that until fairly recently would have seemed extreme.

To make a penis bigger, you can add length, width or both. A new procedure designed to add girth takes fat from another part of your body, usually the abdomen, and inserts it into the shaft of the penis; the head, or glans, cannot be enlarged. Price ranges from $2,500 to $5,000 with about a half-inch added to circumference. Length is added by cutting the suspensory ligament that attaches the penis to your body; this costs about $4,000 and typically adds one-half to two inches to length.

At least one plastic surgeon, Brian H.

Novack, M.D., of Beverly Hills, can combine two operations to make the penis both thicker and longer. Plastic surgeons and urologists who perform both procedures usually offer a reduced-price package deal. The operations are done on an outpatient basis under general anesthetic or intravenous sedation. You should be able to return to nonphysical work in about a week but will have to forgo intercourse for ten days to two weeks.

Just because these procedures are now routine doesn't mean they aren't extremely controversial. "Generally, men who think they have small penises don't," says E. Douglas Whitehead, M.D., a board-certified urologist and the director of the Association for Male Sexual Dysfunction in New York City. "Urologists see thousands of men each year who fear they have a small penis. Often it's in response to seeing some adult video or magazine that features exceptionally endowed men. So most men do not, in fact, need an operation. What they do need is an objective judgment as to the [size] of their penis," he concludes.

Nevertheless, the demand is there. Miami physician Ricardo Samitier developed the procedure by which the penis is thickened via fat injection. He calls it circumferential autologous penile engorgement, or CAPE. (Novack calls his procedure penile augmentation by fat transplantation.) Considerable controversy has surrounded Samitier, who is neither a board-certified plastic surgeon nor a urologist, particularly when a patient died of a heart attack after undergoing the surgery. Samitier lost his license to practice for a short period but has been reinstated.

As to the procedure's viability, critics say the injected fat gradually vanishes from the transplant area as the body absorbs it. And before disappearing, it may clump up into little spheres, a condition known as "balling" or "lumping."

Although everyone seems to agree that the fat will diminish over time, some doctors say it vanishes rather quickly, whereas others, like Harold M. Reed, M.D., a Miami urologist who performs penis-enlargement operations, dispute that. Reed contends that the rich blood supply enjoyed by penile tissue tends to support the injected fat and that, while new injections will certainly be required eventually, the time that passes between them—usually three to six months—will be acceptable to most patients. According to Reed, the surgeon can also control balling.

Perhaps the greatest limitation, Novack points out, is that because only the shaft can be enlarged, the penis can be made only so much thicker: "If I overpower the glans by making the shaft very big while the glans remains small, that's not going to look very good, especially in the flaccid state."

"I can inject about 1/8 to 3/16 inch of fat under the skin," Reed says, which comes out to about an extra 4/10 to one inch in circumference. Whitehead says chances of infection and eventual dispersal of fat make transplantation procedures unwise. He also points out that injecting fat into penile tissue is strictly an experimental surgery, and not recognized by the vast majority of urologists.

The surgery required to lengthen the penis is much more serious. Once the suspensory ligament, which attaches the penis to the pubic bone, is cut, the penis hangs down (or sticks out during erection) farther because a portion of the penis that usually resides inside the body is now outside, or "advanced," to use Novack's term. He considers this procedure major surgery that must be undertaken with extreme caution to avoid complications and/or infection.

The amount of "advancement" varies from man to man, within the range of 3/8 inch to a whopping two inches. Since the suspensory ligament's function is to support the penis, one side effect of the operation is that the erect penis will not point as high as it normally would. Unlike fat injections, there is nothing temporary about this procedure's results; the penis remains at its new length.

Whitehead views the suspensory-ligament operation dimly. While urologists have performed it on a small number of patients for serious medical reasons, he believes that "the risks of bleeding or of cutting the nerves in the area that have to do with penile sensation are too big for a cosmetic surgery."

In all cases, even surgeons who perform these experimental procedures are quick to remind prospective clients that neither surgery is going to create a gigantic penis where there was a very small one before. But the changes will be noticeable, and if the procedures are correctly performed, there is no loss of sensation.

Don't expect to go to a plastic surgeon—even one who performs these procedures—and ask if your penis is too small and get a straight answer. Plastic surgeons take pains not to guide their patients into forming conclusions. Why so circumspect? One plastic surgeon related a story about a prospective patient who wanted a penis-enlargement operation. A few weeks before the surgery, the patient traveled to Thailand, where he met a woman who thought that he (and his penis) were a little bit of heaven. They fell in love, got engaged and he canceled his operation. "When it comes to pleasing a partner, what counts isn't the size but the fit the two of you enjoy," says Novack.

That's what makes the notion of penis enlargement so complex. The fact is that most of us have very little reason to subject ourselves to the risks and side effects of enlargement surgery. But there are men for whom having a very small penis is stark reality and not just a sexual inferiority complex. (The medical term is micropenis, characterized by an appendage less than 3/4 inch long.) For that tiny minority of men, the experimental surgeries of today may foretell the promise of normal and unapologetic intimacy in the future.

8

RELATIONSHIPS

Our relationships can be the most transformational aspects of our lives. Think about how you, or someone you know, has changed as the result of becoming a husband or a father. Intense, ongoing relationships like these can unearth aspects of ourselves that we never suspected we had. Add in our relationships with our parents, siblings and old friends—with everyone's role changing and evolving over time—and you have the incredible mosaic that is our lives. Our relationships, simply, *are* our lives. Relationships are the source of some of our richest experiences. They are also the source of some of our greatest frustrations.

Relationships seem to come easier to women than men. For many of us handling our relationships is a skill; for women, it seems to be a natural talent. Yet these experiences mean just as much for men as women. If relationships are a skill, then they can be learned and practiced. The first step is simply to acknowledge the importance of this aspect of our lives, and to make more time for the people we care about.

Our relationships are of primary importance to our overall emotional health. But if emotional health isn't reason enough to think about how we relate to others, then how about physical health? High stress is linked to almost every serious health problem affecting men. One solution to stress is to get a friend. In a study of about 1,200 men, researchers at Yale, Duke and Mount Sinai Medical Center in New York City found that men who reported having lots of friends had fewer stress-indicating chemicals in their blood than men who didn't have many friends. And the more often a man saw his friends, the less stress he showed.

Dr. Dean Ornish, who emphasizes relationships as part of his program to fight cardiac illness, has even cited isolation and loneliness as a form of "spiritual heart disease"—and a cardiac risk factor. A Duke study that tracked 1,300 patients over nine years who had been given a diagnostic procedure for heart disease found that those who didn't have a spouse or confidant were three times more likely to die within five years. Research is confirming the proverb, "No man is an island." Men like to think of themselves as independent and self-reliant, but we need others in order to have a full, healthy life.

For most men, the primary relationship of their adult life will be with their spouse. But how does a man travel that rocky road from "relationship" to "marriage"—and how will he and his wife meet the challenges they face by being married?

MAKING A COMMITMENT

Exclusivity, monogamy, commitment—these words can get under a man's skin like fingernails on a blackboard. But in any serious relationship, sooner or later they start sounding rich with the promise of emotional depth, stability and blissful disengagement from the dating wars. Is she the one? Is this the time? Do you take it to the next plateau—whether that means living together, getting engaged or marrying—or do you hum along like some other couples, never coming to any hard conclusions about whether the relationship is or isn't going anywhere? When does it all become . . . certain?

Biology provides you one answer, and it's harshly unambiguous: never. Our search for meaning, companionship and loyalty is simply at odds with the fact that in much of the animal kingdom monogamy is the exception; the rule is a frenzied lifelong ricochet from one partner to the next. Consider the birds. Geese and roadrunners mate for life, but most species are pretty casual about forming pair bonds, staying together for a summer, a few days or only for the duration of the briefest of sex acts. (Naturalists saw one North American sage grouse coupling with twenty-one different females in a single morning.)

So we humans, with our urge toward durable little arrangements in cottages for two, are something of an exception. But as Mary Batten points out in her book *Sexual Selection,* even among us the attraction toward lifetime pair bonds is far from universal. Anthropologists, she notes, tell us that a mere fifth of human societies today are basically monogamous.

But suppose you've decided to buck the promiscuous tradition established by our animal ancestors, as most Americans ultimately do. You're dating, you're intrigued, even infatuated, and suddenly the thought of spending one, two or three nights a week together isn't enough. You start envying paired-off friends, their even-keeled lives, their air of settled contentment, maybe even their kids. The absolutes of marriage, or even a live-in arrangement, on the other hand, can be terrifying, too. Yet an agreement to date exclusively, while reassuring, is not exactly the gold standard for intimacy. How do you know when to take a braver leap? And which leap should you take?

One school of thought advises you to lighten up and rely on your instincts. Don't consult a checklist or visit an astrologer. You'll simply know in your gut when the right person comes along. A few years ago, a friend went to a couples counselor when debating the future of a (now defunct) relationship. He was obsessed about some thorny issues. Were they sexually and emotionally compatible? What would he feel like in a year, two years, seven years? Could they afford a house? And what about children?

After he'd fulminated in this vein for about half an hour, the counselor cut him off. "Stop trying to solve the mysteries of the universe," she exclaimed. "Just answer a simple question: Are you committed to this person?" That launched him on an agonized examination of what "commitment" meant. She listened for about ten minutes more, then said: "Are you trying to reach a decision or compile a dictionary? You know what commitment means. Everybody does. Just answer my question: Are you committed to this person?"

There's a refreshing simplicity in this approach. Just sit down and ask—first yourself, then each other—this question: Are we committed? Don't confuse the semantics of commitment with the consequences that may follow: marriage, children and so on. Those are the forking paths you'll choose later, once you've agreed the relationship is a go. Take things step by step. Decide whether you think there's oil down there before you start wrangling over how to build the derrick.

Of course, you may not be content with a seat-of-the-pants approach. After all, there are home testing kits for diabetes and pregnancy. Why not for relationships—something that will come out pink if the affair's for the ages and blue if it's headed for oblivion? Actually, there is such a test, sort of. About ten years ago, the *Journal of Marriage and the Family* published a test called the Relationship Events Scale (RES) to help people calibrate their progress toward couplehood. It's a series of true-or-false statements about the relationship; the more you answer "true," the further along you are.

The RES wasn't designed to help you decide whether to commit, but it can be a reality check on the state of your romance. A few of the statements on the test are fairly obvious in their intent:

- We are or have been engaged.
- My partner has said "I love you."
- I have said "I love you."

But others, deceptively simple, are less obvious. For example:

- I have lent my partner more than $20 for more than a week.
- We have received an invitation for the two of us as a couple.
- We have spent a vacation together that lasted more than three days.

You can ask yourself other indirectly diagnostic questions as well, including ones that bear uniquely on your situation. For example, when you're making plans for major holidays, do you consult your partner before you settle on what to do, or do the two of you decide unilaterally and tell one another afterward? Would you cancel a $1,000 purchase your heart was set on if your partner thought it was a bad idea? The answer to a suddenly asked question of this sort can tell you where your heart is even if you've never come to a conscious conclusion. If you're a halfway competent taker of your own pulse, a week or two of this sort of analysis may tell you whether you want to take the plunge—or a powder.

So, use either the commonsense tack advocated by my couples counselor, or the more analytical approach suggested by the RES test. And get both your partner and yourself to answer, as honestly as you can, this question: Are we a pair, or just two people who get a transient kick out of each other? Answering this question doesn't get you completely out of the woods, though. You still have to decide whether that commitment, if you choose to make it, means marriage or a less formal arrangement. But it's a step. And if it all makes you feel queasy, remember that while the sage grouse inside you may tell you to bolt and play the field, the beauty of being human is that it's up to you whether to listen.

COMMITMENT QUIZ

Answer yes or no to each of the following questions:

1. Do friends you run into automatically ask about your partner?
2. Would you lend your partner your car—no questions asked—for a week at a time?
3. When you think about a trip or vacation, does it seem unimaginable not to include your partner?
4. When you make plans for a holiday (Thanksgiving, Christmas, Passover), does your partner at least sometimes come first, even before family?
5. Are you more often than not invited out together and treated as a couple?
6. If you were to ask your parents or siblings, would they call you and your partner a couple rather than friends or steadies?

7. Would you feel comfortable if you and your partner shared a joint bank account?
8. Suppose you dated somebody else, your partner found out about it and canned you as a result. Would you feel—no matter how sex-bombish, bright or rich the date—that you'd blown it, and trashed something vital to you?
9. If you do make a commitment now, suppose you're still a couple twenty years hence. Imagine unflinchingly what you'll both look like then. Under those circumstances, does something still please you about the idea of sharing a bed with her?
10. Answer the following question in two seconds or less (no thinking allowed): Do you love this person?

To compute your score, count up your "yes" answers. 1 to 3: You're a long way from security. 4 to 6: You're wavering. So buckle down: What's it going to be, boy? Yes or no? 7 to 9: It's time to consider taking the plunge. Perfect 10: Can we come to the wedding?

MONOGAMY

A relationship is like a muscle: it can't remain static and stay strong. When boredom sets in, we have a tendency to assume that something is inherently wrong with the union and to blame someone for it. But we wouldn't condemn exercise itself if we stopped seeing results from our regular workouts. We'd realize that the program simply needs variety, new goals, added intensity – in short, more attention.

The secret of satisfying monogamy is paying attention to ourselves and to our partners. Successful relationships blend friendship and companionship with passion and sex in a cycle of ever-changing intensities. If we're aware of—and have respect for—those fluctuations, we'll have a better sense of how to keep the benefits coming, regardless of where each partner is in his or her own cycle. With a little rearrangement of routine and a bit of modification in behavior, longtime couples can thrive. Here are four ways to fan the flames of romance.

1. The Importance of Touch. Men, more so than women, think of touch as a prelude to passion, and if passion isn't in their minds, they forgo the touch: the kiss, hug or caress. Yet our skin, the human body's largest organ, contains more than five million tiny nerve endings spread over its surface, one-third of them concentrated in the fingers and hands. We're obviously well designed to touch and be touched; both giver and receiver feel pleasure.

Men often are touch deprived as a result of growing up in a culture that discourages males from touching for reasons other than procreation. In her report on male sexuality, researcher Shere Hite asserts that most of the men in her study revealed a yearning for more nonsexual touching by women. Yet many don't know how to give and receive touches that convey intimacy without having intercourse.

Research has shown that being touched decreases anxiety, calms fears, decreases pain, lowers blood pressure, reduces stress and soothes the sick. If touch can do all that, imagine how it can benefit your relationship. When touches are given and received daily—with sincerity—they can lighten the day's load and light a fire in both your hearts. To learn just how erotic sensations other than genital ones can be, try the following experiment. You'll discover that you have the potential to respond much more fully than you currently do—and that you have a huge, untapped erogenous zone.

The exercise: Before you begin, realize that there's a big difference between touching for its own sake and touching as a prelude to sex. The first kind takes place in the present, while the second is programmed for the future. If you focus on reaching the goal, you miss the opportunity to enjoy the moment. In this exercise, sexual intercourse is not your goal—it's the discovery of your capacity to give and receive erotic touch. This discovery in itself can wake up a moribund sex life.

Lay a towel at the foot of a comfortable chair and invite your partner to sit down. Fill a large, deep pan with warm, sudsy water and give her a foot bath. The purpose here isn't to clean her feet, but to enjoy all the tactile sensations possible for both of you. Have her close her eyes, and experiment with fondling, massaging and pouring frothy water over her feet and lower legs, paying attention to each part in its turn. Don't hurry through the process. Notice the different textures of her leg and foot and watch how she responds to various touches. Some other time, she can play the role of the giver and you can relax in the chair, but it's not necessary to get it all done in one session. Just make sure you allow plenty of time for this experience to unfold without a hint of pressure.

2. Don't "Cut to the Chase." Familiarity breeds perfunctory sex. Our society breeds a thirst for instant gratification. Together, they spell doom for long-term lovers. Have you forgotten how much fun it is to look forward to a rendezvous with someone who excites you? It's impossible to be bored when you're anticipating the delights that await you in the foreseeable future. Just because you've seen each other every day for the past few years doesn't mean that you'll never again experience that same thrill of anticipation.

Slow, nongoal-oriented lovemaking can keep you stimulated and intermittently erect all day. By delaying your climax and engaging in "appetizer" sessions, you increase your level of sexual tension. You'll feel more sexually sensitive and become excited more easily. If you and she arouse each other two or three times in the course of a day, you'll start to feel a level of sexual urgency and desire that you might not have experienced in a very long time.

The exercise: Start out in the morning with a lazy, half-asleep warm-up that can be as brief as four or five minutes—just enough time to leave both of you wide awake. Keep the tempo slow and gentle. Later, as you get ready to leave for work, take a few minutes before you're fully dressed for some more unhurried stroking, perhaps enough to bring on the heavy breathing. Over the course of the day, pause to think now and again about the encounter that awaits you. During the evening, while the chores are being taken care of, stop occasionally to give her a sexy little caress (but nothing more). You're free to go for broke when the day's work is done, but a few words to the wise: Don't wait until the eleventh hour to take action, and don't rush the climax.

3. Playing Around. Couples who have fun together are really saying, "I trust you to love me even when I'm being silly." How important is a shared sense of humor? One study reported in *Psychology Today* found that couples who laugh at the same jokes are more likely to remain together. And humor is sexy. It always makes the top five when women list the sexiest qualities in men. It's easy to get bogged down under the weight of daily responsibilities. The solution, strange as it may sound, is to plan a little spontaneous play time. "Planned spontaneity sounds contradictory," says Sarah Catron, Ph.D., former executive director of the Association for Couples in Marriage Enrichment in Winston-Salem, North Carolina. "But you can't be spontaneous if you don't have time to be. Carve out time for yourselves, away from distractions, to do whatever you like. Take an afternoon off and drive, just the two of you. Go to the zoo, buy balloons and feed the monkeys."

The message you give your partner when you reserve time just to play with her is powerful: "I love being with you." During your courtship days, you were all important to each other, and you were eager to make time for enjoying your togetherness. Get back in touch with that desire to have fun.

The exercise: Make a date with your mate. It doesn't have to be elaborate, but it should be something you'll both enjoy. If nothing else, send the kids to their grandparents' and cook a candlelit dinner at home. Ask her to dress up in something special or buy her something sexy for the occasion. If neither of you likes to cook, you can always turn down the lights and order in a pizza. There are thousands of ways to revive the spirit of fun in your relationship. The important thing is to give each other permission to be playful, and then watch what happens.

4. Weathering the Storms. Researchers have discovered that the particular trials of life are far less important than the way people cope with them. Small disappointments can kill one marriage, while another survives great tragedies. Couples in enduring relationships are able to face difficulties with a positive attitude. The partners allow each other respect, latitude and room to grow. The quality of their relationship depends on how they treat each other, in good times and bad. In bad times, strong couples know that their love will survive the storm. Realizing that, they can withstand crises that cause other relationships to collapse.

Survival is rooted in remembering why you two are in the relationship in the first place. You can't desire another person over the long haul without being best friends. During the courtship phase of a relationship, feelings of excitement, of euphoria, dominate. But it's the sharing of fears and concerns that makes for real intimacy.

We don't expect our friends to be our mirror images, but many of us expect our mates to be exactly that. Many partners are far more selfish with one another than they realize. We extend ourselves for our friends, look for areas of common interest, are attentive to the events in their lives. Why should it be a different story with our partners?

Love is acceptance. It isn't a license to remodel a person according to our tastes. The more responsibility you assume for the quality of your life, the happier you—and your partner—become. The friendship you share allows you to feel accepted, respected and loved. Even though passion will wax and wane, and your cycles might not always be in sync, you have no cause for alarm. As the proverb says, there's a time for everything.

MONOGAMY—THREE VIEWS

Life-partner eroticism is the newest trend among married couples. The big question: Can it be done? We asked three purveyors of this trend to tell us in their own words whether lifelong monogamy can be hot for men, and if so, what steps a man can take to stay true.

"Biologically, men are more inclined to mate with several females serially because they have ten to twenty times more testosterone than women," says Patricia Love, author of *Hot Monogamy*. "I took testosterone while writing the book, and there was clearly a different attitude that went along with it, a greater sense of arousal and urgency. I was actually uncomfortable with the feeling."

"Historically, when sex was only for

procreation, it made sense for the man to 'spread his seed.' But maybe sociologically now we're seeing a bifurcation. The world is already populated. Men are searching for something deeper. I see it in my traditional couples workshops: it used to be the women who would drag in their husbands. But for the hot-monogamy workshops I conduct, the men are the initiators. So something is definitely changing."

"This shift is even affecting younger people. Many of them grew up with divorce in unhappy homes, and they saw how painful it was for their parents. They saw their parents and stepparents struggle through two or three marriages. They didn't have healthy models. Some people don't even know how to have a relationship, but they do want to learn. Sex can be a brief encounter between strangers. It can be a mechanical act between people who've grown weary of each other. Or it can be a lasting, healing experience between two people who've become soulmates. That's what hot monogamy is all about."

Harold H. Bloomfield, M.D., author of *Love Secrets for a Lasting Relationship*, knows firsthand about man's struggle to be faithful to one partner. "In my single days, I would have said no way. I believed, as many guys did, that to have an outrageous sex life meant being single. I grew up at a time when most marriages I observed didn't look like places I wanted to be. But now I've discovered that what women have been telling me all along is true: As you give in to overcoming your fears of intimacy, learn to be yourself and open your heart, sex with a life partner really does get better. "

"Now, I'm in my fifties. But I've been talking to a number of men in their twenties, and they don't want the hassle of walking around with rubbers and taking sexual histories of their partners. True, AIDS hasn't changed much behavior among heterosexuals, but it's changing attitudes. There's nothing wrong with saying that there are some negative motivations for staying together. Divorce is expensive, and so is an affair. Some people romanticize and say they have only positive reasons for staying together. But all behavioral choices have their pluses and minuses, and people tend to find really good reasons for the choices they make. As a man matures there's really no reason to create any unnecessary messes in his life. I'm at the point where having one really hot partner suits my sex drive fine."

Susan Page, author of *Now That I'm Married, Why Isn't Everything Perfect*, offers some great advice on how guys can make the transition—using fantasy and other methods—to a monogamous mindset. She also talks about "soulmates." "I spoke with thirty-six couples who are very happy and clearly monogamous, and for the men it was because they were very involved in the lives they shared with their women. This sort of man doesn't sit around thinking about being in another relationship or wondering what he'd do if another woman came along. It's easy for him to pass on a fling because of the real pleasure he gets from being with his mate."

"I believe in giving permission to people to have a rich and varied fantasy life. It's lovely for both men and women to allow themselves to fantasize about a movie star or a co-worker. Some people may be threatened by the idea that their partner has fantasies. But for people who don't find it threatening, I believe that the more you self-disclose about what's going on in your inner life, the more intimate you can become. My husband and I share the sexual fantasies we have about other people and it's not threatening because it's clear that we're loyal to each other."

"The shift toward monogamy parallels a trend in our society toward meaning. You come to recognize that the real, rock-bottom meaning in life comes from the quality of our human relationships, and you can't sever sexual relationships from that scheme. Monogamy is harder for men. I don't like to talk about making a sacrifice in a monogamous relationship or marriage. Rather, it's a tradeoff. You give something up, like your ability to have a heightened erotic experience with a stranger, in exchange for the opportunity to love and treasure and be loyal to your mate. It might be a loss, but you don't just dwell on the loss. You make a choice and recognize the pleasurable and rewarding side of having made that choice."

What makes a monogamous relationship most successful is lack of ambivalence—no hesitation about being with each other. A couple knows they are right for each other and aren't driving through the relationship with the brakes on. "Finally—and I know it's interesting for me to be saying this—it helps a lot for a man to have had a lot of sexual experience before entering into a monogamous relationship."

IN THE HEAT OF THE FIGHT

It's a legendary battle, the war between men and women, the stuff of Greek tragedy, crass melodrama and low farce. But it's also a daily and thoroughly practical real-life challenge. Disagreements and arguments—and the way they culminate in either civilized negotiations or lurid crimes—are the bedrock of relationships. There's no way to completely escape the slow burn that comes from someone always being "in your space." Ask Samson and Delilah. Ralph and Alice. Lorena and John Wayne. (Bobbitt, that is.)

That's a point Los Angeles social psychologist Carol Tavris makes in her book *Anger: The Misunderstood Emotion.* Tavris cites tribal societies where ritualized bickering is a vital institution. Fighting can be aggravating, but as long as it's controlled, as Tavris shows, it provides a way for people to air grievances, smooth down the rougher edges of their interactions, work out the complexities of their communal lives and get what they want—all without resorting to flying crockery or bullets. In other words, the occasional argument can be a means for growing, learning and getting closer. If handled poorly, it can also be the spark that ignites the powder keg within us all.

So the first rule for conducting arguments with your partner is to expect them, and not to treat them as if they were an outrageous assault on the Ward and June Cleaver bliss you perceive to be your birthright. The opportunities for disagreement are legion. For his classic 1979 study, John M. Gottman audiotaped 60 couples on the subject and boiled the 180 tales they told of connubial warfare down to a list of 85 conflict situations.

Gottman further distilled these into a five-item checklist of the most common bones of contention:

- Communication (over such matters as how much time you spend with each other, how you live your daily life together, how you express your feelings);
- Sex (no explanation required);
- Jealousy (ditto);
- Relationships with the in-laws (double ditto);
- Chores (housekeeping, child care, errands and how much money should be spent on each).

So assume, as you must, that you and your lover will sooner or later trip on one or all of these affectional land mines. While researchers have documented that couples' fighting styles change as they age—younger pairs tend to square off, then discuss and even joke about their donny-brooks, while middle-aged and older couples tend to avoid divisive issues altogether—most people still need advice on how to manage their fights, keeping them from destroying a relationship they both wish to maintain.

Again, the experts overflow with advice. None of it's guaranteed, of course, and strategy is usually the first casualty of any conflict. Remember that there are basically two types of arguments. The first, beloved by macho types (and virtually guaranteed by all observers to bring on disaster), is the zero-sum dispute: If you win, your partner loses. And grovels humiliated in the dust. And broods. And schemes. And possibly—if she doesn't first slip antifreeze into your protein shake or your Rolex into the garbage disposal—walks out.

The second kind of argument is the model most conciliation experts say you should aim for. It's framed so both participants emerge from the strife with something to show for the effort. Nobody has to swallow a bitter defeat; nobody has to put up with the loser's corrosive resentments.

Don't, in other words, regard victory as a matter of first dominating the battlefield and then shooting all the captives. Leave your adversary with something gained from the struggle. When you want something, don't merely attack; offer her a quid pro quo, a consolation prize that holds some meaning and entails either sacrifice or effort on your part. Think negotiation, not hostile takeover.

Example: One couple nearly took their relationship to the sanitary landfill over the question of whether the female half of the pair should buy a country house. Marcia, haunted by dreams of romantic country evenings and prize homegrown rutabagas, desperately wanted the place. Bany, a dyed-in-the-wool urban guerrilla, blanched at the prospect of bottomless do-it-yourself disasters, eerie silence and prowling, rabid wildlife. In the happy and long-negotiated upshot, both won. Marcia got the house. But Bany got an ironclad (in fact, a written) agreement that she'd take the dead rats out of the attic, suffer (and fix) the septic system in silence, and let him buy a stereo of barbarian-horde power, which, if installed within the jurisdiction of New York City's noise-control laws, would eventually have landed him in Attica. Now they're happy as clams.

But there's a catch in such beautiful scenarios. The non-zero-sum argument demands that you figure out what your partner wants. No matter how constructive a couple's approach to disagreement may be, the conciliation effort will fail if either can't fathom the other's real motivations. And that's no small problem because men and women don't think alike, don't communicate in the same way and don't take the same attitude toward aggression. In *Men, Women and Aggression,* Anne Campbell points out that men tend to focus on the morality of the rules that govern fighting, while women question the morality of fighting itself. Deborah Tannen— author of the contemporary bible of miscues between the sexes, *You Just Don't Understand*—records it as a revelation when she first read of an exchange between two preschool boys who initiated a friendship with a fight, a situation virtually unheard of among girls.

For men, Tannen points out, the art and practice of argument can be an exhilarating end in itself. For women, it's more typically just an unpleasant if necessary means toward achieving a specific objective. "Men may be more concerned with winning," Tannen says. "Very often in an argument a man would rather die than say 'I'm sorry: I was wrong.' But the woman would be happy to apologize and say she was wrong—as long as she could get whatever it is she wants.

"Another key point," Tannen adds, "is that men seem to assume somebody's got to be on top and somebody's got to be on the bottom, while women feel people can be on an equal footing. She merely wants equal rights; he hears her trying to get the upper hand." Women. in other words, don't regard fighting as a character-builder or a sport—and can become mightily perturbed at the bloodthirsty pleasure men take in the fray. A woman (and historian) who specializes in the annals of relations between the sexes going back to the Middle Ages, puts it even more strongly: "Men always operate from an unspoken, unexamined position of power, wanting to win rather than work something out, and being willing to do anything, no matter how obviously destructive, to win."

Which suggests the final (and perhaps the most difficult) rule for winning an argument with women: Don't try. The tenacity and drive that propel you to dominance on the squash court or in the boardroom may win you victory after victory in the disputes that haunt any relationship. But if you don't heed the lesson that love is neither business nor squash and that a mate is something much more than a pretty wrestling opponent, you may lose the relationship itself.

FIVE RULES OF ENGAGEMENT

1. Conflicts are normal. That doesn't mean you should go out of your way to provoke fights or be in constant bicker mode, but don't panic when disagreements bubble to the surface, either.
2. Winning isn't everything. Sometimes it's a terrible idea. Try to guide the argument to a productive end in which both you and she gain something. Humiliating her with defeat may give you a quick rush, but it's relationship poison.
3. Am I saying what I thought you heard me say? Bear in mind, even when the "discussion" heats up, that men and women often tend to think and express themselves differently. Take the time to make sure you know what she means and wants, and that she knows what you mean and want.
4. Talk less, hear more. Don't let that brilliant, smashing, take-no-captives reply you're thinking up make you oblivious to what she's saying. Don't just appear to be listening while you're waiting your turn to jab: actually listen.
5. Throw down your sword and make concessions. A successful man/woman fight is one that preserves, even strengthens, the relationship. Save your need to dominate for poker, tennis and war.

WHO BATTERS, AND WHY

Fighting is normal in relationships. Abuse isn't. But where exactly is the line between the two? Characterizing a batterer as someone who beats up his partner all the time is like describing an alcoholic as someone who gets drunk every day. Both definitions are inaccurate.

The truth is that domestic violence generally exists on a continuum, and wherever it begins on that continuum, it often escalates over time, sometimes with deadly consequences. According to a report in the *Journal of the American Medical Association,* domestic violence is characterized by "a pattern of behaviors, where the victim is coerced by her intimate partner. The behaviors may involve deliberate and repeated battering with injuries, sexual assault, psychological abuse, progressive social isolation, intimidation and deprivation."

Not only are there different types and degrees of abuse, there are different kinds of abusers. Some rarely batter, others hurt only the people they love, and still others will abuse anybody. Often these people have grown up in abusive households where they learned that hitting is the way to resolve problems. Some grew up in overly controlling families where they were frequently shamed or put down and never learned to talk things out. Batterers are usually insecure people who hide their fears by acting tough, bullying and attempting to control the weaker people in their lives—namely, women and children. In some instances, flying off the handle may have a genetic component.

But the underlying cause of battering, whether it's genetic, environmental or pathological, is probably irrelevant when actual abuse is going on and lives may be in danger. Mark Miller, MFCC, a Santa Clarita, California, psychotherapist who set up a men's program to treat the partners of abused women, expresses skepticism about the value of looking for the "whys"- in domestic violence. "Batterers first have to stop the battering behavior," he says. "Then they can start looking into their childhood for the reasons."

Early indications that someone may be on his way to becoming an abuser:

- Embarrassing the woman, treating her like a child, being critical or sarcastic, belittling her
- Making her feel guilty, being a nitpicky perfectionist
- Being maliciously unpredictable, raging over small things
- Being excessively suspicious and jealous, accusing her of actual or fantasized infidelity
- Having an extremely low tolerance for frustration
- Insulting her family and friends, undermining her accomplishments, trivializing her ambitions
- Refusing to let go of an argument, following her around to continue it, waking her up to confront her
- Intentionally isolating her from family and friends
- Depriving her of money

- Switching from charmer to snake in a split second
- Slamming doors, hitting the wall near her, punching holes in walls, breaking things, throwing things that land near her
- Driving dangerously fast with her in the car
- Stalking her, pulling phones out of walls, cutting phone wires, taping phone conversations
- Cutting up her clothes, throwing out her possessions, preventing her from going to work or school
- Demanding that she account for her money and time, opening her mail, locking her out of the house
- Lashing out at a pet
- Brandishing a weapon, threatening suicide, sleeping with a weapon under the pillow, threatening to hurt her children and relatives, shooting a bullet into the ceiling.

What Friends Can Do

If you suspect your friend is a batterer, here's a list of steps you can take toward doing the right thing:

Assess your own values. If you're not sure that battering is bad, stop reading right here because you're not going to do anyone any good. In fact, you may need to examine your own beliefs and actions.

Assess the situation. You've noticed some telltale behaviors; now check things out further. If you see suspicious-looking bruises or other indications of battering, you might ask the woman directly, "Is he hitting you?" But don't assume no means no; she may be in denial or in fear for her life. Discreetly ask friends or other family members if they've seen any signs of abuse.

Assess your reasons for inaction. If you've established that your friend is abusing his mate but you're not saying anything to him, ask yourself why. Are you afraid of his anger? Are you afraid of what mutual acquaintances will say? Is your motive for holding back selfish? Is it about looking good and avoiding discomfort? If so, are you man enough to overcome these hesitations and do what you know should be done?

Confront your friend. Be direct without being antagonistic. The fact that you're his friend gives you all the clout you need. He cares what you think of him. If he has children, make sure he's not abusing them. (If he is, report him immediately.) If it's "just" spousal abuse, point out how his battering affects his kids, how they're really scared and hurt and how they'll start imitating him if he's not careful. "Ask him outright, 'Do you want your daughter to grow up to be abused or your son to be an abuser?'" suggests psychotherapist Mark Miller. If you take this approach, be prepared to lose the friendship if he's not capable of confronting the reality of his behavior head on.

Point out legal consequences. He should know he could end up imprisoned. "In some places, even if the woman doesn't ultimately press charges and doesn't have bruises or marks, he could still be jailed for domestic violence," Miller says.

Look for addiction. "In most battering situations, I would be very surprised if there were no alcohol or drugs involved on one or both parts," Andrews says. "If you suspect that's what's behind your friend's behavior, tell him to get help."

Confront the woman. This may not be appropriate in all cases, especially if your friend is the jealous type, but in some instances it can work if she gets counseling or attends a self-help group. "I've seen recoveries happen when the partner of the batterer goes for help first," Miller says. "Often, when the woman says, 'I'm not going to take it anymore,' that's when the guy snaps out of it."

Be available. If your friend listens to you, seeks help and manages to stop the battering behavior, you can offer to be around to help him through the shakes. "You can say, 'Hey, if something happens and it escalates, take time out. Call me. Come over to my place. Or we'll meet for a cup of coffee,'" Miller suggests. "Just offering to go jogging to help your friend let off steam can do wonders."

Understand the syndrome. There can be relapses of abusive behavior, just as there are with drug or alcohol addiction. "It's a sick cycle," McGrath explains. "It's not at a crisis point all the time. There's a buildup of tension, then comes the explosion, then there's the honeymoon period when he's sunny and promises to be different. Then it happens again. The cycle can take months. In between, everybody forgets there's a problem."

Have resource information handy. Research the topic and have some book titles written down in case your friend decides he's ready to investigate his situation. Also write down the names of therapists who specialize in domestic violence, along with related self-help groups, counseling centers and men's groups.

"Today there's a lot of work being done on teaching batterers techniques to help them control their anger," McGrath says. "By noticing bodily clues like sweating palms and a churning gut, men can learn to recognize their anger before it's too late. They learn how to take 'time out,' how to keep an anger journal in order to analyze what sets them off and how to use 'self-talk' to replace a thought that makes them angry ('She's not doing what I want') with a new message ('She's doing the best she can')." Your friend should also know that sometimes prescription medications can help when abusive behavior is related to a biochemical imbalance.

Be realistic. "The recovery from battering is a long process and takes commitment," McGrath says. "Many men don't have that commitment and drop out of counseling programs, so statistically the chances that stepping in to try and help fix things aren't that high. But that doesn't mean you shouldn't do it. While there are no guarantees, there's always hope."

"I'm optimistic," Andrews says. "I think that just making the batterer aware of the possibility of change can alter his attitude a little bit. When people start making positive inner changes, however small, one of the first things they do is turn around and start making positive changes in their environment, so that bit by bit larger changes begin to happen." At some point, your friend is going to have to confront his demons. Whether he does it inside a prison cell or a therapist's office may very well depend on you.

BITTER BETRAYALS

Adultery is one of those subjects: people either salivate or flip out at the very mention of it. Did she or didn't she? Have you or haven't you? Should you or shouldn't you? You could fill Carlsbad Caverns with the available books on the subject. Fiction? Try Flaubert's *Madame Bovary*. Fact? Annette Lawson's excellent 1988 study, *Adultery*. How-to manuals? Casanova's interminable *Memoirs* is a famous example. A trip to the library—or a session with a marriage counselor—will make you realize just how much research has been done on the subject, how many statistics unearthed, trends tracked.

The demographics of spousal wanderlust have been changing in ways that ought to give you pause if you're male. Back in the 1940s, Alfred Kinsey found, not surprisingly, that husbands were likelier to cheat than wives. By the late 1980s, though, Annette Lawson detected a mind-warping change: Her research suggested that young married women were actually philandering more often than their husbands.

But sterile, clinical surveys can't begin to capture the agitation and fury that come along with the experience of adultery, no matter if you're the betrayer or the betrayed. Love's not science, it's life. Even though experts make countless useful generalizations about the subject, the emotions here are too volatile for these rules to be very helpful. As soon as you join two humans, their quirks synergize and there's a quantum leap upward in complexity and danger. So, if you contemplate fiddling with something as loaded as a live-in relationship (with or without the benefit of marriage vows), you can throw out the rule books and advice columns.

Tim, a real-life expert on the subject (his name, like those that follow, is fiction), put the would-be adulterer's dilemma particularly forcefully. "You're like a four-year-old who takes the controls of a Boeing 747," he said. "You may have a thrilling ride, but it'll be nothing compared to the landing." This is what people who've been in the trenches seem to agree on: If you choose adultery, you're drawing a wild card. A fling may rejuvenate you and send you back to your marriage feeling refreshed. It may be the messy but inevitable *coup de grace* that polishes off a relationship that's already on its deathbed. Or it may be a plain old disaster.

Andrea, an insurance executive whose twenty-year marriage foundered after a cheating episode on her husband's part, offers some philosophical advice: "This is the messiest thing you'll ever do—and one of the riskiest. Don't kid yourself. When you get involved in it, it's as if it never happened in the world before, and it's going to shake things up more than you think." Remember: There are three people in a triangle, and the destabilizing influence of an affair may drive any or all of them over the edge. And that includes the dupe—the person who doesn't (or isn't supposed to) know what's going on. In this poker game, in other words, there are three wild cards, starting with:

1. Your paramour. The person you're having it off with is obviously sexual dynamite, but she may also be a ticking bomb. Be forewarned: The explosion can come when you're unprepared, and in a form your worst nightmares couldn't have imagined. Tim's case illustrates: A dozen years into a relationship with Marcy, he embarked on what he thought was a casual once-a-week arrangement with their friend and neighbor Francesca (herself fresh from a divorce). They were, Tim thought, urbane, sophisticated, thoroughly cool. Until, at Marcy's New Year's Eve party, Francesca administered a not-so-furtive grope at his crotch. He spent the next two weeks explaining to Marcy, but what, really, was there to explain? Two months later, he moved out.

Why did Francesca do it? The very secrecy of their liaison may have frustrated her, kindling an irresistible urge to blow Tim's cover. Or maybe she was drunk. Or who knows. She didn't have much of a relationship to lose, after all. Don't paint her as a villain in the piece, however; the yen to go public if you've snagged someone who bewitches you is universal. And the revelatory gesture needn't be so blatant. Sometimes subtle body language is a giveaway.

Your extramural lover isn't the only imponderable. Also consider:

2. Your partner. You cheated, remember, because you thought the relationship was tired, stagnant, frustrating. Might she not be thinking the same thing? Maggie M. simply picked up vibes from her lover, Daniel, sensing that he'd strayed. (In fact, she was right.) But before the affair came to light, and without quite knowing why, Maggie found her own eyes wandering. "Maybe I'll dabble," she remembers thinking, "just because it might create a crisis and that will resolve things." As it happened, she didn't yield to the temptation. Now she wishes she had. "You don't know what fault lines an affair is going to expose in your main relationship," Andrea says. "It may force your partner to confront issues she's never faced before. And you can't control the consequences."

Well, suppose your lover is the soul of discretion and your spouse doesn't choose to entertain the mailman while you're delighting the meter maid. You're still left to cope with what may well prove to be the most volatile ingredient in this witch's brew and the one that can most easily destroy you along with your primary relationship:

3. Yourself. Remember, the same confessional urge that drove Francesca may unconsciously be motivating you. Chances are your spouse can read you fairly well. Are you flaunting your adultery without realizing it? Forget about the new crotch-accentuating underwear you bought yourself, or the long blond hair you didn't brush off your collar. Have you changed your gift-giving pattern? (Suddenly more expensive is a dead giveaway.) Or, because your illicit connection is making you cocky, are you routinely tangling with your wife over minor issues you'd have hesitated to bring up before? (The opposite, not tangling over issues you normally fight about like cats and dogs, is also a tip-off.)

"My birthday was a watershed," Maggie recalls. "Daniel wanted to make me dinner; I wanted to have some people over afterward for cake. But he was hours late starting the cooking, so we were still eating dinner when the guests came. We rushed through dinner, the guests rushed through the cake and went home, Daniel left the kitchen a mess, and then we had a fight about how late he was, during which I broke my toe." The meaning? "He'd never admit all this was anything but an accident," Maggie says, "but in fact it told me he was mentally out of the relationship and that we were washed up. The actual revelation that he was having an affair was an anticlimax. All it did was finally break us up."

That reality, perhaps, is the scariest and hardest-to-face underside of an affair: Your desire to have one may be a disguised sign of dissatisfaction with your main relationship. While a small percentage of couples—experts say about 5 percent—might be able to tolerate extramarital affairs, those are still poor odds, which suggests that succumbing to the itch has potentially fateful consequences.

Of course, you may give in to temptation, be forgiven and emerge with a marriage or living arrangement stronger than the one you started out with. Or you could end up with a new and even more appropriate partner. But don't count on it. Don't, in other words, just assume your fling is an innocent tumble in the hay, only to realize in the end that it was a leap off the marital cliff.

FRIENDS AND LOVERS

A generation or two ago, while you might have traveled the rocky path from friendship to love affair, you probably wouldn't have told anybody about it. Both chumminess and passion abounded, of course, but if you were somebody's lover, you were in a relationship that was by definition secretive, if not downright illicit. You didn't chat it up with friends or see relationships similar to it discussed in mainstream magazines. And when infatuation dimmed, you didn't meet her on Thursdays for tennis or Scrabble, or to share a drink at the local brewpub. You went your separate ways, and she became a memory or a journal entry.

But then, in the sixties and seventies, came the relationship revolution, which culminated in the *When Harry Met Sally* phenomenon. One of the best-ever date movies, it follows Billy Crystal and Meg Ryan from college acquaintanceship to friendship to love and marriage years later. And in the process it draws a map of the uneasy border lying between affectionate camaraderie and love.

Crossing this uncharted territory, Harry and Sally exchange endearments, crossed signals, misunderstandings, even fisticuffs. You'll appreciate their confusion if you've been there yourself. You're not glued to someone by the epoxy bonds of marriage, yet you're more than passing acquaintances or transient beneficiaries of a fling. How do you know just what you are? At what point is it wise for a friend to become a lover? And if a relationship starts as infatuation but then grows moldy—think *Seinfeld's* Jerry and Elaine—how do you ease into friendship?

All the relationship experts consulted agreed on one point: It's easier (and probably more common) for friends to mutate into lovers than for lovers to stay amicable once the passion has ebbed. The key difference between the two slates is that love, whether gift or curse, is a thunderbolt, a mystery, a visitation from the gods. That means it's a quantum jump beyond the calmer (and more pedestrian) experience of friendship. "Friends can become lovers," says Tom Adamski, a New York City–based family and couples psychotherapist. "But I don't think it's really a natural occurrence, because it's usually magic that draws us to lovers."

Of course, it's possible for the prose of camaraderie to blossom into the poetry of love. "Sometimes magic can happen through negotiation," Adamski concedes, "but a lot of people would consider that boring. Magic, after all, defies the eye—we see past what we don't want to see in the person and get a little obsessed."

Nonetheless, it's clearly possible to work into love gradually, and there are some real advantages to doing so, says Carol Dougherty, a certified social worker with a couples practice in New York City. "It gives you a chance to get to know the person without the when-are-we-going-to-go-to-bed question popping up," she says, "and it always skews a relationship if one person wants to be sexual before the other: 'If I go to bed too quickly, will he think I'm cheap?' It can be good to have that whole element removed." Dougherty remarks that gay and lesbian couples (particularly the latter) seem to have an easier time making the transition from friendship to love than male-female pairs do, if only because they generally find friends and lovers among the same people.

"The single life, male or female, just doesn't seem to be about having friends of the opposite sex," Dougherty says. That's too bad, though not inevitable; she suggests that you might move more easily and smoothly from friendship to love if you're generally accustomed to regarding women as friends, and don't exclusively associate an opposite-sex relationship with passion.

Cooling love down into mere amity is often a taller order: You may be able to light the fire, but can you douse it without smashing the windows, flooding the house and wrecking the furniture? Both Adamski and Dougherty agree that doing so, while difficult, is possible. "People who are in the process of breaking up don't often say they want to stay friends," Dougherty says. "But it does happen."

But don't expect it to happen overnight. "In all separations," Adamski cautions, "there has to be a healthy period of anger." And Dougherty advises that the best way to turn a dying love affair into a living friendship is not to push too hard. "Make it okay not to be friends right away," she advises. "Realize that you're going to progress through your emotions at a different pace and that a breather is necessary."

So you have to face certain ambiguities. While there may be a natural harmony between love and friendship, the passage from exclusively one to exclusively the other can be ticklish. As Adamski points out, if someone's a friend but you want her to be a lover, you're proposing sex not out of simple lust but in a context of intimacy, and that can complicate things as much as it may enrich them. "Intimacy means exposing our vulnerabilities without the fear they'll be used against us," Adamski explains. Thus it's hard to add sex to (or subtract it from) intimacy without blowups. Remember the scene in the movie when Harry and Sally have sex? She's contented; he's stunned. Later, at a wedding, she does an about-face, clobbering him with a right cross for (she says) using sex as a weapon.

Such are the risks. Both Adamski and Dougherty agree that transitions require patience and tact, and caution against expecting them to be quick or trouble-free. Harry and Sally finally accelerate from the neutral of friendship to the overdrive of love on a romantic (and climactic) New Year's Eve. And downshifting's possible, too: It's not unusual to hear a divorced man admit, "I couldn't stand her when we were married, but I love her as a friend."

OF HUMAN BONDING

"Going male bonding again?" Bet you don't like the sound of it and never did, which is why the only time you usually hear "male bonding" is when it rolls from a woman's smirking lips. After all, there's something sacred about that rendezvous you're headed for, even if it does celebrate beer and basketball instead of relationships and emotions. As unrevealing or unemotive as these casual encounters may be, they provide the only social contact many of us make with others of our gender.

"I think male company is important," says thirty-six-year-old George Shadroui of Washington, D.C., "but at this stage I'm really not thinking about finding male friends. I'm thinking about finding a woman. I go to the gym and play basketball a couple times a week, but that's it for hanging out with guys."

For others among us, male friendships start to dwindle once we find a mate and begin spending all our free time with her. The competitiveness among men and our fear of appearing vulnerable also make many of us wary of confiding in any but our longest-held friends.

And then there's that homophobia thing. As Irma Kurtz writes in her book *Man Talk: A Book for Women Only*, "If any pair of men were as exclusive as two women best friends, they would be marked as homosexuals." So, we gather to shoot hoops, drink beer, watch football, play cards. We emote for home runs and winning three-pointers, leaving the impending divorces, terminal diseases and other not-so-fun stuff in the bleachers.

That's why psychologist Herb Goldberg, Ph.D., author of five books on men, including the bestseller *The Hazards of Being Male*, describes men as generally dysfunctional in their social contact with other men. In fact, Goldberg says, male bonding itself is a complete misnomer. "It has become nothing more than a trendy term," he says. "Men may gather to share an activity, but without the activity or without the TV or without looking at women, they really don't have much to say to each other. I don't think men generally feel very comfortable around other men." Goldberg defines real male bonding as "a deep connection, particularly emotional, when men offer support and empathy, real caring, for each other. This doesn't happen in bars. It's very rare."

Of course, you could argue that if deeper connections are so rare, a casual get-together in a bar is better than nothing. In fact, says psychologist Ritch Savin-Williams, it's not only better than nothing but perfectly fine. "Men often bond based on activity rather than on emotional, face-to-face exchange," says Savin-Williams, a professor of development and clinical psychology at Cornell University. "Just because men don't usually sit down and share their lives with each other as women tend to do, this isn't to say men don't form intimate friendships. You don't have to talk to feel emotionally close to someone. Men just don't have the same need to exchange feelings verbally. "

You could do what folks have been doing since Freud and blame male taciturnity on your forefathers. But according to Lionel Tiger, the Canadian anthropologist who coined the term male bonding, you'd have to follow your family tree back about a million years. Indeed, in *Men in Groups*, his still influential 1970 book, Tiger finds the seeds of bonding among our caveman forebears, whose tradition of gathering for the hunt, he says, became genetically ingrained. In this way, says the anthropologist, the male-male bond became "of the same biological order for defense, food-gathering and maintaining social order as the male-female bond is for reproduction."

Tiger says we are innately drawn together in groups, our guttural sporting cheers for the home team perhaps harking back to our chants during those meaty pursuits of millennia past. "Make that quarterback eat some turf," in other words, could be a rough extension of "Let's get that woolly mammoth." Gail Kennedy, Ph.D., a biological anthropologist at UCLA, says that while "there is no scientific evidence we've found to support [Tiger's male-bonding theory] I don't doubt there may be some very deep genetic basis to it. Still, I think the origin has been overwhelmed by our culture. I mean, it's hard to take a group of men hunting woolly mammoth on the frozen plains and find a link with a bunch of guys getting together to drink beer and watch sports all day."

Whether or not there's a connection, beer-commercial-style bonding may be more complex than meets the eye. After all, everyone who's ever watched "Cheers" knows that once the beer gets flowing, guys often start opening up and emoting. As psychologist Ken Druck writes in *The Secrets Men Keep*, "We can be sentimental, tearful, silly and affectionate with other men if we have been drinking beer. And later if we are embarrassed by our actions, then we can always claim we had 'one too many' and none of our buddies will think the worst of us."

Which is why some people suggest men are drawn to beer and sports, seeking the pseudo-intimacy they provide. Of course, psychologists like Goldberg would prefer these encounters were not alcohol-related and that a more thorough forum for issues and feelings were created.

The contrary school, though, says that talk is cheap, emotions ephemeral and that men simply bypass discussion of these constant undulations. A woman may be able to share her thoughts comfortably with a group, but most men do have a best friend to, in effect, unload on when problems persist. The other men, those you gather with to watch a game or cross-train or whatever, may be no less valuable for the simple camaraderie they provide. As Savin-Williams explains, "The female pattern of friendship has become the way we seem to measure all friendship. Male friendship should not be measured against the female."

Nonetheless, perhaps we accept ribbing from a spouse or girlfriend about male bonding because deep down we know our best friendships are behind us. Remember the middle-aged protagonist, played by Richard Dreyfuss, in *Stand by Me*? He concluded that his best friends ever were those he had when he was ten years old. "There's some real truth to that, an unfortunate truth," Savin-Williams says. "We do look back nostalgically on those times when we were so expressive of our feelings with our friends."

FOR BETTER BONDING

Fred had Barney. Wally had Lumpy. Lenny had Squiggy. Do you miss having a really good buddy? Here are a few unscientific ways of recapturing those friendships of yore.

1. Join a team. Bowling, softball, basketball, whatever. Few bonds are as strong as those forged in sweat. Every town has a recreation department. Call for start-up dates.
2. Bond on the run. Running is the perfect non-team sport for making friends. Talking and sweating at the same time is the ultimate comfort zone for most men.
3. Head for the mountains. You may be uneasy about asking a guy you think is pretty cool to join you in a weekend resort town. But camping, pitting man against nature (or, at least, against public campgrounds), is beyond misinterpretation.
4. Pick a sensitive flick. For more revelatory conversation, take a potential pal to see something like *Field of Dreams*. If you do this, however, you have to make sure you avoid eye contact for at least sixty seconds after the movie ends to give your tears time to dry.
5. Hunt for a giant screen. Invite a prospective buddy to a sports bar to watch the home team with you. Why fight it? Beer plus sports equals male friendship.

GAY RELATIONSHIPS

For gay men in America, this is both the best and worst of times. On the upside, being openly gay has never been more accepted. Homosexuals can have open relationships—and in some cases, even marry—in many parts of the country. Some states and private companies extend spousal benefits to gay couples, conferring a legal acknowledgment and acceptance of these relationships that has never existed before. The public acceptance of gay men has never been higher, giving them a real choice about whether they will live their lives "out" or not.

Then there is the other part of this equation. While some states affirm the rights of gay people, others (notably Colorado) have tried to legislate homosexuality out of existence. Spousal benefits and marriage are a reality for gays in some places, but many more still face laws on the books against "homosexual acts" like oral sex (these laws also apply to straight people, but are almost never enforced except in cases of rape). The freedom to be openly gay exists primarily in major cities, which also have the highest incidence of "gay bashing" physical attacks. And then there is AIDS.

What would your life be like if perhaps half of your friends had died over the course of the last fifteen years? For gay men, those grim statistics aren't just theoretical. AIDS hit the gay community first and hardest, killing tens of thousands of homosexual men since the early 1980s. As if watching so many friends and lovers die wasn't horrible enough, gays also had to listen to evangelicals characterize AIDS as a "punishment from God" for their lifestyle. There is enormous bitterness among gays (and many others) over what they see as a slow response to the AIDS crisis by government health organizations. It was this aspect of AIDS that radicalized many gays, and encouraged them to become both "out" and vocal. But for all the media hype about the "gay nineties," homosexuality continues to be feared, misunderstood, demonized and attacked.

GAY/STRAIGHT FRIENDSHIPS

By Bruce Fierstein

Can a straight man and a gay man enjoy a close friendship? C'mon. On the face of it, doesn't this seem to be a real no-brainer? Halfway through the nineties, isn't it obvious that gay men and straight men can be friends? Yet as I thought about it—and talked to a half-dozen straight friends—I realized that maybe the answer isn't so simple or obvious.

I'm a straight, married, white male. I also wrote *Real Men Don't Eat Quiche*, which was widely misinterpreted to be both a) antigay and b) pro-Neanderthal. (In fact, it was neither. But you'd be amazed to find out how many "thinking" people condemned it without bothering to read past the title.) I have gay friends, just as I have straight friends. And just as there are homosexuals I greatly admire, there are also one or two I'd like to run over with a truck. (Most notably a gay decorator who embezzled $5,000 from my wife and me and, when caught, used his lover's AIDS treatments as an excuse. Only his lover didn't have AIDS. The decorator was just a thief who happened to be gay.) Do I condemn all forms of prejudice? Yes. Do I think anybody has a choice about being gay? Absolutely not.

So fine. That's all well and good (at least I think so), but these are just generalities. Politics and platitudes are nice, but friendships—one-on-one relationships—are based on trust, respect and honesty. And I think that the problems which stifle many gay/straight friendships are the falsehoods and misunderstandings we all bring to the table. Mostly, I think they fall into three areas: 1) sex, 2) sex, 3) sex. The following true/false questions might be illustrative.

1. All gay men look at you as a possible sexual partner. *False.* Have I been hit on by gay men? Sure. By every gay man I've met? Absolutely not. (And after a polite rebuff, the men who were interested just dropped it.) Look at it another way: Are straight men hot for every woman they meet? Of course not. Thus, this shouldn't be an issue. As a gay friend once kidded me, "Sorry, honey, but you just don't do it for me."

2. All straight men are a little bit gay. *Also false.* Unfortunately, I've sat at a dinner table with a smug gay man who claimed that all straight men are threatened by gays because we're repressing our own homosexual tendencies. With apologies to Sigmund Freud, I don't buy it. I've never been interested in or curious about having sex with a man. And the fastest way to kill any possible friendship is to impose your own beliefs and prejudices on somebody you barely know. In other words: I'll

accept you as a homosexual if you'll accept me as a heterosexual.

3. Sports and sex are the basis of all male bonding, and gays just can't fit into a heterosexual group. *False again.* I've worked on construction crews with Asians, Hispanics and African-Americans; inevitably, we found common ground by a) bitching about the boss and b) teasing each other about our sexual exploits. You hear that having gay men in this situation makes straight men uncomfortable. From my own experience, though, I know this isn't true. On one construction crew, we did have a gay man. One morning he showed up and, when he was asked why he was in such a good mood, he shrugged and said, "I got laid last night." Everyone cracked up, and whatever distance we felt from each other disappeared. In other words, lighten up. We're never going to be friends unless we start looking at each other as people and not as political statements.

Still, gay/straight friendship isn't easy. I've found it's easier to be friendly with someone who's openly homosexual and proud of it. If friendships are based on honesty, this is the fundamental truth. I don't care if you're gay. But I do know we're never going to achieve any kind of friendship if we're lying or hiding things from each other.

About a year ago, I was driving out to a film set with a gay man. We got stuck in traffic and, having time to kill, both began to talk about our sexual orientations. I got to ask the question I'd always been curious about: When did you first know you were gay? ("In seventh grade," he responded. "When everybody else had crushes on

girls, I was attracted to the math teacher.")
His frankness was not only interesting, but enlightening. I learned something about what makes another person tick.

Truth, honesty and understanding. As Humphrey Bogart said to Claude Raines at the end of *Casablanca*: "This could be the beginning of a beautiful friendship."

FAMILY RELATIONSHIPS

We all know what families used to be. The archetypes are familiar to us from sources as diverse as the *Little House on the Prairie* books and *Father Knows Best*. The question is: What is a family now? To be sure, the traditional "nuclear" family—homemaker mother, working father, children—is still with us as the most common variety, but it has been joined by other types of family as society has changed.

A family today might mean a divorced father raising two kids as the primary parent. It might refer to children who shuttle back and forth between working, separated parents. One family might consist of a child being raised by a set of grandparents, while another might be a traditional married couple parenting several adopted children. A family today can include stepchildren or stepparents, a woman raising a baby she conceived through artificial insemination or a gay couple having a child by adoption or artificial conception. Clearly, the "family" is a much more diverse institution than it was even a few years ago.

What do all of these families have in common? Though "family values" has become a freighted term, there are certainly common ethical threads that should be found in these various arrangements. To get the most from your family relationships, regardless of the type, these five elements are the most important:

1. Commitment—the idea of a "pact" that binds spouses to each other, parents to children and children to parents, and extended family members to one another. Without turning the clock back to the era of "until death do us part," there is a renewed emphasis on finding ways to rehabilitate troubled marriages rather than end them—especially when children are involved. After a divorce, there are stronger expectations that both parents remain faithful to the unbreakable covenant that binds parents to their children.

2. Care—the physical and emotional support of spouses and family members for one another. Care builds on the sense of commitment and requires the ability to empathize with and understand one another. To the traditional family's emphasis on physical and moral care of children, we now also expect parents to understand and foster the emotional lives of their children—and each other. As lifespans increase, the care of parents by adult children will become an even more important aspect.

3. Community—the importance of the family's ties with its neighborhood, local community, state, nation and world. The responsibilities go both ways—the family to the community and the community to the family. This value reflects efforts to mend the split between the private world of the family and the public world of the community and its institutions. Ultimately, the family can be no healthier that its community—and communities no healthier than their families.

4. Equality—the belief that women and men should have equal say in family matters and should stand as equals in the larger community, and that children should be given influence commensurate with their age and developmental abilities. This is the litmus test for the new emphasis on "family values." Will they become part of an effort to reverse women's gains towards equality with men, or will they instead become a vehicle for creating a new relationship between family members and their community?

5. Diversity—the support for all family forms that embrace the values stated above and provide for the well-being of their members. This is the chief new value underlying the "new family," and it will be hard to build a new consensus on family values without incorporating the value of diversity. Such family types as the never-married mother with children and gay and lesbian families are here to stay in a world that accepts the rights of citizens to form nontraditional family arrangements. This does not mean, however, that anything goes; all families should be judged by how well they provide commitment, care, equality and community for their members.

Family relationships were never simple, but are becoming increasing complex. But add a healthy dose of love to the above elements, and there's nothing that a family can't be—and can't do.

Creating Quality Time

James Colvin understands the impact of sports on relationships. A psychotherapist and minister, he's also a 2:25 marathoner. He runs so well that he literally ran away from his first marriage. "I was fairly young and clearly not with the right person," says Colvin. "I wasn't willing to face it, so running was a way to escape. Any sport can be an avoidance of reality."

Most of us first get into a workout groove, or begin playing recreational sports, when we're young and unattached. But the man who gives up sports often regrets it, and the man who refuses to give up his sport often pursues it at the expense of his family life. Is there any middle ground? Sure. Sometimes, the solution is to convince your mate to develop an interest in what you do. If you hit a stumbling block, then just back off.

Making peace, and compromising, is something thirty-five-year-old Todd Edelson, a former NCAA weightlifting champion and currently a serious cyclist, learned early in his marriage. They lived well enough with their differences (he rode; she read) until the birth of their two sons. Leisure time became a distant memory, so Todd figured out how to squeeze in road work by literally adding the boys to his workouts. Carrying one at a time on the back of his bike, he pedaled a mile and a half uphill—until they became too heavy to pull. "They loved being on the back of the bike," says Edelson, who has since graduated to teaching them to ride their own two-wheelers. Another good strategy: focus on sports like hiking, nature walks or in-line skating are good for the entire family.

The more serious you are about your sport, as a general rule, the harder you're going to have to work to maintain a happy household. Colvin cautions that it's very difficult to be a high-performance athlete, a good husband, a good father and hold a job. If you're serious, ask yourself if the investment is worth the price. If the answer is yes, he adds, "Give yourself permission to pursue what you love to its conclusion. Give it your best shot. But be realistic about your goals and what can be derived from accomplishing them."

Another issue to ponder is what your mate can expect when she accommodates your exercise habit or joins you. "Reciprocity is very important," says Colvin. Edelson, for example, frequently takes his sons out biking or on all-day hikes, which gives his wife time to herself.

The ultimate key to avoid becoming married to your workouts, says Colvin, is communication. "In essence," Colvin advises, "what you need to say is, 'This is important to me, and you are important to me. I'd like you to share it with me.'" And of course, there's nothing to stop you from taking up a sport or activity that's important to your significant other. Ultimately, with time and communication, a balance can be found.

9

THE MIDDLE YEARS AND BEYOND

It surprises me to discover, when I remove my shoes and socks, the same paper-white hairless ankles that struck me as pathetic when I observed them on my father. I felt betrayed when . . . the other day, and not for the first time, there arose to my nostrils out of my own body the musty attic smell my grandfather's body had.

—JOHN UPDIKE

Getting older might be a drag, but it's certainly better than the alternative. Besides, where is it written that it has to be a drag? In the past, aging was accepted passively. While there where always a few Dorian Gray types out there, most men simply shrugged and let nature take its course. Today, we know that it isn't necessary to go quietly into that dark night: we can fight the aging process tooth and nail (hopefully, with our own teeth). It's not a battle that we will win, but simply engaging in the fight can make all the difference in determining what the last half of life will be like.

If you want to determine what kind of hand you'll have to play in your later years, look to your family. What did your father's father die of? Which diseases recur in your mother's family? This information let's you know where you're starting, but how you conduct your life will greatly determine where you end up.

In this chapter we'll examine family medical histories and describe how to chart the health of your own family tree. But the bulk of the information here focuses on what changes you can make to slow the aging process and to be healthier today and tomorrow. There's a great deal of evidence that you can increase the quantity of your life. More importantly, the same changes that increase longevity also increase life's quality.

THE AGING PROCESS

As a species, man's "life span" is about 100—that's the age at which an average man would die if there were no diseases, predators or accidents. That figure hasn't changed throughout the years. Man's "life expectancy," however, continues to fluctuate. This is the age at which an average man can expect to die in a given country, when factors like environment, accident and disease rates, infant mortality and the quality of health care are figured in. For a resident of the United States, life expectancy was 47 years at the turn of the century; today it's about 75.

Say you're a typical American male of age 30. You've already lost six and a half pounds of lean body mass since your prime, which occurred roughly ten years ago. Lean body mass is composed of muscle, bone and vital organs—in short, everything that's not fat. What's in its place? You guessed it: six and a half pounds of fat.

Your body chemistry has changed, too. It doesn't burn the calories it once did. Your cardiovascular system has become less efficient. Your heart has already started to deteriorate, pumping fewer beats per minute. There are no outward signs, but your glucose tolerance, which is your body's ability to control blood sugar, has started to decline, putting you on the path to diabetes in about twenty years' time. High blood pressure is creeping up on you, particularly if you haven't been exercising enough, putting you on another fast track to heart disease.

"We don't just wake up when we're sixty years old and find out that we have diabetes, 40 percent body fat and reduced strength," says William Evans, Ph.D., co-author (with Irwin Rosenberg, M.D., and health writer Jacqueline Thompson) of *Biomarkers: The Ten Determinants of Aging You Can Control.* "Aging is a gradual and continuous process."

You can do a lot about that process. It's possible for you to slow down, stop and in some cases reverse changes in what he calls biomarkers, the body's internal, biological markers that determine how old your body really is. The secret, says Evans, is incorporating a realistic exercise and nutrition program into a busy work and personal schedule—no easy task, as you already know. But the payoff is compelling. "The important message," he says, "is that the earlier you begin in terms of prevention, the greater the effects are ultimately going to be."

Biomarker One: Muscle Mass

Evans and Rosenberg, in addition to holding faculty positions at Tufts University, work at the U.S. Department of Agriculture's Human Nutrition Research Center on Aging in Boston. Rosenberg, who directs the center, is a physician with a special interest in nutrition and metabolism. Evans heads the center's Human Physiology Laboratory and is the exercise advisor to the Boston Bruins and the New England Patriots. Their broad experience has led them to conclude that muscle is the key to slowing down the aging process. Not only does increased muscle mass boost your strength, but it also allows you to more easily burn body fat, increases your aerobic capacity and triggers your muscles' use of insulin—reducing your chances of developing diabetes.

Most physiologists believe you inevitably lose muscle cells as you grow older. Some studies show a loss of up to 30 percent of them between the ages of 20 and 70. You can compensate for this by increasing the size of the remaining cells through strength-building exercises.

The formula for strength is to work in the range of 60 to 80 percent of your 1-RM (or one resistance movement)—absolutely the heaviest weight you can lift with a single movement or muscle contraction. If you try to lift that weight a second time, you don't succeed because your muscle is too tired. If, for example, the most you can curl with a single movement is 60 pounds, you need to lift between 36 and 48 pounds for two or three sets at 8 to 12 repetitions for each set.

Biomarker Two: Strength

Like muscle mass, strength can be regained even if you've been dormant most of your life. But the strength you restore by exercise is different from the strength you felt in your teens to mid-twenties. Most of the muscle cells you lose are those that compose the fast-twitch fibers used for high-intensity exercises like sprinting or lifting. Those that remain, the slow-twitch variety, are essential for endurance and low-intensity movement.

The more you exercise, the more you forestall the loss of fast-twitch fibers, though some decline is inevitable. This explains why world-class sprinters, who need tremendous bursts of power, peak in their late teens or early twenties, but world-class marathon runners, for whom endurance is the key, can still compete into their late thirties.

Overall, the amount of strength you can both regain and maintain is still considerable, regardless of your age or physical condition. Evans and Rosenberg point to their work with 60- and 70-year-olds whose lifting ability, on average, increased from 44 to 85 pounds.

Biomarker Three: Basal Metabolic Rate

Your body is constantly building and destroying tissue, releasing heat and energy, a chemical process known as metabolism. Your basal metabolic rate (BMR) is the measure of this process when you are at rest—when you first awaken in the morning, for example. It's an important sign of how many calories your body is consuming because even at rest, your body needs fuel.

On the average, a person's BMR declines about 2 percent per decade starting at the age of 20. And as the BMR falls, so does the number of calories you need. At 30, you probably need about 100 fewer calories a day than you did ten years earlier. But if your eating habits haven't changed and you're not exercising as you did when you were younger, then that reduced BMR, those excess calories and that lighter exercise load all add up to more fat.

You can compensate by building muscle, which restores your BMR by forcing your body to burn more calories. Unlike fat, muscle is active tissue that requires extra caloric fuel to maintain itself.

Biomarker Four: Body-Fat Percentage

With a reduced BMR unmitigated by regular exercise, you probably would gain fat even if your body weight didn't change much. On the average, a man's body is composed of 18 percent fat at the age of 25. This increases to 38 percent at age 65.

To reverse this process, you shouldn't be overly concerned about losing weight unless you're obese. The primary goal should be shedding fat by gaining muscle. If you do that, your overall weight may not change significantly. Muscle tissue weighs more than fat, and that means someone covered with muscle could weigh more than he did when he was once covered with flab.

To change your ratio of fat to muscle, the best prescription always has been exercise and better eating habits. Diet alone may reduce the fat on your body, but you'll probably lose just as much muscle, if not more. A low-calorie diet can also rob you of nutrients, vitamins and minerals that you need to stay healthy.

Biomarker Five: Aerobic Capacity

Aerobic capacity is your body's ability to process oxygen, getting it from your lungs into your blood and, through the bloodstream, to all parts of your body. To do this effectively, you need healthy lungs, a strong heart and a good vascular (blood vessel) network.

If you're the average man of 30, your aerobic capacity has already started to decline. By age 65, it could be 30 to 40 percent smaller than it was when you were 20. As time passes, Evans and Rosenberg say your heart becomes less responsive to the surge of adrenaline that occurs with exertion. This deterioration is best reflected in peak heart rate, which typically drops from 200 beats per minute for a 20-year-old to 160 for a 60-year-old.

Exercise helps in two ways: It increases the density of your capillaries, raising the amount of oxygenated blood that can reach muscle cells, and it allows those muscle cells to put that oxygen to better use—converting energy stored in carbohydrates and fat into physical activity. As you grow older, muscle mass becomes more important for maintaining your aerobic capacity. Consequently, weight training is just as vital as walking, running or cycling.

Biomarker Six: Blood-Sugar Tolerance

The sugar in your blood, generated by the foods you eat, is called glucose. No matter how much or what you eat, your body tries to maintain a constant blood-glucose level. If you eat too little food, your liver compensates by manufacturing extra glucose. If you consume too much, your pancreas secretes insulin, which stimulates muscle cells to use glucose.

As you grow older, develop more fat and lose muscle, this balancing act can collapse. It takes more insulin to stimulate inadequate muscle tissue. Unfortunately, as you age, your pancreas starts to have trouble pumping out additional insulin. In fact, the pancreas can burn out, requiring insulin therapy to offset diabetes. Evans and Rosenberg say a diet low in fat and high in fiber (which means more raw vegetables and whole grains), along with regular workouts, can help reverse this trend.

Building muscle is particularly important since muscle burns up glucose, transforming it into energy. Muscles also store glucose as a reserve fuel called glycogen. If your muscle cells are inadequate, the glucose is circulated back to the liver and converted into fat.

The effects of exercise can be short-lived, and nowhere is this more evident than with muscles programmed to respond to insulin and burn up glucose. One week without strength building, says Evans, and the muscles' insulin sensitivity returns to pretraining levels.

Biomarker Seven: Cholesterol Levels

Cholesterol is a fatty substance that flows through the bloodstream attached to proteins. This combination of cholesterol and proteins is called lipoproteins. Not all lipoproteins are harmful. In fact, some are essential for your survival.

First, the bad guys: low-density lipoproteins (LDLs) are the kind of cholesterol that causes a waxy plaque buildup in the coronary arteries of the heart, a contributing factor to heart disease. Fortunately, high-density lipoproteins (HDLs) act as a scouring agent, cleansing the arteries of plaque buildup. If you want to protect yourself from heart disease, you must not only lower your LDL-cholesterol level but also raise the HDL cholesterol. A diet low in fat and cholesterol will take care of the first. A steady dose of aerobic exercise will help the second, as will reducing your overall body fat, quitting smoking and limiting your alcohol consumption to no more than six to eight ounces per week.

Biomarker Eight: Blood Pressure

Abnormally high blood pressure, called hypertension, affects about 60 million Americans and is a leading cause of strokes and heart attacks. Heredity plays a big role here. But it's not the only cause of hypertension. Smoking, obesity, too little exercise and too much fat and alcohol can contribute to the problem.

A common belief is that a low-salt diet is the first line of defense. But only 10 percent of the population has blood pressure that's truly salt responsive, Evans and Rosenberg report. Overall body composition, though, seems a key ingredient in everyone's blood pressure. Too much body fat will trigger blood pressure problems just as it contributes to glucose intolerance. Again, it's important to replace a lot of those fats in your diet with carbohydrates.

Moreover, vigorous workouts have been cited as effective for preventing and treating hypertension. The Institute for Aerobics Research found that people who stay fit have a 34 percent lower risk of developing hypertension. Other studies show that those who already have hypertension can lower it through aerobic exercise, although the results may not be long lasting.

Biomarker Nine: Bone Density

On the average, you can expect to lose about 1 percent of your bone mass each year. More important than mass, though, is bone mineral content. Deficiencies in calcium and other minerals could leave your bones brittle, more easily fractured and harder to heal. You have two types of bone in your body: cortical bone—compact, solid-looking bones found mostly in your forearms and shins; and trabecular bone—the lattice of branching, bony spicules found mostly in your spine, hips and thighs. More trabecular bone is lost with aging, although the decline is more of a problem for women than it is for men.

Repeatedly placing stress on your bones through aerobic exercise like walking, running or cycling can reverse this deterioration, causing the bones to absorb more calcium from the blood and grow stronger. Bone loss also seems related to muscle loss. In their studies, Evans and Rosenberg found that weight lifting, because it maintains or increases muscle mass, is also an important way to preserve and even increase bone density.

Biomarker Ten: Internal Temperature

Your body comes with a built-in thermostat that keeps your internal temperature within a degree of 98.6 Fahrenheit—even if it's hot or cold outside. In hot weather, sweat acts as a cooling-off mechanism. In cold, shivering is the body's way of generating heat. Unfortunately, your ability to sweat and shiver declines with age.

As your heart grows older, it pumps less blood to the skin, through which internal heat finds its escape in the form of sweat. With heat trapped inside, your internal temperature can soar to dangerous levels. The kidneys' ability to control internal water balance also declines with age, increasing the risk of dehydration. Exercise compensates for your heart and kidneys' reduced capacity by improving your ability to sweat and increasing the amount of water in your blood, allowing you to lose more through perspiration.

Shivering is a simpler process involving the rapid contraction of muscles to generate body heat. Loss of muscle mass means a reduced ability to shiver. By building up muscle through strength training, you improve your ability to do so. Aerobic exercise and weight training, then, keep you fitter in fair weather and foul.

The Anti-Aging Prescription

If you want to slow down the aging process, the conclusion of the biomarker section is clear: Exercise keeps you young. And not just any kind of exercise, either. Your body is a complex piece of work, and it thrives on variety. Aerobic conditioning and weight training are twin components in reversing the effects of age. If you were to simply lift weights to build muscle, you'd be neglecting the needs of your cardiovascular system, which has a primary role in four of the 10 biomarkers and a vital supporting role in the other six. On the other hand, if you did only aerobic work, such as running or cycling, you wouldn't reap the anti-aging benefits of building muscle mass.

The research conducted at the USDA's Center on Aging has convinced Evans and Rosenberg that the highest level of "biomarker fitness" is gained on an anti-aging program that consists of five aerobic workouts—such as brisk walking, cycling, running, swimming or jumping rope—and three weightlifting sessions per week, for a combined total of seven hours tops. Once you reach that point, you can maintain your peak fitness with three aerobic and two strength-building sessions, for a weekly total of four to five hours. On that kind of program, you don't need to count calories. Just cut back on saturated fats and eat plenty of vegetables and whole grains.

But to affect your biomarkers, Evans explains, the exercise frequency and intensity have to be consistent and strenuous enough to get you huffing and puffing, but not torturous. Don't do too much too fast. "We see this all the time with men in their thirties and forties," he says. "They think they can gain it all back overnight. If you start out too fast, you're likely to be hurt or discouraged." To ensure that you don't overtrain, Evans suggests, "Take days off to let the muscles recoup. Otherwise, you negate the benefits you've gained."

How much can you control your life expectancy? A lot, according to numerous studies. One, involving almost 7,000 adults in Alameda County, California, showed that there was a difference of eleven years in life expectancy between people who maintained healthy habits and those who didn't. The habits were simple: a regular eating schedule that included breakfast, proper body weight based on height and age, seven to eight hours of sleep regularly, no smoking, little alcohol and regular exercise.

As significant as longevity is, both Evans and Rosenberg stress that quality of life, what they term "health span," is as vital as a longer life expectancy. Your health span is the period of life characterized by vigorous activity and general physical well-being. If you follow an exercise regimen throughout the years, you could achieve the ideal: a health span that comes close to matching your longer life, leaving you fit and self-reliant almost to the end.

Age isn't destiny: If you stay in shape, it's possible to be a rock at 70, and just as easy to lapse into mashed-potatodom at 20 if you don't exercise. On average, you achieve your maximum lifetime muscle strength somewhere between ages 20 and 30, then gradually lose 10 to 20 percent of it by the time you're 65. Your maximum heart rate, aerobic capacity, reaction time and movement speed also all decline with time. If you're a fit 20-year-old male, about 10 percent of your total body mass is fat; by 55, it's typically 25 percent. We won't talk about what happens to your brain-cell count.

But there's a significant crack in the tombstone raised by such somber statistics. Remember, they're averages, which means they describe what typically happens to a large group of aging men. That may say something about Americans' health habits in general, but it doesn't mean you have to be the average Joe. Here's what can happen if you buck the trend:

- In a Stanford University study published in the Journal of Gerontology, a group of seniors (average age just over 68) embarked on a yearlong weight-training regimen. During the first three months of the program, those who worked out 3 times a week, doing 3 sets of 8 reps at each of 12 stations, had strength increases of up to 97 percent. They also enjoyed muscle size leaps of up to nearly 70 percent.
- A recent study conducted by the NASA/Johnson Space Center and the

Cooper Institute for Aerobics Research in Dallas found that if an average 30-year-old man's body fat percentage increases by 50 percent (not at all unusual) and he remains sedentary, by age 70 he will lose nearly half his aerobic capacity. On the other hand, if he keeps his body composition at 20 percent fat and exercises even a little, he will cut that loss in half. If he stays lean and exercises aerobically three times a week, he will lose only 7 percent of his aerobic capacity.

- In another recent Cooper Institute study of men from 20 to 82, those who merely went from sedentary to moderately active reduced their risk of dying by 44 percent.
- The 26-year-long Harvard alumni study found that men who expended at least 1,500 calories a week in "vigorous" activity (brisk walking qualified) were 25 percent less likely to die during the study, even after accounting for age, smoking habits, high blood pressure, diabetes and family history.

Anybody who's considering embarking on a serious workout program should get a check-up first, but unless you're incapacitated by illness, age isn't all that cruel. "For somebody starting at 40, there'd be almost no difference from the routine of somebody starting at 30," says Eric Martellini, a fitness consultant at New York's American Fitness Center with a background in sports immunology. "In general, a 50-year-old should start a little slower. You might get to the same cardiovascular level as somebody who's been working out for 25 years, and your range of motion will increase, but you probably won't achieve the same strength and endurance levels. And at 60, as long as you have no physical impediments, I'd focus on increasing your flexibility and range of motion," Martellini says.

"Your body has a very acute memory," he adds. "If you stop exercising, say, between 45 and 60, you may not get back to where you were 15 years earlier. But you will be able to outdo somebody who's never worked out." That's not to recommend repeated bouts of self-indulgence followed by repentant frenzies of exercise: While slips, even long-term ones, can be coped with, consistency remains a virtue.

Of course, you can't compare a 25-year-old's body to a 65-year-old's. But a 65-year-old who's achieving his full potential can be better off than a 25-year-old who goofs off.

CHEMICAL WARFARE AGAINST AGING

The longevity "miracle" of the moment is a hormone that has become so faddish, health food stores are having trouble keeping it in stock. Blood levels of melatonin, which is secreted at night by the pineal gland in the brain, rise from birth to about age six, then decline. At age 45 people produce only about half as much melatonin as they did at six.

Some years ago, an Italian immunologist began injecting mice with enough melatonin to maintain peak levels throughout their lives. Those that got extra melatonin lived one-third longer, the equivalent of 25 years in human terms. Since then, studies have shown that melatonin improves sleep, combats jet lag, boosts the immune system and acts as a powerful antioxidant, which may help prevent cancer, heart disease and possibly Alzheimer's disease. Marketers are also touting it as a life extender. Here's just some of what melatonin may be able to do:

- Cancer prevention and treatment. At the University of Texas, when live tumors were induced in mice, those that received melatonin developed substantially fewer tumors. When melatonin-taking mice were zapped with high doses of radiation, the death rate was half what it would have been without the hormone. In an Italian study, 10 milligrams daily of melatonin extended the survival of people with lung cancer.

- Cataract prevention. In rat studies, melatonin has been shown extremely effective in preventing the clouding of the lens of the eye that often accompanies aging.

- Immune-system enhancements. Several animal studies have shown that melatonin increases laboratory animals' ability to resist deadly diseases such as viral encephalitis.

- Insomnia. Several studies show that taking as little as 1 milligram of melatonin at night brings sound sleep to chronic insomniacs. (The hormone also reportedly increases the frequency of erotic dreams.)

It's still too early to know if melatonin is a major longevity booster. Most of the research has been performed on animals, not people. But the results have been intriguing, and the human tests to date have produced similar results.

By most accounts, melatonin appears safe at recommended doses—1 to 10 milligrams a night—but side effects, interactions with other drugs and long-term effects are still unclear. A month's supply costs about ten dollars in health food stores—if they have it in stock.

Another hot, potentially life-extending item is DHEA (dehydroepiandrosterone), an adrenal hormone involved in the synthesis of estrogen and testosterone. While testosterone has been used for men (and women) to fight the loss of libido that can come with aging, DHEA is a controversial new hormone-replacement therapy that may protect patients from the depression and loss of energy that can accompany the last third of life.

So far, DHEA looks extremely promising. Lab mice treated with the hormone drop body fat, increase muscle mass and live longer. Human studies at the University of California at San Diego have linked men with naturally higher levels of DHEA to a sharply decreased heart-disease rate. In one study of men who took DHEA experimentally, 67 percent showed increases in their ability to sleep, handle stress and in their overall wellbeing. Human Growth Hormone has shown many of these same benefits, but must be injected twice a day at a cost of $800. DHEA is in pill form, and costs about $30 per month.

Though preliminary results are promising, DHEA is a long way from being accepted by the medical community as an age tonic. Still, some doctors around the country are prescribing it—and many patients find the result to be nothing short of life-altering. Time will tell if DHEA really can relieve the symptoms of aging, or whether it will join the list of anti-aging substances that were mere flashes in the pan.

BODY IMAGE THROUGH THE AGES

Chronological aging is a constant, unrelenting process. It just can't be stopped. But some physical aging can be slowed, and the visible evidence hidden. Men have a real advantage here because our skin is thicker and shows the effects of age more slowly. Facial and body hair also protect the skin (and hide a multitude of sins). And if you shave regularly, the exfoliation keeps your skin renewed and healthier in appearance.

Genetics dictate many of the physical aspects of getting older. Fairer skin, for instance, doesn't age as well as darker skin because it lacks protective pigments—and there's not much you can do about that. Still, there are ways to detour nature's march. If you exercise regularly, avoid sun damage, don't smoke (it causes wrinkles, among other things) and eat a healthy diet, you're already on the path to aging gracefully. If you don't already do these things, start now. Then consult the chart for ways to improve your appearance at any age.

HOLDING BACK THE YEARS

	20s	30s	40s	50+
SKIN CHARACTERISTICS	Skin is generally clear. Main problems are oiliness and acne. Collagen, the substance that helps skin maintain elasticity, begins decreasing by 1 percent per year.	First signs of crow's feet. Wrinkles from sun exposure appear if you haven't been using sunscreen. Elasticity declines; eyelids begin dropping. Gravity-induced wrinkles as well as solar lentigos (flat brown freckles) often emerge. Blood vessels may appear on the top layer of skin. Skin becomes duller.	Sleep lines form in the forehead. Nasolabial folds (the lines between the corners of the nose and mouth) deepen. Solar lentigos increase. Skin becomes dryer and elasticity decreases. Double chin may appear.	Wrinkles increase, especially around the mouth. Lips thin, nasal tip droops, jowls increase and nasolabial lines deepen. Oil gland activity decreases, making skin dryer and flakier. Skin loses pigment. Sun and age spots increase.
SKIN OPTIONS	Use mild soaps to reduce oils. More drying soaps tend to be antibacterial and can irritate sensitive skin. If you have acne, ask your dermatologist about Retin-A or Accutane. Most important: Use a sunscreen (at least SPF 15) whenever you go outside. It can delay the onset of wrinkles and help reverse the effects of sun exposure in adolescence.	Keep using sunscreen for protection and to help reverse any earlier damage. Ask your dermatologist about exfoliants like Retin-A or glycolic acid to remove dead top layer. Hyfercation, a brief office procedure, can zap surface blood vessels. Use a hypoallergenic moisturizer to mask lines and wrinkles by hydrating the skin.	Continue sunscreen, exfoliant and moisturizer use. Sleep on your back to combat facial wrinkles. Avoid large weight fluctuations; skin stretched by fat doesn't always return to its previous state.	Continue sunscreen, exfoliant and moisturizer use. Sun protection is particularly important since pigment loss lessens natural protection. Camouflage thinning lips with facial hair. Cryosurgery (liquid nitrogen) or bleaching cream can eliminate sun and age spots.

	20s	**30s**	**40s**	**50+**
HAIR CHARACTERISTICS	Still a full head, but a normal daily loss of 75 hairs begins. Male pattern baldness may begin to develop.	Scalp produces less oil, and hair loss increases. Graying may occur. Hair grows in ears and nose. Male pattern baldness hits its stride for some.	Loss quickens and crown thins. Graying continues. Eyebrows thicken.	Thinning continues, but male pattern baldness may stabilize in the 60s. Scalp becomes dryer, hair more brittle.
HAIR OPTIONS	Be gentle with your hair. Hold the blow dryer away from your head and keep it moving. Use conditioner and a wide-toothed comb to prevent excess daily loss.	Minoxidil treatments may help combat balding. Keep up gentle hair care and cut back on shampooing (there's less oil to wash out). Pluck or trim unwanted hairs.	Minoxidil treatments may help slow or reverse hair loss. Continue gentle handling. Cut hair short to make it appear fuller.	Wear hats in the sun. Use gentle preservative- and fragrance-free shampoos and conditioners to prevent drying.

THE AGING ATHLETE

At which chronological crossroads of his life do we begin referring to a sportsman as an "aging athlete"? We all played touch football on the college quad with Joe Shmoes whose midsections were already expanding by spring of their freshman year. Perhaps aging commences at 25—the age before which "you don't need to stretch."

How you define an "aging athlete" is relative to how you define your limitations. In this era of sophisticated conditioning and sports-specific training, it's now possible to actually improve in your sport as you get older. If you have any doubts, check out a few of these "aging athlete" profiles:

- Butterfly swimmer Pablo Morales had an Olympic silver medal at 19, was a burnout at 23, but somehow figured he wasn't done yet. In a sport considered the domain of teenagers, Morales came off a three-year layoff to finally secure his gold at 27.
- In 1992, runner Jim Spivey was 32 and still America's top miler.
- Nolan Ryan, 46, still throws a 92 mph fastball.

Anomalies will always exist—a generation ago, pitcher Warren Spahn won 23 games at the age of 42, while George Blanda played professional football until he was 48. But when they're as plentiful as they are today, they constitute a major trend.

Elite athletes are prolonging their careers thanks to improvements in equipment and facilities and breakthroughs in coaching and sports medicine. But now we know that recreational athletes can make similar strides in their sports. These days, it's entirely possible to get older and better.

A recent entry in a research journal called *Sports Medicine* offered this shocker: "Static and dynamic muscle strength seem well preserved to almost 45 years of age." In other words, strength can remain on a plateau or can even increase until the mid-forties. And the news gets even better: The study, performed at the University of Toronto, shows that strength deteriorates by only 5 percent per decade after 45.

What this and other studies tell us is that a man with a fitness plan involving a carefully thought-out program of diet and exercise can, to a degree, slow down or even reverse the debilitating effects of aging on athletic prowess. The Toronto study says it "remains uncertain how far any age-related losses of muscle function are an inevitable consequence of aging, and how far they merely reflect the age-related decrease in physical activity." The rapid physical deterioration we saw in adults of our parents' generation is far from an inevitability.

All athletes should realize that when training, sometimes more isn't better. Suggestions from the pros follow.

- Break your training into distinct seasons. College and professional team sports aren't at full tilt twelve months a year, and neither should you be if you want to preserve your athletic career.
- Learn the virtues of rest. If your emphasis is on competitive performance, your mission is to be ready for superlative effort on contest day. This requires freshness. A runner or cyclist with a race on Saturday, for instance, might train lightly on Thursday and do nothing on Friday. Develop sufficient self-knowledge and self-confidence to realize that your conditioning base won't vanish overnight.
- Don't pay attention to guys who brag of eleven-year streaks without having missed a day of workouts; these guys are maniacs, and they're probably in constant pain.
- Many people, once they leave competitive sports in college, quit weight training and just do the cardiovascular work. The American College of Sports Medicine recommends weight work twice a week to build muscle, in part because "muscle is ten times more metabolically active than fat."
- Then, of course, there's also the issue of injury prevention. Frank Shorter, 1972's Olympic marathon champion, observes in *The New York Road Runners Club Complete Book of Running* that "it's not so much that you're prone to injury as you get older, it's that the amount you've done builds up. Everybody has a saturation point. Then you get hurt." Cross training allows minor injuries to heal while you stay active. Shorter, for instance, has stayed fresh with run-bike biathlons, "an area in which I can still improve." He does 40 percent of his aerobic training on the bike "to relieve the stress" caused by pounding the pavement.
- Athletes of all inclinations are getting into the pool, but not necessarily to swim. Flotation devices permit zero-impact workouts, which are great for cyclists, runners, basketball and football players, and anyone else who needs to minimize stress while staying in top shape.
- As a cross trainer, pay attention to the benefits you may need but might not get from your primary sport. Running stairs is an excellent aerobic exercise, and it'll increase your range of motion, too. In-line skating may seem like an obstructive nuisance to sportsmen competing for the same space. But, in fact, it's a serious cross-training tool for runners, hockey players, cyclists and other sorts of endurance athletes.

- Your primary sport can be less of a chore if you have specific goals, even in training. How many twenty-foot jump shots can you make in a row? Can you swim one more lap than you did in your last arduous workout? How many times can you punch the light bag in regular cadence?
- Don't let your motivation shrivel up. If your own is stale, get it from others. Think about teams, training partners, classes, personal trainers.
- Athletes in so-called "individual" sports may, as they age, begin to crave company. Triathlete Art Murphy, 27, enjoys biking with a team because "you ride faster in the pack. It's easier to let someone else take the lead for a change." And time passes faster. "I remember going for 100-mile rides by myself, That's six hours. Your mind starts to wander and your body aches and you say, 'What am I doing this for?'" Murphy says.
- Teammates and training pals are a boon, but the aging athlete may also desire advice, tips, guidance—a coach. Outside evaluation helps, as does the notion that someone else cares and encourages. Many amateur sports clubs pool their dues to hire a coach.

An aging athlete (whether he's 25 or 65) should appreciate that training for his sport is the one thing he can control. If the rest of your life is a struggle, the pursuit of your athletic goals—ever higher, ever farther, ever better—remains a constructive chase. Being an athlete offers a challenge to one's apparent limits.

There's much we can do to retard the body's aging process. And when the inevitable athletic slide does start, there are still plenty of good reasons to stay in the race.

ADVICE FOR AGING WEIGHT TRAINERS

by Arnold Schwarzenegger

Any athlete can improve his sports performance through strength training, regardless of his age. I've lifted weights for almost thirty years without injuring myself. Here's some practical training advice to keep you healthy and fit.

The Warm Up: The older you are, the more time it takes to prepare the muscles and connective tissue for a serious workout. You should always stretch your muscles before you train. Stretching improves circulation, enhances flexibility and helps to prevent injuries. And that increased flexibility is another way to increase your range of motion for lifting, triggering muscle-fiber stimulation, growth and strength.

High-Intensity Training: Heavy weights aren't the only ticket to building strong and powerful muscles. The aging athlete should rely on creativity instead of heaving heavy iron. A few high-intensity training alternatives:

- Forced reps: Enlist a training partner to help you squeeze out one or two more reps after you've reached the point of momentary muscle failure.
- Supersets: Do two exercises back-to-back for opposing muscle groups like biceps or triceps), or when training the same body part (bench presses and flyes for the chest, for example).
- Giant sets: Do four to six different exercises—one set each—in sequence. With this method, stick with working one body part at a time.

All three techniques allow you to use a somewhat lighter weight, stay in the proper groove to prevent injury and still work hard enough to build muscle mass.

Recovery Time: Proper exercise form demands adequate recovery time between workouts, especially as you get older and become more susceptible to nagging injuries. Never train the same body part two days in a row. A three-day-a-week program hitting all major muscle groups is ideal.

Proper Diet: I like to eat four to six small meals a day, and split up the calories as follows: 60 percent carbohydrate, 30 percent protein, 10 percent fat. Stay in this range, and you'll be able to maintain energy, build muscle and stay lean for a lifetime.

SEXUALITY THROUGH THE AGES

It's ironic, isn't it? During late adolescence, that awkward period of runaway hormones, hasty orgasms and erections that possess a mind of their own, our sex drive peaks when we can least control it. With a certain relief, as we enter our more sexually subdued twenties, that freneticism becomes a thing of the past.

But being beyond that libidinous heyday is no piece of cake either.

With each passing decade, our physical sexuality inevitably diminishes: The desire for it wanes, the orgasms seem less intense and the erections become less resilient. Even though regular exercise greatly reduces the impact of aging, if you plan on remaining sexually active into your seventies and beyond, you'll need to be psychologically prepared for the changes Mother Nature has in store.

The physical aspect of a man's libido declines gradually throughout adulthood because the testicles produce diminishing levels of the male hormone that fires his sex drive. Researchers have discovered, for example, that in men as young as thirty, testosterone levels begin to ebb and surge in regular monthly cycles. As we enter our fifties and sixties, the overall hormone level drops and the fluctuations become more pronounced.

The dampening effect this has on sex drive is apparent in the average rate of sexual activity among men in different age groups. According to McGill University associate professor Yosh Taguchi, M.D., author of *Private Parts,* "For men in their twenties, the average frequency of ejaculation or intercourse per week is four to five times; two to four times a week during the thirties; once or twice a week during the forties; none to once a week during the fifties and from the sixties on, once or twice a month." Taguchi also notes that two-thirds of men in their sixties and one-third of those over seventy remain sexually active.

With the passing of years, men also exhibit changes in their physical response to orgasm. When you were twenty, for example, your erections probably retained their rigidity for several minutes after a climax, maybe even longer. Men in their thirties and forties, however, find that erections relax almost immediately following orgasm.

The characteristics of arousal and climax eventually change as well. By the time they reach their fifties, men begin to notice that ejaculations are less powerful and contain smaller amounts of semen. The intensity level of the orgasm itself may diminish, too.

This isn't all bad. That somewhat delayed sexual response makes us more erotically compatible with women, who tend to reach their own sexual peaks in their late thirties. Middle-aged men often require additional foreplay to become physically aroused, and they need longer periods of intercourse before they climax—all of which makes them very popular with the ladies.

These changes are so subtle that they're almost imperceptible to the man who's younger than forty-five. They're also not carved in stone: As researchers are beginning to discover, men who remain physically and mentally fit throughout adulthood remain sexually much younger than their years.

In the general population, which is mostly sedentary, men first begin to notice distinct changes in sexuality between the ages of 45 and 55. However, a recent study performed by Maria Simonson, Ph.D., of Johns Hopkins University, revealed that men who were physically active didn't exhibit appreciable differences until they were in their sixties. "The men who noticed changes at 65," Simonson explains, "and who felt young and good and could perform were the ones who, around 50, had started jogging, walking or working out at a gym. A lot of them quit smoking. They were trimming down, too. One man lost 65 pounds."

Simonson adds that not surprisingly, the changes which did occur were generally positive. "For instance, it took them longer to climax," she says. "But they weren't sweating it out and waiting; they were deliberately prolonging the act. They enjoyed it more and were more relaxed."

According to Simonson, much of the success enjoyed by the men in her study was the result of maintaining a positive mental attitude. "It's 50 percent physical and 50 percent psychological," she notes. "A lot of men are taught from early on that the older they get, the less real pleasure they'll receive and the less they'll be able to perform. That's what drags them down."

Researchers in the field of sexuality and aging now believe that many performance problems previously attributed to age actually have psychological origins. A man may lose interest in sex, for example, because his relationship with his wife has changed or because other areas of his life—like his health and his career—are problematic.

What often happens, says Los Angeles psychologist Linda DeVillers, Ph.D., who specializes in the treatment of sexual dysfunction, is that once a man starts feeling old, he perceives the physical changes affecting his body as beyond his control, and he panics the first time he has difficulty gaining an erection. The resulting fear and loss of confidence snowball into full-blown sexual dysfunction. "If a man doesn't learn to cognitively reframe his sexual experiences as he grows older, he risks complications," she adds. "There's a lot of self-fulfilling prophesy in these performance problems. It's amazing how much depends on what's going on between your ears."

Joy of Sex author Alex Comfort showed this in a study of the "refractory period" following orgasm, the recovery time during which a man can't regain an erection. Previous research had concluded that the refractory period lengthens with age, and that men older than fifty might not be able to have another erection for a full day. More than half of the men that age in Comfort's study were able to ejaculate a second time within ten minutes.

The point is, factors associated with age do slow us down. But barring such medical problems as prostate cancer or impotence caused by illness, a man's libido can remain highly charged if he takes care of his body and his mind. Sexual vitality is as much a mental state as it is a physical one. As DeVillers suggests, check between your ears.

MALE MENOPAUSE

The change. The Silent Passage. Menopause—thank God it doesn't happen to men. Or does it?

If you've been paying attention to the media lately, you might be forgiven for thinking so. Since the seventies, some experts have publicly speculated that males do indeed undergo something akin to the female "change of life," and that the bell tolls at roughly the same age: somewhere between 40 and the early 50s, with the typical onset occurring around age 48.

But the subject flared up with renewed ferocity in recent years with a much-discussed *Vanity Fair* article by Gail Sheehy, titled "The Unspeakable Passage: Is There a Male Menopause?" Since then, the topic's been debated in *Reader's Digest*, on *Sonya Live* and in a feature on ABC's *20/20*.

In one sense, it's all piffle. Strictly speaking, the word "menopause" means one thing only: the cessation of menstruation. This happens rather suddenly in many women as ovaries begin to produce less estrogen. Ovulation ceases. Menopause, in other words, is an estrogen thing—and in that respect, at least, it's strictly female property. As a man, you're in the clear.

Sort of. While we don't experience menopause as such, men do go through a passage that experts prefer to call "viripause" or "andropause." Either term describes the consequences of a gradual fall in testosterone levels common in aging men (they typically undergo a 30 to 40 percent dip between the ages of 48 and 70). But most endocrine-system specialists and medical experts on aging are at best hesitant to liken this to menopause, because the two processes are so dissimilar.

"If you ask an endocrinologist whether there's such a thing as male menopause, the answer will be yes and no," says S. Mitchell Harman, M.D., Ph.D., a specialist in the field at the National Institutes of Health. "No, because a sudden drop in [hormone] levels doesn't typically happen in men. Yes, because there is a modest downward trend in total testosterone, and a slightly more prominent decline in available testosterone. But this doesn't happen to everybody, and except in the rarest cases it doesn't go down to pathologically low levels."

Testosterone, after all, is largely responsible for the development of most of the male secondary sex characteristics that emerge during puberty—the deepening voice, the ability to ejaculate semen, the hairy chin, the bulging muscles. It's been associated, both anecdotally and in some research, with the male lust for dominance and social status.

Indeed, some physical consequences have been associated with the gradual age-related drop in testosterone levels. "Certain men may have a decline in muscle strength and function," Matsumoto says. They may also experience an increase in body fat and a decrease in bone density as testosterone tapers off.

But contrary to popular wisdom, declining testosterone levels don't necessarily mean reproductive meltdown or even a sluggish libido. "Most studies suggest that sexual functioning isn't always related to [male hormone] levels," Matsumoto adds. And men, unlike women, can remain fertile until they're 80, 90 or even beyond.

Of course, whether you're wallowing in testosterone or starved for it, aging is stressful and full of predictable pitfalls. Your body changes over time, even if it doesn't suffer the relatively sudden transition of menopause. Aging has cultural as well as physical ramifications, and our youth-oriented society can be merciless to any form of weakness or disability. And here, predictably, meno/andro/viripause blends in with an even murkier and more discussed phenomenon: mid-life crisis.

Faced with mortality and the inevitability of at least some physical decline, it's scarcely surprising if you occasionally wake up in a fog of terror, convinced you're on your way over an athletic, sexual and mental Niagara. But remember: Napoleon dumped Josephine, married Marie Louise, fathered a son and invaded Russia, all well after he'd turned 40; you don't normally run out of testosterone on your 39th birthday. And even if you do, the hormone can be replenished artificially at your doctor's office.

Which leads to an interesting question: Should you take preventive measures? Are we entering a world in which men—on the off-chance they're among the few fated to experience a sudden, dramatic drop in testosterone production—begin replacement therapy in advance as a kind of machismo insurance?

"I hope not," says Emory University's Joyce Tenover, M.D., Ph.D., who has conducted a number of studies on the subject. "To take it, you have to either wear a scrotal patch, which isn't cosmetically great, or get injections, which isn't fun." And, paradoxically, receiving extra testosterone reduces the amount you naturally manufacture, which can have some nasty consequences if, for example, you're thinking of having children. (Testosterone treatments have, in fact, been looked at as a possible form of male contraception.)

Finally, while surplus testosterone may strengthen your bones and bulk up your muscles, it's also been linked with acne, antisocial behavior and heart, liver and prostate trouble.

"It's not a good idea to think about starting to replenish your testosterone levels at age 40," Matsumoto says. He and Tenover agree that it's more important to worry about extremely low testosterone levels in men of any age. However, Matsumoto concedes, "functioning declines with age, and anything within reason you can do to preserve it is worth doing."

So if you're 48, say, tired, flabby, brittle of bone, frail of muscle and besieged by frayed nerves and a flagging libido, consider talking to your doctor about testosterone replacement. But remember that these are ills all flesh is sometimes heir to, and their occasional appearance doesn't mean you've been mowed down by "viripause," "andropause" or "male menopause." There may well be less to those labels than meets the eye.

Men may not be doomed to a hormonal midlife crisis, but the way we age is inextricably tied to something just as mysterious: our genes. The aging process may well be determined from the moment of conception, when our individual genes are formed. While there's a great deal of influence we can have on our own health throughout life by the choices we make, it can be instructive to look to the family tree for clues to what our genes may have in store for us.

DOES HEREDITY EQUAL LONGEVITY?

On a hunch, thirty-year old Daniel Maier sat his paternal grandmother down a few years ago and asked some key questions about his family's health history. He was surprised to learn that his grandfather, who had died at eightysomething in a car accident, suffered from leukemia late in life. Talking to his mother, Maier later found out that her father had died of malignant melanoma.

"I had never considered myself at risk for cancer and had always checked 'no' on the doctor's office forms," Maier says. "My doctor told me that because my grandfather got his leukemia so late in life, I probably don't have to worry—but we still keep our eyes open for anemia, an early sign. And now I'm much more careful in the sun," which can trigger melanoma.

That's the whole purpose of tracking your family's health history—"to prevent disease or treat it early," says Michael Fleming, M.D., a family physician in Shreveport, Louisiana. However much you may not want them, many health problems—certain cancers, heart disease, diabetes, schizophrenia and more—pass from generation to generation via the genes. "The most important indicator of your health and fitness is your genes," says Maier, news and information director for the American Medical Association in Chicago.

Genes are made of DNA, chains of chemicals that control every process in your body. Half your genes come from Mom, half from Dad. "When something goes wrong with a gene," says Margaret Wallace, Ph.D., a genetic researcher at the University of Florida in Gainesville, "it may cause or predispose you to disease."

In some cases, if you get the defective gene, you almost certainly get the disease. This is true for familial hypercholesterolemia (very high cholesterol that becomes apparent in childhood) and neurofibromatosis ("Elephant Man disease"), both of which, fortunately, are rare. Others, including prostate and breast cancer, which seem to run in tandem through families, are far less inevitable. An as-yet-identified genetic defect may be behind both, theorizes David F. Anderson, Ph.D., of the University of Texas M.D. Anderson Cancer Center in Houston.

Another group of diseases, usually specific to certain ethnic groups, surfaces only if you acquire the problem gene from both parents. These include Tay-Sachs disease, cystic fibrosis and sickle-cell anemia.

PLAYING THE ODDS

For a more precise approximation of your risk factor, here is a table listing many common physical and mental-health problems affected by, but not directly linked to, genes. The risks are based on having one parent with the disease and increase if it affected or affects additional primary relatives.

Problem	Lifetime Risk (Percent)
Alcoholism	10–20
Alzheimer's	19

Problem	Lifetime Risk (Percent)
Asthma	4
Colon cancer	10
Diabetes (Type II)	5–10
Duodenal ulcer	30
Glaucoma	4–16
Migraine	45
Schizophrenia	8–18

Finally, there are male-specific diseases that the mother passes on. She doesn't experience the illness, but her sons have a 50–50 chance of acquiring the defective gene. The most common are hemophilia, color blindness and Duchenne-type muscular dystrophy.

Researchers have recently found that genes even play a role in such common disorders as allergies, heart disease, diabetes and many others. As studies of identical twins show, whether you actually develop the disease may depend on outside factors such as your diet, where you live, and what viruses and toxins you're exposed to.

To compile a history that's more definitive than the vague recollections of relatives, you will need old medical and government records. A living relative can probably obtain whatever records you need on him- or herself, if the person is willing. "The information in a medical record belongs to the patient, so the patient should be able to get a copy," Fleming says.

Getting the medical records of a deceased person presents more of a challenge. "Family members have the right to take to the grave whatever information they choose," explains Pamela Wear, executive director of the American Health Information Management Association in Chicago. "To get medical records, you need permission from the executor of the estate," who decides whether to release them. It's possible to beat the system by finding a cooperative physician or attorney to request the records.

Or, as Dan Maier points out, "One legally available document is the county coroner's report. The cause of death should be on that." Check with the Bureau of Vital Statistics, located in your state capital.

Additional places to check include newspaper obituaries, insurance company records, census records (check the National Archives in Washington, DC, or branches in major cities), the public library and military records (you can obtain a request form from the National Archives). (To obtain the pamphlet "Where to Write for Vital Records," write to: Superintendent of Documents, U.S. Government Printing Office, Washing-ton, DC 20402.)

With your research done, arrange your pages or index cards in the shape of a family tree. Then transfer your information onto one piece of paper, making squares for males and circles for females. (Or enter it into your computer database.) Include illness and causes of death, drawing a line through a deceased person's circle or square.

What do you see among family members nearest you? Any conditions that struck early in life or that hit several family members at the same age? Any that appeared on one side of the family? Do you see disease in someone whose lifestyle should have spared him—say, your grandfather the vegetarian had low blood pressure, exercised a lot and still had a heart attack? All of these are evidence of genes at work.

For more definite answers than your family tree provides, gene testing can pinpoint inherited defects that may presage disease. It should be noted, however, that ethicists cite instances in which insurers and employers have used the prospect of undergoing this testing as grounds for discrimination. It seems, for now, that means interested people need to weigh the benefits of knowing whether their genes are programmed for certain hereditary diseases against potential prejudice on the part of the powers that be.

We don't yet have tests for all diseases, but more and are becoming available, according to Paul R. Billings, M.D., Ph.D., chief of general internal medicine at the Palo Alto Veteran Affairs Medical Center in California. Currently available tests include those for Huntington's disease, cystic fibrosis, Lou Gehrig's disease and others. (To learn more about such diseases, contact the individual foundations that deals with them.) In adults, researchers usually look at blood cells; these tests cost anywhere from $100 to $1,000.

Whether you've gleaned knowledge from your family tree alone or from gene testing, your task is simply to watch for symptoms and stay clear of behavior that might magnify your risks. You need not become obsessive and live life in fear. It's as simple as maintaining some awareness to maximize your longevity.

APPLIED RISK

So what are you supposed to do if your family tree reveals you're at risk for these common health problems?

- Allergies. If you suspect you have allergies, your life will improve greatly if you have yourself tested for specific allergens (triggers) and avoid them or use antihistamines. In the case of severe allergies, especially those that set off an anaphylactic reaction involving your entire body, identifying allergens could save your life. Some people even believe that allergies can cause depression, learning disabilities and other quasi-physical symptoms.
- Asthma. Forget over-the-counter remedies. Your wheezing and coughing may indicate a serious condition that needs medical treatment.
- Colon cancer. You will want to start yearly testing for blood in the stool at age 30, not the generally recommended 40. Eat less fat and more fiber, advises Manrie Markman, M.D., director of the Cleveland Clinic Cancer Center.
- Diabetes. Your genes may have made you prone to diabetes, but you can still help prevent it by exercising and watching your weight. Frequent blood-sugar tests will let you know the minute disease sets in.
- Glaucoma (high pressure in the eye). Get your first test at least by age 40, not the recommended 50, especially if you have diabetes or high blood pressure.
- Heart disease. Have your cholesterol checked every one to five years, eat a low-fat diet and exercise regularly. Cholesterol-lowering drugs can reduce some of your risk.
- Migraine. To prevent a migraine, avoid triggers—certain foods, emotional stress, flickering lights, high altitudes, irregular sleeping and eating patterns—says Alan M. Rapoport, M.D., medical director of the Headache Inpatient Unit at Greenwich Hospital in Connecticut.
- Prostate cancer. Start undergoing the digital (finger) exam, as well as PSA blood testing, not in your early fifties as is usually suggested, but in your forties, maybe even thirties. (For more information, see the section on prostates in Chapter Three.)
- Rheumatoid arthritis. Early diagnosis and treatment may mean less damage to joints, says David S. Pisetsky, M.D., Ph.D., a medical advisor for the Arthritis Foundation. The same low-fat, high-fiber diet that helps prevent heart disease may help too, says Pisetsky, author of *The Duke University Medical Center Book* of arthritis.
- Skin cancer. Have a whole-body check yearly and—of course—avoid sunlight or use sunscreen.

By setting up a family tree, you can help determine your own disease risks and adjust your lifestyle so as not to enhance those risks. Start by interviewing your blood relatives—obviously, you share no genes with in-laws or step-relatives—going as far back as your four grandparents. (If you can gather data on great-grandparents, it can't hurt and may help.)

You'll need a tape recorder and a list of questions. Make a copy of the questions for each family member, with one page or index card for each interviewee. If you wish, use a gold star or different-color paper or cards for first-degree relatives (such as parents and siblings), since they carry more genetic weight. Don't forget yourself! Your own written history can offer insights that memory alone won't provide.

If you're entering information about relatives who are long dead, some answers may be hard to translate into modern medical language. For example, a "nervous breakdown" could have been anything from alcoholism to schizophrenia to depression—and nobody in the family is talking. The best you can do is log "mental illness." "Consumption" is the old word for tuberculosis or sometimes pneumonia. "Dropsy" meant congestive heart failure. "Brain fever" could indicate meningitis or encephalitis. "Softening of the brain" referred to dementia, cerebral hemorrhage or stroke. "Summer complaint"—diarrhea and vomiting—is now known as gastroenteritis. "Mortification" meant gangrene, trauma, infection, diabetes or aneurysm of the aorta.

Ask your relatives these questions:

1. When were you born?
2. What conditions or diseases threaten your health? Hypertension, high cholesterol? (Make your own note about obesity.)
3. At what age did they come on?
4. What major operations have you had?
5. At what age? At what hospital?
6. Do you have allergies?
7. Do you smoke? How much?
8. Do you drink alcohol? How much?
9. Do you exercise? How much?
10. What is your diet like?
11. (For women) Have you had any miscarriages? Stillbirths? Children with birth defects?
12. Have you had any mental problems—alcoholism, anxiety, major depression, schizophrenia, psychiatric treatment or hospitalization, suicide attempts?

Now ask those questions about relatives who have died, plus these:

1. What are their dates of death?
2. What did they die of?
3. Where?

GROWING THROUGH GRIEF

You can learn a great deal about your own history and health by investigating your family tree, but one lesson is bound to come through loud and clear: death is an inescapable part of life. Along with the births and weddings that punctuate our family histories are major illnesses and unexpected demise. These losses often catch men unprepared—and unable to deal with the acute, painful emotions that accompany them. Men, as a rule, don't know how to grieve.

Western culture celebrates success and encourages the expression of triumphant emotions—the high five, for example, or the ticker-tape parade. But our many losses often get stuffed into a figurative back pocket, unacknowledged, unexpressed and unresolved. Instead of airing the natural feelings aroused by losing something we value, we're far more likely to play the strong, silent type and simply carry on as best we can. But it's in the last half of life, when there are bound to be important losses, that men most need to grieve.

"Men find it hard to show grief—they try to cover it up and act brave," observes Catherine Thompson, Ph.D., a psychotherapist and grief counselor in Pittsburgh. "But if you bottle it up—if you don't express it emotionally—your body will experience it in some other way. "

Grief is a collection of spontaneous emotional responses to the loss of something significant. It can wear a lot of hats, being felt as disappointment, rage, sadness, frustration, pain, fear, guilt or anxiety. Frequently, it involves a baffling combination of them all. Mourning, on the other hand, is an intentional response to loss. As Mark Goulston, M.D., professor of psychiatry at UCLA, points out, "The main task of mourning is learning to live with the fact that life will never be quite the same again. It allows us to release our pain to make room for growth."

Every culture develops mourning rituals that encourage people to process extreme grief—such as that resulting from the death of a loved one—so it doesn't disrupt the community. But the "lesser" hurts and setbacks of life tend to pile up, unheeded. A key client cancels his account. Your cousin is diagnosed with cancer. You tear a ligament. The home team unexpectedly loses.

The intensity of grief will vary with the loss that triggered it, but the basic stages are remarkably similar. Typically, we experience shock ("I can't believe this!"), denial ("Hey, no big deal—I'll be fine!"), anger/resentment ("This isn't fair!") and depression/withdrawal ("Just leave me alone."). These initial stages seldom follow a linear progression, and everyone experiences them differently. Mourning completes the process by first acknowledging the legitimacy of the emotions, and then helping us move beyond them and toward resolution.

Thompson notes that, in our culture, "there's a tendency to rush through the process—to be strong and get back to normal." Furthermore, men associate grief with weakness: we fail to admit its emotions, even to ourselves. Unfortunately, men who act "strong" actually become vulnerable to additional grief, loss and pain.

The human system needs time to fully process the experience of loss. If we fail to invest in it, we create a backlog of "raw" emotion—bottled-up pain that can come flooding out at inopportune or inappropriate times. Eventually, this backlog can even reveal itself in sleep disorders, substance abuse, reckless or antisocial behavior and susceptibility to injury. It can suppress the immune system and promote a variety of disorders, from cancer to heart disease.

Grief isn't a gender issue: Men and women both feel it, but their efforts to cope are markedly different. "If a woman suffers a loss," Slaby explains, "another will approach and offer to help. Women welcome the attention. They give themselves over to the need to grieve. With men, a friend is likely to say, 'Gee, let's get together to play some racquetball one of these days.' The net effect is that women tend to be more emotionally literate and to have extensive social networks available for support."

As a result, men commonly get stuck in denial, withdrawal and anger. "Socially," adds Goulston, "this increases our isolation. We start to lose friends." In short, we consistently cut ourselves off from opportunities to create the very support system that enables us to recover.

What can you do to help yourself grow through grief? Start by acknowledging the importance of mourning. When confronted with a loss:

- Take stock. Things have changed. Ask yourself: Where does this leave me? Where do I go from here?
- Adapt your response. Old habits don't serve new circumstances. You need to shift emotionally and physiologically. Spend more time with family. Accept help you'd normally decline—professional or otherwise. Vent your feelings through physical action and strenuous workouts. But don't overdo it: "If any type of activity is used to block or escape deep feelings," Thompson cautions, "it can actually lead to reckless and harmful extremes."
- Take your time. Don't rush the process. Healing isn't a sprint, it's a marathon.

These basics will generally facilitate a steady recovery. But if anger, anxiety or withdrawal persist for more than a few weeks, you should consider professional counseling. And don't wait for grief to seem chronic before seeking comfort. As Goulston observes, "Just letting your anguish be heard is a tremendous first step."

"Men who do make the effort to mourn," Slaby emphasizes, "find it helps them grow through a wide range of challenges. It's a learning experience. One of the most fundamental and rewarding strategies is to begin investing in friendship, and consciously working through the grief arising from each of life's many small losses so you're prepared for the larger jolts. Don't wait to create your support system. Do it now. "

10 FITNESS

IS THE FITNESS BOOM BUST?

The eighties was the Fitness Decade. Jogging went from an obscure pastime to a national obsession. Jane Fonda went for "the burn"—and everyone, it seemed, went with her. Dozens of periodicals were created to inform readers about the best ways to work out, and mainstream magazines suddenly began to cover the trend. Fitness, in short, became a cover story.

Cut to the nineties. Many of those fitness headlines have disappeared. So, apparently, have many of the fitness devotees. What happened to the much-hyped "fitness revolution?" Why have our short-lived fitness traditions started down the road to extinction? The entire United States is apparently on a fitness slide. Some facts:

About 33 percent of Americans were obese (20 percent over their ideal weight) in 1995, up from 25 percent in 1983, according to Centers for Disease Control statistics. (In some Native American communities, that figure more than doubles.)

After peaking in 1990, the number of frequent fitness participants in the U.S. declined by 4.8 percent in 1991 and again by 2.7 percent in 1992, according to American Sports Data. In 1995, about 60 percent of Americans only exercise sporadically—or not at all.

In 1986, 53 percent of adults said they made a point of ordering healthy foods when dining out. By 1992, the percentage dropped to 47, according to the National Restaurant Association.

Meat and egg sales are rising for the first time in years. In 1994, Americans consumed on average 64 pounds of beef per person—the highest consumption level in five years.

There currently seems to be a wholesale backlash in the works against the kind of self-denial people associate with diet and exercise. The ubiquitous trend-monger Faith Popcorn has dubbed this the "pleasure revenge": after a decade of denial of the flesh, Americans are indulging in their weaknesses.

Sales of junk food, red meat, alcohol and even cigarettes are up; purchases of potato chips, for example, are up 6 percent in 1994 and 1995, while the bland-but-diet-friendly popcorn has dropped by 3 percent. Even cigars—the very symbol of a debauched lifestyle—suddenly became all the rage.

As Wendy Kaminer, a public-policy fellow at Radcliffe, summed up the trend for *The New York Times* in 1995, "People ate their bran muffins for five years and nothing changed. They didn't lose weight, they still got fired and they're still unhappy." Indeed, tough economic conditions often send people reeling for the refrigerator. Perhaps the economic discues of recent years have sent people to the more immediate pleasures of couch and ice cream. Hard times, it seems, aren't conducive to maintaining a hard body.

Something's going on here. To find out what, let's look at the numbers through the eyes of folks who are on the cutting edge of the fitness movement.

Take Nike. The Oregon-based sneaker giant continues to grow every year, but spokesperson Keith Peters agrees the climate has changed. "People aren't wearing running shoes with jeans the way they used to," he says. In the eighties the jock look was de rigueur. We wore sneakers with everything, including suits, and then often scrapped the suits for flashy warm-ups. Today, the grittier street look is in, with kids trading in their tennis shoes and cross trainers for Doc Martens.

While we big kids may not be going grunge, we are making outdoor-shoe makers like Timberland very rich. Sales for the New Hampshire-based company were up almost 50 percent in 1993. "I'd say the trend is definitely away from the athletic look," says Timberland's Elise Klysa.

You could say that changing fashion doesn't necessarily indicate changing fitness habits, but Nike's Peters isn't very argumentative. "I would agree people are taking a mellower approach to things," he says. "They may be less intense about what they're doing and do it less frequently than in the eighties, but I think there's still a large group out there doing at least something occasionally." Peters uses running as an example. "Ten or fifteen years ago, people were pretty obsessive about it," he says. "Today, there may be a new wave of people trying the marathon, but I don't think they're as competitive. They do it to achieve a goal and for fitness, but they're just not as mondo about it."

The sport of triathlon is a good example. Born in the early seventies, it hit its stride in the eighties, a time when Americans seemed to be pursuing optimal fitness: Oh, to be triple the athlete, to have the swimmer's muscular upper body, the cyclist's chiseled legs, the runner's wind. A national triathlon series was born.

Well, the twelve-year-old Bud Light Triathlon Series died in late 1993. Membership in Triathlon Federation/USA, the sport's governing body, has dropped from a late-eighties high of 32,000 to 18,400 last year. "We've been pretty flat," admits the federation's executive director, Steven Locke. He blames the economy, since race entry fees average about $50, but expects to sanction more races in the future, with the economy showing definite signs of improving.

Money, though, is only a small part of the problem, according to chiropractor Martin Skopp of Alexandria, Virginia. Skopp, 32, was an avid triathlete throughout the eighties, racing at about 170 pounds. His last race was in 1988. Now he tips the scales at 196 pounds. "It was just a reorganization of priorities," he explains. "I've had less of a desire to compete and really push myself than to just stay relatively fit. My life has become more balanced, although now I would like to swing the pendulum a little bit in the other direction."

A balanced life, particularly the kind that involves a spouse and kids, is apparently slowing down a lot of athletes. The Baby Boom ended in 1964, meaning the youngest of that 78 million-strong generation is in the early thirties, which is about the age when balance starts becoming a central issue in one's life. This, then, could be a logical explanation for the fitness slide.

"I could see some credence there," says Locke. "As you get older, you have more time constraints. I guess we have to hope the next generation replaces us." But with American schoolchildren reportedly the world's most slothful, the future of fitness here doesn't seem all that bright.

So much confusing or downright contradictory information on health and fitness is being disseminated that no one is quite sure what works and what hurts. "We used to hear more about the harmful effects of things," says John Poteet, associate director of continuing education at the famed Cooper Institute for Aerobics Research in Dallas "Now it seems like all you hear is that anything in moderation won't hurt you. Everything's loosened up. You can drink alcohol, eat a little red meat."

One recent advisory that has more credibility than most: The American College of Sports Medicine (ACSM), the Centers for Disease Control and Prevention and the President's Council on Physical Fitness have agreed that strenuous physical activity is not the only form of fitness that will improve health. Their report states that basic physical activity, from walking the dog to mowing the lawn, offers the same basic health benefits as, say, training for a marathon.

"We used to think that the guy who runs would naturally be in better health than the guy who doesn't. That's no longer the case," says Michael Pollock, Ph.D., a member of the ACSM committee that analyzed the research (much of it provided by the Cooper Institute) leading to the landmark opinion. "Moderate physical activity [for instance, walking thirty minutes a day, four or more days a week] offers the same benefit in deterring heart disease and other ailments as more demanding activities."

Pollock says that the report is directed primarily at the 78 percent of Americans who barely make it from the couch to the refrigerator. "It's not meant to discourage those people who enjoy working out," he says. "A lot of people will never exercise, but now at least they have hope, a reason to do something."

People thinking that maybe they can get behind this fitness-backlash thing should know, for starters, that they're not going to get chiseled calves and washboard abs just strolling through town. Pollock offers another reason to keep pumping: "Psychologically, the value of being physically fit can be great. Athletes know the feeling."

The Cooper Institute's Poteet believes most Americans relate in some way to that feeling, which is why he maintains that fitness is not lagging and never will. "We have 3,200 members in our club here [which operates out of the research facility]," he says. "People may not be as fervent as they once were, but they're still coming. They want the same results."

So while many of us are slowing down, it doesn't seem like we're giving up. Those of us who've discovered the intrinsic benefits of working out know that fitness is truly its own reward. Fitness doesn't have to be the cover story in *Time* to be fundamental to your life.

In this chapter we'll explore the best ways to work out, with a special emphasis on the an area that remains a mystery for many men: the weight room. But before we get there, let's begin with a stretch.

STRETCHING

Ask anyone who trains seriously if he thinks warming up and stretching are important, and he'll say, "Sure." But watch that guy in the gym and you'll notice that he probably does neither. Or maybe he performs a few stretches and assumes he's simultaneously warming up. Time, after all, is tight. If he only has his lunch hour to train, and skipping a warm-up might mean an extra set of each exercise, he'll probably choose muscle building over muscle loosening.

Most guys who work out don't really understand why they're supposed to get their muscles warm and limber. Warming up not only allows your muscular system to get ready for the upcoming exercises, it also heats your circulatory system. When your blood vessels get warmer, they allow more nutrients to reach the muscles you're working. The higher temperature also helps your brain and nervous system function better, improving the connections between mind and muscles and speeding up reaction time.

This is pretty crucial when a heavy weight is heading for your foot. That, of course, is the biggest reason for warming up: The warmer you are, the easier it is to prevent injuries. Most tweaks and twists occur early in your workout, generally when you're still working with relatively light weights. And it's just a short hop from minor pains to real injuries, which can set your training back weeks, if not longer.

How much warm-up is necessary? A lot depends on how hard you intend to work your body. If you're only planning to do a few light exercises, you can usually get away with just a cursory warm-up. But if you're going to try to move heavy weights, or do such high-skill exercises as power snatches or clean-and-jerks, you'll need to prepare longer.

The weather is also a factor. In the colder months, muscles (like everything else) are harder to warm up and easier to tear. In warmer weather, you can usually get away with a shorter preworkout routine. Age, too, is a major factor. Older men need to spend more time preparing their muscles, primarily because flexibility decreases as a body ages. Also, nagging old injuries need extra warm-up time.

The proper warm-up has two phases: The first is designed to elevate your body's core temperature and increase all of your muscles' elasticity. Using a stairclimber, stationary bike, rowing machine or treadmill will serve this purpose. So will calisthenic exercises, such as jumping jacks. Or you might do a series of abdominal and lower-back exercises. A simple routine of crunches, twists with a broomstick and back raises can get your midsection thoroughly warmed up, and from there the rest of your body will quickly follow. How do you know when you're properly warmed up? Make perspiration your barometer. If you haven't started sweating, you haven't done enough.

Once you've broken a sweat, it's time to move into the second phase of the process, when you prepare the specific muscles you're going to train that day. For example, if you're going to work your legs first, do a few warm-up movements for them. Try this circuit: Do one set (15 repetitions) each of leg extensions, leg curls and leg adductions (pulling your legs closed on the inner-thigh machine). Use a very light weight; the object here isn't to build new muscle but to move some warm blood into those you already have.

The area most endangered by short or nonexistent warm-ups is the shoulder girdle, which includes your chest, upper back and rib cage muscles along with your shoulders. Most guys—even weight-room veterans—think nothing of starting off a bench press routine with heavy weights. They believe that if they work at warming up they'll run out of energy before they get to their maximum poundages. But this isn't how your body works. It gains energy from being properly warmed up. A good rule to follow: The initial weight on the bar can never be too light, but it can be too heavy.

Also, if you've been injured, take extra time preparing that area. If, for example, your shoulder girdle often gives you trouble, spend a few minutes working with light dumbbells or even small weight plates before starting your regular workout. Again, the more blood you get into the area, the lower your chance of injury.

You'll notice that nothing has been said yet about stretching. That's because many believe the best time to stretch is during and after your workout (although there's nothing wrong with stretching as part of your warm-up, too). Stretching between sets helps your muscles respond better to the exercises, particularly when you're working your shoulders and hamstrings, which sometimes tighten up during strenuous exercise.

Stretching doesn't have to be particularly complex. For your shoulders, you can simply pull on a rack between sets, or hang from a chin-up bar. Your hamstrings will get a nice stretch if you bend from the waist and allow your upper body to hang for a few seconds. Another benefit to this kind of stretching is that it keeps you working during the otherwise dead time between sets.

If you can't do a complete stretching routine immediately after your workout, set aside some time later in the evening. You can stretch while you're watching the news, for example. Give your entire body a good loosening up, paying special attention to the body parts that tend to give you the most trouble. This will alleviate post-workout soreness and help your body get ready for its next training session. On top of all that, a relaxed body will sleep easier than a tight, sore one.

One last thought about warming up and stretching: Don't think of them as activities that take time away from your training routines. Rather, consider them the exercises that make your training routines possible. A good warm-up not only prepares your body for the upcoming workout, it gives your mind a chance to think about what you want to accomplish. This makes for a much better workout. Same with the stretches afterward:

You can use the time to focus on how the exercises you just did made your body feel, what seemed to work and what didn't, and how you're going to approach things the next time you train.

All of this may seem like a lot of time and effort now, but as you make steady progress in the gym, and as you see others get hurt or fall into training ruts, you'll realize it's all worthwhile.

THE WEIGHT-ROOM LEXICON

If you've been training with weights for any length of time, you're probably familiar with the basic terminology. You know the difference between a barbell and a dumbbell, a *set* and a *rep*. Chances are you know what all the exercises are called (it's probably been years since you referred to a cable crunch as "the thingy with the rope") and you've tried a few different movements for each body part.

Before starting a program, it helps to know the language of lifting. The gym is home to a subculture of sorts, and its denizens speak a lingo that—to the uninitiated—sounds as foreign as Latin (in fact, some of it *is* Latin). If you can't talk sets and reps, bi's and tri's, poundages and weight limits, you might miss some valuable advice being offered to you. If you're making the leap from an intermediate to advanced weight trainer, you'll find a whole new world of exercise theories, techniques and descriptions for which you'll need this vocabulary. The following is a guide to some of the terminology commonly used by uncommonly large people. So let's look at some definitions:

Burns: As its name implies, this is a technique you don't want to practice too often or without forethought. In other words, it hurts. At the end of a set, you knock out three to six partial reps, bringing the weight through about half its normal range of motion. This floods the muscle with blood and lactic acid, swelling its capillaries and increasing its size. But there's a price you pay: Lactic acid produces a burning pain. It only lasts a few seconds and presents no danger, but it lets you know you're pushing the envelope.

Cheating: This is what experienced lifters deliberately do to trick their muscles into giving them an extra rep or two when they're doing sets to failure (i.e. total exhaustion). But it doesn't mean using bad form, like lifting your butt into the air on a bench press or arching your back like a question mark on biceps curls. Say you're doing one-arm concentration curls on a cable machine. You might cheat on the last rep or two by using your free hand to help pull the cable, all the while keeping continuous tension on the muscle you're working. In other words, it's the same as having a partner assist you on the final reps of a set.

Confusion: While you may not like surprises in your personal life, your muscles desperately need them. Muscles stop growing when they get used to a training system. That's why you need to keep them confused, constantly varying the exercises you do and the ways you do them. Switch from barbells to dumbbells or from dumbbells to barbells; from flat benches to inclines and vice versa; from free weights to machines and back again. When a routine starts to feel stale, it's time to adjust.

Curl: Any movement that involves pulling the resistance in toward the body with either the arms or the legs.

Cycling: Cycling your workouts means you aim for different goals at different times of the year. For example, you may do your heaviest training to bulk up during the winter months, then switch to higher-rep, lower-weight workouts in summer, when you want your muscles to look as sharp as possible while you're wearing shorts and T-shirts. Then you might close out the year with maintenance workouts that better accommodate the hubbub of the holiday season. Varying your workouts like this not only provides variety but also helps prevent overuse injuries.

Giant sets: This is a technique that helps give your muscles more definition. You do four to six consecutive exercises for a single body part—chest, back, front of thighs—with little or no rest between them. You don't want to do it too often, but if you've been spending a lot of time trying to bulk up, giant sets can help you shape what you've built.

Limit weight: The heaviest amount of resistance you can lift for one repetition. Also called one-rep max.

Negatives: Each movement has two parts: the positive portion, when you're lifting the weight, and the negative phase, when you're returning it to its starting position. If you simply focus on doing that second portion of the exercise slowly, you'll get some of the benefits of negative training. To get the full benefits, you need a training partner to help you lift a weight that's too heavy for you to raise on your own. You then return the weight to the starting position as slowly as you can. This is an intense form of exercise, and you shouldn't do it too often.

Peak contraction: During a normal set, you bring the weight up in such a way that the muscle you're targeting only spends a second or two in its state of peak contraction—in other words, when it's working the hardest. You can avoid this by never fully "locking out" on any given rep. For example, say you're working your shoulders with seated dumbbell presses. Most guys lift the weights through a full range of motion, clanking the dumbbells overhead at the end. Not only does the noise bother those around you, that final motion allows your shoulder muscles to relax, as your straightened arms are now supporting the weight. If you stop short of that point, you keep your deltoids in a continuously contracted state, forcing them to work harder and, thus, grow.

Poundage: The amount of weight or resistance that you will be using on any given exercise.

Press: Any movement that pushes the resistance away from the body with either the arms or the legs.

Pronated: Lifting with the palms down.

Pyramiding: While most grammarians would hate to see "pyramid" turned into a verb, it's what serious weight trainers use to describe how they start an exercise with a light weight and high reps and then gradually add weight while subtracting reps. Since the early sets warm up your muscles and the latter sets push them to their utmost, pyramiding allows you to train hard with less risk of injury.

Rep: Short for "repetition," this word describes the contraction and/or extension of a given muscle group against resistance from a starting position of full extension to a completed position of full contraction. You finish a rep by returning to the starting position.

Routine: The sum total of reps, sets and exercises in any given workout or training session.

Set: A series of repetitions (anywhere from 1 to 100 or more). Generally, a brief rest of between 30 to 90 seconds is taken after performing a set to allow the trainee to catch his breath and provide time for the targeted muscle group to partly recuperate.

Staggered sets: Working small body parts—calves, forearms, abdominals—doesn't require a lot of energy but takes as much time as working bigger muscle groups. Staggered sets allow you to do both at the same time: While you're resting between sets of bench presses, for example, you might knock out a quick set of crunches or toe raises. Not only do you get through your workout faster, you also keep moving, which means you burn more calories.

Stripping: For our purposes, stripping means using one or two spotters to peel weight plates off the bar, allowing you to extend a set past the point of failure. Say you're doing this with bench presses, and your spotter is standing behind you. You do as many reps as you can with a heavy weight, the spotter peels off a plate from each end of the bar, you knock out as many reps as you can with that weight, then he takes more weight off, and you keep going until you're out of plates. To strip effectively, you need to load the bar with smaller plates that can be easily and quickly removed without radically unbalancing it, and you need to avoid the temptation to do it too often. It produces results, but it requires a lot of recovery time, too.

Supinated: Lifting with the palms up.

BASIC TRAINING: STARTING A WEIGHT PROGRAM

Not everyone who picks up a barbell wants to be Mr. Olympia. But it's a safe bet that a lot of us would like to look a little more like Mr. O than we do now. Whether weight training is an end in itself or a means to better performance in softball, basketball, tennis, golf or any other sport, undertaking a program is a commitment. For starters, you have to increase your ratio of muscle mass to body fat, and that means making changes in your diet as well as your regimen.

What follows is a guide to starting a weight-training program, or improving the one you're already following, especially designed by the editors of *Men's Fitness*. But before we launch into the program, let's dispel a few myths about weight training. First, some potential lifters are put off by the thought of going to a hard-core bodybuilding gym, only to be verbally abused by some Herculoid in a tank top barking out, "No pain, no gain!" In truth, you don't need a) the hard-core bodybuilding gym, b) the Herculoid or c) the verbal abuse.

All you really need, as you'll see, are some basic, inexpensive pieces of equipment that'll fit in your garage or basement, knowledge of which weightlifting exercises will produce the surest gains, and the motivation to improve your physique or build more strength and endurance for your sport.

But before we get into all that, let me offer a simple cautionary note. The first few months on any new weight-training program offer a number of pleasant surprises. Your muscles begin to grow. Your body begins to change. The hard work begins to yield dividends. This quick success, though, is actually a trap. Buoyed by the lure of increased muscle size, many lifters make the tactical error of increasing the volume of their workouts. In a matter of months they stop growing, and maybe their bodies even shift into reverse.

The reason is overtraining. No trainee, regardless of his level of development, needs to work out more than three days per week. The three-day-a-week program is a proven mass builder, both for beginners and advanced lifters. (Overtraining will be examined further later in this chapter.)

Note: Always assess your current physical condition before starting any new training program. Once your doctor gives you the green light to train, then—and only then—should you proceed.

The program you're about to embark on will, if followed to the letter, improve your health, strength and body composition. If you're drastically underweight, be prepared to gain up to 30 pounds of rock-hard muscle mass. If you're overweight, with no discernible shape, be prepared to become firm, develop a V-taper, lose inches from your waist and tone your chest, back, shoulders, legs and arms. Or if you're a recreational athlete who's at or near your ideal weight, be prepared to pursue your sport with more power and stamina.

This is a three-day-a-week regimen with a day of rest in between. At the end of the weekly cycle, you'll get two days of rest before you start over again. No matter how good you feel, you should never train the same muscle groups more than three days a week. You'll thank yourself down the road when you don't suffer from overtraining.

The alternate-day schedule is set up this way for two reasons. First, exercise physiologists have determined that the human body needs a minimum of 48 hours of rest between workouts to recover from the training session. Second, the rest gives the muscles time to overcompensate for the forces of resistance by increasing their mass. When they don't work, they grow.

Exercise form is crucial to your success. If you're a beginner, enlist a personal trainer (or a friend who knows what he's doing) to walk you through the routine. There's no substitute for on-site instruction. Start with moderate poundages: in other words, weights you can lift 12 to 15 times with good form. If you have no idea how much that is, it's better to experiment with lighter weights than with heavier ones. If you pick up a barbell and find you can curl it 20 times when you planned to do a set of 12, consider it a warm-up and increase the weight for the next set. Remember, you want to teach your muscles to handle the movements, not force them to rip apart while heaving weights they've never touched before.

The Routine

1. Squat (two sets of 15 reps): Squats are the key to creating an impressive lower body. You'll build both power and mass in your quadriceps and glutes. But it's crucial that you do this exercise correctly. *Correct form*: Stand erect with a barbell across your shoulders. Taking a deep breath, bend your knees and lower your body until your thighs are parallel to the floor. Rise from this position while exhaling. Repeat for the required number of repetitions. Option: Rest your heels on a weight-plate to keep your back straight. As soon as you finish your first set, immediately do a set of pullovers (see below). This immediate transfer from one exercise to another is called *supersetting*. During the rest of the routine, take a 60-to–90 second break between sets.

2. Pullover (two sets of 12 reps): There are two ways to develop a bigger chest: Stimulate the pecs with exercises that add size (like bench presses) and expand the rib cage with stretching exercises (like pullovers). *Correct form:* Lie on a bench holding a light barbell at arm's length over your chest. From this position, slowly lower the weight until it almost touches the floor behind you. Try to keep your arms locked throughout the movement and return the weight to the starting position.

3. Bench Press (two sets of 15 reps): The bench press has its shortcomings, but it's still the perfect exercise for building a base of muscle mass. *Correct form:* Lie on a bench with a barbell over your chest. Slowly lower the bar to your upper chest. Once the bar touches your chest, slowly press the weight back up to the starting position and repeat.

4. Standing Barbell Military Press (two sets of 10 reps): An excellent deltoid developer. As a bonus, it also stimulates growth in the trapezius and

the triceps. *Correct form:* Bring the barbells to your shoulders and then slowly press the weight upward until your arms are fully extended over your head. Slowly lower the bar back to the starting position and repeat.

5. Barbell Bent-Over Row (two sets of 10 reps): Most of the emphasis here is on the *latissimus dorsi*—the back muscle that gives you a V-shaped torso. *Correct form:* Bend over at the waist so that your torso is almost at 90 degrees. From this position, grasp the barbell with a palms-down, shoulder-width grip. Now slowly pull the bar up toward your torso until it touches your lower chest. Feel the contraction and slowly lower the bar to the starting position—your arms should be fully extended. Repeat.

6. Standing Barbell Curl (two sets of 10 reps): There are many variations, but when it comes to building strength and size in your biceps, the standing barbell curl is your starting point. *Correct form:* Stand erect with a palms-up, shoulder-width grip on the barbell. Your arms should be fully extended, with the bar directly in front of your thighs. Now slowly lift, or curl, the barbell up to shoulder height using only the biceps muscles; simply bend the muscle as you curl the bar up. From the fully contracted position, slowly lower the bar to the starting position. Repeat.

7. Deadlift (two sets of 15 reps): If you're new to the gym you might want to work up to this slowly, but when performed correctly it's a terrific way to build strong glutes and hamstrings. It's also great for the spinal erector muscles of the lower back. *Correct form:* Stand erect, with your feet just under the barbell. While bending your knees, grasp the barbell with your hands just a little wider than shoulder-width and your knuckles facing the wall in front of you. Slowly stand up, straightening your legs, and continue lifting until your back is perfectly straight. Lower the bar to the floor and repeat.

8. Crunch (two sets of 20): If you do only one ab exercise, this should be it. The actual range of motion is small, but the crunch can really sculpt the muscles at the top of the abdomen. *Correct form:* Lie on your back on the floor, your hands behind your head and your knees at 90 degrees to keep your lower back flat on the floor throughout the movement. Now curl up slightly and try to bring your rib cage as close to your pelvis as possible. Hold the position for a two-count, then slowly lower yourself back to the starting position and repeat.

Monday	EXERCISE	SETS	REPS
Chest	Bench press	3	8–15
	Incline dumbbell press	3	8–15
	Machine or cable flye	3	8–15
Shoulders	Shoulder press (machine)	2–3	8–15
	Dumbbell lateral raise	2–3	8–15
	Barbell upright row (optional)	2–3	8–15
Triceps (optional)	Cable pushdown	2–3	8–15
	Lying dumbbell extension	2–3	8–15

Tuesday

Abs	Superset: Crunch/leg raise	3	25–50
Back	Let pulldown	3	8–15
	Seated row (machine)	3	8–15
	Lower-back machine	3	8–15
Biceps	Preacher curl (machine)	3	8–15
	EZ-bar curl	3	8–15

Wednesday

Abs	Crunch	3	25–50
Legs	Leg press	3	8–15
	Leg curl	3	8–15
	Leg extension	3	8–15
	Standing calf raise	3	8–15

Thursday

Chest and Back	Superset: Incline press (machine)/ bent-over row (machine)	3	8–10
	Superset: Dip (machine)/pull-up (machine)	3	8–15
Shoulders	Military press (machine)	3	8–15
Triceps	Dumbbell kickback	3	8–15

Friday

Abs	Superset: Crunch (machine)/leg raise (machine)	2–3	15–25
Legs	Sissy squat (with a rope)	3	8–20
	Superset: Leg extension (machine)/ seated leg curl	3	8–15
	Calf raise (on leg-press machine)	3	8–15

WEEK TWO

Monday	EXERCISE	SETS	REPS
Chest	Barbell incline press	2–3	8–12
	Chest press (machine)	2–3	8–12
	Pec deck	2–3	8–12
Shoulders	Seated shoulder press	2–3	8–12
	Rear deltoid machine	2–3	8–12
Triceps	Overhead triceps extension (machine)	2–3	8–10

Tuesday

Abs	Superset: Crunch (machine)/ leg raise (machine)	2–3	15–25
Back	Wide-grip pulldown (to the front)	3	8–12
	T-bar row (machine)	3	8–12
	Hyperextension (machine)	3	8–12
Biceps	Seated dumbbell curl	3	8–12

Wednesday

Abs	Superset: Crunch (machine)/ leg raise (machine)	2–3	15–25

Legs	Leg curl (machine)	3	8–12
	Leg extension (machine)	3	8–12
	Lunge (while holding dumbbells)	3	8–12
	Seated calf raise	3	8–15

Thursday

Chest & Back	Superset: Wide-grip pulldown/ incline press (machine)	3	8–12
Shoulders	Shoulder press (machine)	3	8–12
	Dumbbell lateral raise	3	8–12
Triceps	Lying triceps extension (with barbell)	2–3	8–12
	Barbell curl	2–3	8–12

Friday

Abs	Superset: Crunch (machine)/ leg raise (machine)	3	15–25
Legs	Giant set: Leg press (machine)	3	8–12
	Lunge (while holding dumbbells)	3	8–12
	Leg curl (machine)	3	8–12
	Donkey calf raise (machine)	3	8–12

WEEK THREE

Monday	EXERCISE	SETS	REPS
Chest	Barbell decline press	3	8–10
	Dumbbell bench press	3	8–10
	Dumbbell incline flye	3	8–10
Shoulders	Shoulder press (machine)	2–3	8–10
	Reverse flye (with cables)	2–3	8–10

Triceps	Triceps pushdown (with a rope)	2–3	8–10

Tuesday

Abs	Superset: Crunch (side-to-side)/ leg raise	3	25–50
Back	Seated cable row	3	8–10
	Lat pulldown (machine)	3	8–10
	Lower-back machine	3	8–10
Biceps	Standing dumbbell curl	3	8–10

Wednesday

Abs	Superset: Crunch (side-to-side)/ leg raise	3	25–50
Legs	Squat (machine or barbell)	3	8–10
	Abductor (machine)	3	8–10
	Adductor (machine)	3	8–10
	Standing calf raise	3	8–10

Thursday

Chest & Back	Superset: Dumbbell bench press/ dumbbell row	3	8–10
	Superset: Wide-grip pulldown/ cable crossover	3	8–10
	Cable upright row	3	8–10
	Reverse curl	3	8–15

Friday

Abs	Superset: Crunch/leg raise	2–3	25–50
Legs	Superset: Leg press (machine)/ sissy squat (holding onto a rope)	3	15–20
	Leg curl	3	8–10
	Hack squat	3	8–10

THE 20-MINUTE WORKOUT

The preceding "Basic Training" workout is simple and effective, but it does have one drawback: it can take some time. Isn't there a routine that you can squeeze into a lunch hour?

Men's Fitness enlisted personal trainer John Richling to create a weight-training program that'll give you noticeable results in the shortest possible time. How short? How does twenty minutes a day, five times a week sound? (It's okay to do this routine that often since you're not training the same muscle groups every day.) That's only twenty minutes to get buff, with enough of your precious lunch hour left to actually eat lunch.

"I've seen at least a dozen other twenty-minute workouts in the past, and they were all very incomplete," explains Richling, a former body-builder who now teaches classes in breathing, stretching and posture at Gold's Gym in Venice, California. "Those workouts don't take into account the supporting muscle groups. I've chosen six exercises a day, using machines, free weights, barbells, dumbbells and cables so that no area of the body is neglected."

In other words, this is not one of those "better than nothing" training routines. Richling has meticulously mapped out a three-week program that can be adjusted to maintain your present shape or to make muscular gains. You want more mass? Increase the weights and lower the reps. Looking to define the mass you already have? Then up the reps and decrease the weights.

Instead of strict one-body-part-per-day workouts, Richling has opted for more of a push-pull system that stresses the upper body on Monday, Tuesday and Thursday and the legs on Wednesday and Friday. You're lifting progressively heavier as you move into the second and third weeks. But these sets and reps aren't written in stone; the program is designed in such a way that you can adjust the weights depending on your goals.

To make all this work, you have to become a perpetual-motion machine for twenty minutes a day. "When you're in the gym, you can never be idle," Richling says. "A body in motion stays in motion. If I'm sitting on a piece of equipment between sets, psychologically I'm telling myself, 'This machine is for sitting on.' That's going to make me lackadaisical. It's going to waste my time."

Efficiency—no wasted time or movement—is the foundation of Richling's training program. "My philosophy is what I call the 'eye of the turtle': slow, consistent, progressive steps forward. That's why I always stress slow and continuous tension through the full range of motion. You can never sacrifice form for the sake of lifting a heavier weight. You may make short-term gains, but they won't last."

Richling firmly believes in warming up before hitting the iron. Spend about five minutes on a stationary bike, and stretch out the body parts you're working between the sets. As for aerobic training, he recommends 20 to 30 minutes of cardio work three times a week for starters, increasing to five times a week after you've been with the program for a month. You can add the aerobic work to the end of your workout, or do on your days off and before or after work.

Note: If terms like "lat pulldown" or "incline flye" are new to you, have a qualified person at your gym show you the ropes. Better still, have a personal trainer go through the exercises with you to check your form and help establish your weight ranges.

The 20-minute workout

Richling recommends that you start off doing two sets per exercise. Then, as you learn to work more efficiently, progress to three sets. He's also provided optional exercises to be worked in when time permits. Allow for 20 to 60 seconds of rest between sets. After the third week, repeat the cycle.

Note: A superset—crunches and leg raises, for instance—is two exercises done back-to-back with no rest between sets. A giant set is a superset consisting of four or more exercises.

BODY LANGUAGE

Think the gym equipment has perplexing names? Try your own body. Here's a guide to the peculiar abbreviations used for muscles at the club.

1. *Abs*: (Rectus abdominus) Front of the abdomen.
2. *Bi's*: (Biceps) Front of upper arm.
3. *Brachy*: (Brachialis) Outside of upper arm.
4. *Delts*: (Deltoids) The point of each shoulder.
5. *Flexors*: (Forearm flexors) Inner forearm.
6. *Glutes*: (Gluteus maximus) Buttocks.
7. *Hams*: (Hamstrings) Rear of thigh.
8. *Lats*: (Latissimus dorsi) V-shaped muscles on back.
9. *Obliques*: (External, internal) Sides of the waist.

---

10. *Pecs:* (Pectorals) Upper front of ribcage.
11. *Quads:* (Quadriceps) Front of the thigh.
12. *Tri's:* (Triceps) Back of the upper arm.

To make consistent progress in the 20-minute workout plan, Richling stresses the need for proper breathing techniques and precise body alignment and posture. "The most essential source of power is your breathing," he says. "The next time you see some guy struggling with a weight, look at the tension on his face. He's probably holding his breath."

A few guidelines on these finer points will help get the most out of your twenty minutes per day:

Always breathe from your diaphragm. When inhaling, your diaphragm (not your stomach) should go out; when exhaling, your diaphragm should go in. It sounds simple, but many people still breathe from their chests. Check yourself the next time you're in the middle of a set.

Pick a spot in front of you to focus on. Keep your eyes fixed on that spot for the entire set to minimize any inefficient—or even dangerous—movements that can throw your posture out of whack.

Keep your mind on the business at hand. "You can't dwell on what's going on back at work if you're focused on getting the most out of each rep, enjoying a total pump in only twenty minutes," Richling says.

MAXIMIZING AEROBIC POWER

If you already include aerobics (as you should) as part of your routine, do you know if you're doing the right kind? The type that's best for you depends on your training goals and expectations, as well as which sports you like to pursue. Picking the right aerobic workout—or the right series of workouts—can greatly increase your cardiac capacity and your endurance.

For example, imagine this scene at a typical mountain bike race: A hundred riders line up for a 100-yard pedal that ends where the actual course begins: a 12-mile loop of technical single-track, a roller coaster of steep verticals and frame-mangling downhills. If you treat those first hundred yards as your "warm-up," you may as well get off your clipless pedals and do a tap dance, because it's a safe bet that whatever position you grab upon entering the narrow single-track is going to be pretty damn close to where you'll end up at the finish line. So even though this is an endurance event, explosive power matters.

Mountain bikers do all sorts of intense training to prepare their bodies for handling multiple shifts between aerobic energy (the kind that relies on oxygen and is used for long, steady endurance activities lasting more than seven minutes) and anaerobic energy (the intense, muscle-driven sort of activity that leaches glucose from your muscles and can only be maintained for about seven minutes at a time). Because of this, mountain biking serves as a good model for other endurance and sports challenges. An in-shape mountain biker might be going aerobic over a steep, steady incline and then shift to anaerobic energy when he hits an even steeper vertical stretch.

This science is all in a day's work for Ed Burke, Ph.D., an associate professor of exercise physiology at the University of Colorado at Colorado Springs and a former Olympic cycling team coach. He currently trains off-road cyclists, helping them achieve a state of conditioning that lets them instantly draw upon their reserves of power. In workouts consisting of ten hard, continuous intervals (spurts of high-intensity exercise followed by a brief recovery period), Burke pushes the cyclists to approach their maximum heart rate—about 180 beats per minute—within thirty seconds. "They'd better know what it feels like," he says, and by that he means uncomfortable. Because to succeed at a high level, especially a competitive one, you need to become familiar with exerting yourself at the upper extremes of your capabilities.

Intervals have another purpose. According to Johnny G., an ultra-distance cyclist who created an intense stationary bike workout known as Spinning, intervals are meant not only to make you work close to your maximum heart rate, but also "to give your body the ability to go from its endurance zone to recovery in as brief a time as possible," ideally no more than fifteen seconds.

In other words, say your intervals consist of one minute of intense exertion followed by one minute of recovery. On a stationary bike, that would mean pedaling superhard, then slowing down to a very easy level for one minute before charging up again. The idea is you're training your heart to handle intense exertion, right?

Well, sort of. If, during the hard-pedaling phase, you take your heart rate up to 180 beats per minute, but during your minute "off" it only drops to 160 or 170, you haven't accomplished that much in terms of performance. Your body is still expending an enormous amount of energy— at a level that it can't maintain for very long.

On the other hand, if you've conditioned yourself so that during recovery your heart rate drops to 120 (the level of someone who is exerting himself only moderately), you've got that much more energy to draw upon in your next interval. If you can't recover that efficiently, the trick is not to push hard at the high end, but to bring your target heart rate down to a more manageable number that will allow for a speedy recovery. Then, as you make gains, you can increase your target heart rate for intervals.

If you want to know how this translates to sports, imagine a game of full-court basketball: You want to be able to sprint to the other end of the court, but that would be purposeless if you didn't also recover enough energy to catch a long pass, dribble and lay it up and in.

Here's what you must know to increase your energy and endurance, whether you need it to charge across a soccer field, chase down a shot in tennis or run a hilly trail.

1. Learn to Measure

The easiest way to measure cardiovascular gains is with a heart rate monitor. A wireless model costs about a hundred bucks, depending on the (usually superfluous) bells and whistles it features. Strap the conductor around your chest, put on the wristwatch-display, and you've got the most important workout tool available: physiological information. If you're a diehard low-tech guy, you can simply use your finger: Touch your neck or wrist to feel the pulse, count your heartbeats for six seconds and multiply by ten to determine beats per minute.

2. Know What to Measure

Here are two important numbers you need to become familiar with:

Resting heart rate (RHR)

What it is: An excellent indicator of overall fitness, your RHR tells you how efficiently your heart is working when you're at rest.

What it tells you: Many athletes' RHRs are in the range of 40 to 50 beats per minute. Generally speaking, the lower yours is, the fitter you are. (Johnny G.'s is 32.) If you're in otherwise good shape, yours might begin slowly dropping into the low 50s after following this routine for a couple of months. But look out for fluctuations—a rising RHR can indicate overtraining or the onset of a cold or flu. In both cases, you'll need to lay off for a couple of days to recover. If you don't, you're begging for an injury.

How to measure it: Check your RHR within five minutes of waking up for five consecutive mornings, then average the figures. Many athletes measure theirs every morning.

Maximum heart rate (MHR)

What it is: A function of age, not fitness. "A fit twenty-year-old and a couch-potato twenty-year-old will pretty much have the same maximum heart rate," Burke says. The standard formula is 220 minus your age. So if you're thirty years old, your MHR is about 190. But that's just an estimate; a third of all people have MHRs that are nine beats higher or lower than this figure.

What it tells you: MHR is the reference point for your cardio training. For example, your aerobic zone is generally 65 to 80 percent of your MHR, and your anaerobic zone is 80 to 100 percent of your MHR.

How to measure it: Do your activity for eight to twelve minutes, steadily increasing the intensity of your workload until you feel you're nearing total exhaustion. Note your heart rate; that's your MHR.

(WARNING: Doing this can cause sudden death if you're predisposed to certain types of heart disease. So if you're not reasonably fit and not sure if you have any underlying cardiac problems, check with your doctor before taking this self-test. You should also consult your doctor first if you're just beginning an exercise program.)

Tip: If you're involved in several different sports, such as swimming, running and biking, your MHR will be different for each. It's generally highest while running and lowest during swimming. For the sake of accuracy, determine your MHR for each sport.

3. Design a Program

The following workouts serve as the backbone of a good general cardiovascular workout, or they can be tweaked to address specific sports and athletes.

"Aerobic base" workout

Description: Your bread-and-butter workout, this is the only type you'll do for the first four or five weeks.

Purpose: To build and maintain your tendons and increase your efficiency in using oxygen, both of which are important for endurance activity.

Intensity: Moderate to low-difficult. Maintain a heart rate that's about 65 to 80 percent of your MHR.

Frequency/duration: Three times a week, for 30 to 60 minutes. Give yourself an additional 5 to 10 minutes to warm up and cool down.

Tip: Go for variety. Do some bike workouts, some on the track, others in a pool. Alternate indoor workouts with outdoor ones.

Interval workouts

Description: Sometimes called splits or repeal an interval workout alternates a brief burst of activity with a similarly brief recovery period. You can add these in the fifth week.

Purpose: By alternating anaerobic "sprints" with "recoveries" in one workout session, you can make phenomenal gains. Intervals build endurance and muscle quickly. But because they carry a higher risk of injury, they shouldn't be performed very often. So do them just once a week until they feel comfortable, and never for more than six weeks in a row.

Intensity: Intervals are anaerobic workouts generally done at 80 to 100 percent of your maximum heart rate. They can be tweaked by playing with three variables: number of intervals, intensity and recovery time. You can experiment on your own or consult a good training book for more information on tailoring them to your needs and your sport.

Duration: Always begin with an extended warm-up, the equivalent of at least one or two miles, or 10 to 20 minutes. Then break into a standard workout of 6 to 10 sets, either one minute on/one minute off or two minutes on/one minute off at a lower intensity. During your recovery minutes, you can either continue jogging (or biking, etc.) at an easy pace (active recovery) or simply stop altogether (rest recovery).

Tip: Choose a target zone that allows you to recover in no longer than one minute. Then, take some time to build into each sprint and start the clock once you've reached that zone.

Tag intervals

Description: An advanced, intense workout that combines intervals with long high-aerobic-zone workouts. This is a variation on a workout used by Dave Fariner, coach of such champion mountain cyclists as Julie Furtado and John Tomac.

Purpose: Trains your body to shift between anaerobic and aerobic energy.

Intensity: Work at 80 to 85 percent of your MHR throughout, but pepper the workout with 5 to 10 evenly spaced "tags" at 95 percent of your MHR.

Frequency/duration: Once a week, 60 to 90 minutes. When you do a tag, build to 95 percent over one minute, hold that rate for 10 seconds, then gradually work back down to 85 percent.

Recovery workout

Description: An easy, steady pace.

Purpose: Maintains cardiovascular benefits while allowing heart and muscles to rebuild.

Intensity: 65 to 75 percent of MHR.

Frequency/duration: Once a week, 60 minutes.

Tip: The biggest challenge is to avoid going over 75 percent of MHR. Stay down!

Finally, you can do *fartlek* (Swedish for speedplay), workouts in which you essentially pick up the speed on an even course at your whim. For example, if you run on a trail with trees, or a street with lamp posts, you might use these landmarks as markers to let you know when to start a burst of moderate-to-high intensity exertion every few minutes, followed by a recovery of two to three minutes.

The most important thing to remember about cardiovascular training is that consistency beats intensity, even if you're doing a minimal (three days a week) program, such as one that includes two long aerobic-zone workouts and one interval workout. The idea is that you can increase your cardiovascular endurance without making a shambles of your personal life or even cutting into your weightlifting routine.

"I look at the big picture," Burke says. "If you're spending time on the weights, you're already getting a fair workout. Then maybe you've got the stresses of marriage and family. Instead of hammer, hammer, hammer, accept that making gains is a longterm process. Think in terms of a three- to five-year program, not a three- to five-week one." Eventually, whether you're hitting the trails, the tennis courts or the soccer fields, you'll have the endurance you once thought belonged to the chosen few.

EXERCISE ADDICTION AND OVERTRAINING

Some people take a good thing way too far. Exercise can make a dangerous transition from outlet to obsession.

If this strikes a familiar chord, you may well be addicted to exercise. Over the past fifteen years, dozens of studies have shown that exercise addiction is a very real and common phenomenon, particularly among competitive athletes, but more recently among noncompetitive fitness buffs as well. Fortunately, being an exercise addict need not have the negative connotations generally associated with physical or psychological dependencies. The real issue is whether your addiction to physical exertion is helping or hurting you.

Successful athletes—particularly those involved in individual, as opposed to team, sports—generally excel because, in addition to natural talent, they possess a high degree of motivation, determination and persistence in pursuit of their goals. Although they may display the classic signs of dependency, becoming anxious, agitated and guilt-ridden if they miss a workout, their form of addiction is beneficial since the result is the achievement of a positive goal.

The noncompetitive athlete may also be "positively addicted," a term coined by William Glasser in his 1976 book *Positive Addiction*. For a dedicated fitness enthusiast, a regular, intensive exercise program pays well-documented dividends: an improved sense of well-being, enhanced self-esteem and confidence, and the reduction of stress, tension and anxiety levels.

Only in the past few years has research been devoted to addiction in nonathletes. In a recent Australian study of sixty male and female health club members, half classified as addicts (they exercised at least five days a week for a minimum of fifteen hours total) and half nonaddicts (less than five days and five hours a week), researcher Mark Anshel found that the addicts were "markedly more restless, eager, self-confident and acutely stressed" than their nonaddicted counterparts, both before and soon after their workouts. The addicts were also far more depressed, anxious and even angry about having missed a workout than the nonaddicts.

"There are definite positive consequences of a regular exercise program, but there is a limit," says sports psychologist Charles Garfield, Ph.D., author of *Second to None*, a study of the positive effects of exercise on job performance. "The addict feels that if X amount is good, then twice the amount is even better. The reality is that twice as much may be doing damage to his system." Garfield describes the archetypal addict as "a person whose lifestyle is one of excess, whose personality is addictive by nature." That image is fleshed out by Tom Kennon, Ph.D., sports psychologist and assistant clinical professor at UCLA's Neuropsychiatric Institute. "The type most likely to become addicted is compulsive in most aspects of his life. He likes structure, order and predictability and is obsessive, almost superstitious, about the way he leads his life."

What leads to this type of behavior? Says Kennon, "The media have idealized the body, and we have been conditioned to believe that the perfect body is a sign of success and that if we have one we will be successful, popular and so on. Especially in these economic times, frustrations are transferred." Indeed, several studies have shown that compulsive exercisers may be compensating for deep inner feelings of inadequacy, unattractiveness and lack of approval from significant others. In addition, the exercise junkie suffers from acute bouts of uncomfortable emotions, such as anxiety and tension, and uses excessive physical exertion as a means to curb these feelings.

Because his drive to work out is so strong, the negatively addicted individual will often ignore illness or injury in order to fulfill his exercise requirements. Most athletes will push through the pain barrier when training or competing but are aware of the difference between pain and injury. The typical exercise addict, on the other hand, "is relatively new to extreme exertion and is not conditioned, has not built up a [pain] threshold like an athlete," says Garfield. "The result is often injury."

Injury isn't the only side effect associated with negative addiction. With excess exertion comes an energy drain that is slow to replenish, a waning concentration and a short attention span. Exercise becomes compulsive when an individual "is driven to exercise as though it were life and death, but it is also drudgery," says Garfield. This is a sure sign that the fine line between positive and negative addiction, or dedication and addiction, has been crossed. Garfield explains, "When the activity becomes the driving force without realistic positive return, and comes at the exclusion of other activities or relations, there's a serious problem."

As with any addictive behavior, acknowledgment of the problem is a major steppingstone to recovery. The solution lies in restoring a balanced perspective. Unless you're a world-class athlete in training, an exercise program is just one part of a life that should also include family, friends and career. Physical activity is a good way to blow off steam and escape from the rigors of the day, but it isn't a panacea for problems. If you suffer from excessive stress and anxiety or have a chronically poor self-image, seek help from friends or professionals. Allow yourself more rest and more frequent social interactions, and replace the old philosophy of "no pain, no gain" with the wiser "train, don't strain."

TEN WARNING SIGNS OF ADDICTION

1. Do you consistently exercise more than fifteen hours a week?
2. Do you feel restless, agitated and uptight before a workout?
3. Does missing a day cause you to become even more stressed and agitated?
4. Do you feel guilty if you miss even a single workout?
5. Is exercise your primary relief from the stresses of daily life?
6. Does exercise take priority over other activities and social relationships?
7. Are you reluctant to take time off because of illness or injury?
8. Do you feel compelled to work out even when you're tired?
9. Are you satisfied with what exercising does for you?
10. Are you having fun?

If you answered yes to questions 1 through 8, and no to questions 9 and 10, you are most likely negatively addicted. It's time to back off and refocus.

Overtraining is a highly relative term. What would leave one person on death's doorstep wouldn't cause a ripple of pain for a professional athlete. And what's too much for you now might be a moderate training session in a year or two. But the general signs of overtraining are the same for all of us. You can be pretty sure you're training too hard if:

You're in pain all the time. Soreness is sometimes the price you pay for challenging yourself athletically. But let's say you're on a Monday/Wednesday/Friday training schedule, and on Wednesday you're still stiff and achy from Monday's workout. You have three sane options: 1) Do different exercises, working body parts that aren't sore from the previous session; 2) do a very light aerobic routine, gently raising your heart rate so extra blood moves into the muscles and speeds the healing process; or 3) just take the day off and come back fresh on Friday.

You're sleeping less, or not as well. A good workout should make you sleep like a baby. Tossing and turning, or having trouble falling asleep, means you may be overdoing it.

You notice that a cut or bruise is slow to heal. When your body stops repairing itself, it may mean that it's too tired to do so.

You get more colds and/or cold sores than usual. These ailments come from viruses that a well-rested body's immune system can fend off.

Your resting heart rate is faster than normal. If you know what your resting heart rate is supposed to be and you notice your current pulse is more than 10 percent higher, your body desperately needs more rest.

Your normal workout suddenly seems much tougher. You're supposed to be moving forward, not back.

You really, really, really don't feel like working out on a scheduled gym day. No problem. Take some time off, and go back to the gym when it seems appealing again.

You just don't feel good. Overtraining symptoms can sometimes feel like a mild case of the flu. You're a little dizzy, a little disoriented, have a little trouble concentrating, and in the middle of walking up a short flight of stairs you just want to stop and take a nap. This may or may not signal illness, but it's definitely a sign that you need to take a few days off from your training program.

MIND FITNESS: CROSS-TRAIN YOUR BRAIN

As exercise addiction indicates, there is a strong connection between our emotional states and our workout habits. Fortunately, the positive greatly outweighs the negative. Got a difficult problem to solve? Work out, and your thinking improves. Feeling stressed, angry or upset? Work out, and your spirits lift. You exercise not just to get fit, but to feel and perform better in the rest of your life. Now researchers are discovering ways to capitalize on that connection.

In fact, the mind/body connection is the hottest topic in fitness today. At the annual international convention of the International Association of Fitness Professionals, the forum resounded with acclaim for the mental muscle. In seminar after seminar, experts emphasized the mind's role in enhancing workout results, reducing stress and providing balance for living in the nineties. Here's a roundup of techniques advocated by the pros to help you make every workout a visit to the mind gym.

Look at how you spend your day. Is your work logical, demanding, result-oriented and filled with deadline pressures? If so, you're working in a left-brain-dominant mode. You need the balance of a right-brain-dominant workout activity, something noncompetitive, expressive: running, in-line skating and t'ai chi are good choices.

If, instead, your work is artistic, creative and process-oriented, you're working in right-brain mode. Your workout needs to be left brain-dominant: structured, logical, result-driven—such as counting sets and reps, doing intervals, perhaps working with a goal-oriented trainer.

If you're a right-brain person working in a left-brain job, or vice versa, it's especially crucial to cross train your brain through exercise related choices. This will help your work as well as your workout. "For you to do your best, you've got to use the powers of brain hemispheres," says Diana McNab, a Livingston, New Jersey-based sports psychologist who specializes in mind/body training techniques. "You've got to combine the two. It's a matter of balance."

Cardiologist James Rippe, M.D., director of the University of Massachusetts Exercise Physiology and Nutrition Laboratory, and Ruth Stricker, owner of The Marsh, a health club near Minneapolis, have discovered you can intensify the psychological benefits of low-intensity exercise to the level of moderate exercise when you keep your mind engaged.

Mental strategies that keep you in the "here and now" will intensify the psychological results of your workout, says Rippe. Some examples: exercise to music you find meaningful; visualize yourself as a powerful animal, an aerobic engine or another image that works to pump up your enthusiasm; use meditation or yoga; focus on breathing in and breathing out.

If distracting thoughts pull you out of the here and now, focus on what you're doing. For example, if you're walking or running, say, "Left

". . . right . . ." when each foot hits. If a distracting thought pops up, says Rippe, don't judge it. Just let the thought pass, then get back to left-right.

Here's a new take on an old idea that will turn each workout into an interesting challenge. To get started, answer these questions, preferably in writing: What are your workout goals? What benefits will you get by reaching your objectives? What barriers keep you from reaching them? What steps can you take to overcome those barriers to success?

Now take this process a step farther. Define your goals for each workout session, and for each exercise within that session. "I determine before a workout of any kind what the purpose or goal of that session is," says John Martin, jujutsu instructor with Combat Arts Institute in the Chicago area. "Then I make sure all preparation leading to the session, as well as every activity within the session, is consistent with that goal."

A mental workout before a physical workout will help you train your mind to handle every challenge, from keeping the ball away from your opponent to cycling switchback curves down a killer hill, says sports psychologist and world-class triathlete JoAnn Dahlkoetter, Ph.D. Here are her mental-rehearsal steps:

Breathe deeply. Bring yourself into a relaxed state.

Visualize the event in detail, especially the most difficult parts.

Imagine how you'll overcome the toughest challenges. Mentally rehearse your options.

Imagine what you'll tell yourself throughout the event. Include positive affirmations in short, simple statements in the present tense, such as, "My breathing is deep. My pace is smooth. My arms are relaxed. I am confident. I am successful."

"Act as if it's already happening the way you want," says Dahlkoetter. "The more specific your imagery is to the event, the better." This process gives pieces of information to your brain, which transfers them to your muscles, enabling your body to use that information. The key is to practice these techniques on a regular basis—train your mind just like you train your body.

Rehearsal is especially effective when training for a triathlon, long-distance bike race or other endurance event. Go to the site at least six weeks ahead and study the course and all the conditions along it. Memorize as many details as possible. Then practice these rehearsal techniques for ten to fifteen minutes each day until the event.

"Weightlifters and gym rats could spend half as much time in the gym if they were 100 percent focused on what they were doing," says McNab. Use your powers of concentration to help your body achieve the benefits you desire. If you go to the gym to zone out, you may be limiting the effectiveness of your workout—and lengthening the time it takes to see tangible results.

Whether you're sculpting your whole body or training your cardiovascular system, get more bang for your buck by visualizing the muscle group you're exercising. This doesn't just make you concentrate and work harder; it elicits an actual physiological response, too. Visualization also works for fat burning. "Get into your target heart rate," says McNab, "and literally visualize the fatty acids coming out of your love handles and being excreted from your body." Focus on the neuromuscular connection you want, she says, and your results will skyrocket.

Just as you wouldn't walk away from a physical workout without cooling down, slow your mind with a few minutes of stretching, meditation or affirmation. Yoga, t'ai chi and aikido are excellent mind-stretchers, and one class of any or each will teach you the basics. "The latest research is that the best time to meditate, still the mind or get peace of mind is after a physical workout," says McNab.

Breathing itself is a good finisher. "Fitness for your brain has to do 99.9 percent with your breathing," says McNab. She recommends deep abdominal breathing, inhaling through your nose, exhaling through your mouth. "The first 30 percent of that breath goes straight to your brain. The other 70 percent goes to the rest of your body," she says.

Many world-class athletes believe so intensely in mind/body performance enhancement that they travel with psychologists. "At the highest level of any sporting event, it's mental," says Rippe. "People who have found ways of engaging the mind and turning it into a friend, instead of an enemy, are the ones who win."

One class of athletes—both recreational and competitive—is emblematic of the way engaging the mind positively can bring amazing physical results: the physically challenged. Exercise is key to their self-esteem, emotional health and physical well-being. But beyond the benefits they get from exercise, they give even more: they provide an enormous inspiration for the rest of us.

PHYSICALLY CHALLENGED ATHLETES

Times have never been so good for the physically and mentally disabled athletes of this world. In the past dozen years, rigorous professional competitions have emerged, with superstars like David Kiley, the king of wheelchair sports, and Jim Abbott, born without a right hand, who's become a top pitcher in the American League. Advanced technology has produced new prosthetic limbs and wheelchairs that put a keener edge on the competition and reduce the risk of injury from intensified action. Companies that develop such products support disabled athletes with sponsorships and offer top prize money at athletic events.

That's the good news. The bad news, according to the disabled athletes themselves, is that they still have to fight to be taken seriously. News coverage of their sports is minimal. The media aren't entirely to blame, according to Charlie Huebner, media director for the Paralympics, which offers international competitions for the physically disabled. Huebner says some disabled-athletes organizations "just aren't sophisticated yet" at promoting themselves. And while some of these groups, he says, hire the best coaches for their top athletes and mainstream them into able-bodied competition, others lag far behind.

Disabled athletes face a more immediate challenge from their own families and friends. Keith Brigman, a coach with Special Olympics, says family support is especially important for mentally challenged athletes who want to compete. But, Brigman says, "Only 10 percent of the parents take any pride in these things and really get out and support their kids."

For the physically disabled, there is often the wrong kind of support: the patronizing variety from friends and spectators. "These guys don't want to hear they're inspiring," says Jon Ross of the Achilles Track Club of Southern California. "What they want to hear is, 'Wow, those guys are hot!'"

And hot they are. They do have obstacles to overcome, but so does everyone else, disabled and able-bodied alike. If they can persist and achieve, he says, what's stopping people on the sidelines from doing the same?

While challenged athletes are increasingly found in gyms and competitive events like marathons and even triathlons, there are organizations that provide activities geared especially for them. Many of these groups are good sources for events and activities in your area.

ARCHERY

AMERICAN WHEELCHAIR ARCHERS
RD 2, Box 2043
West Sudbury, PA 16061

BASKETBALL

NATIONAL WHEELCHAIR BASKETBALL
   ASSOCIATION
Stan Labanowich
110 Seaton Building
University of Kentucky
Lexington, KY 40506

BOWLING

AMERICAN WHEELCHAIR BOWLING
   ASSOCIATION
3620 Tamarack Dr.
Redding, CA 96003

CANOEING/KAYAKING

AMERICAN CANOE ASSOCIATION
7432 Alban Station Blvd.
Suite B–226
Springfield, VA 22150

EQUESTRIAN

NORTH AMERICAN RIDING FOR THE
   HANDICAPPED ASSOCIATION
P.O. Box 33150
Denver, CO 80233

FLYING

FREEDOM WINGS INTL.
1832 Lake Avenue
Scotch Plains, NJ 07076

INTERNATIONAL WHEELCHAIR AVIATORS
11 17 Rising Hill
Escondido, CA 92029

GENERAL

EASTERN AMPUTEE ATHLETIC ASSOCIATION
2080 Ennabrock Rd.
North Bellmore, NY 11710

NATIONAL HANDICAPPED SPORTS
451 Hungerford Drive
Rockville, MD 20850

UNITED STATES CEREBRAL PALSY ATHLETIC
   ASSOCIATION
34518 Warren Rd.
Westland, MI 48185

HOCKEY

A 1 TIME
913 S. Washington
Redwood Falls, MN 56283

OUTDOOR ACTIVITIES

C.W. HOG
P.O. Box 8118
Idaho State University
Pocatello, ID 83209

QUADRIPLEGIC SPORTS

UNITED STATES QUAD RUGBY ASSOCIATION
241 8 West Falicreek Ct.
Grand Forks, ND 58201

RACQUET SPORTS

INTERNATIONAL FOUNDATION FOR WHEELCHAIR
   TENNIS
2203 Timerloch Place
The Woodlands, TX 77380

INTERNATIONAL WHEELCHAIR TENNIS
   FOUNDATION
Pallsier Road, Barrons Court
London W 14 9EN, England

NATIONAL FOUNDATION OF WHEELCHAIR
   TENNIS
940 Calle Amanecer
San Clemente, CA 92672

NATIONAL WHEELCHAIR
Racquetball Association
535 Kensington Rd, Lancaster, PA 17603

SCHOLARSHIPS/ATHLETE AWARDS

GOVERNOR'S COMMITTEE FOR EMPLOYMENT
   OF DISABLED PERSONS
P.O. Box 826880-MTC 41
Sacramento, CA 94208

SKIING

SKI FOR LIGHT
1400 Carole Lane
Green Bay, WI 54313

SOFTBALL

NATIONAL WHEELCHAIR SOFTBALL
   ASSOCIATION
1616 Todd Court
Hastings, MN 55033

SWIMMING

U.S. WHEELCHAIR SWIMMING
229 Miller St.
Middleboro, MA 02346

TABLE TENNIS

AMERICAN WHEELCHAIR TENNIS ASSOCIATION
23 Parker St.
Port Chester, NY 10573

TRACK AND FIELD

ACHILLES TRACK CLUB
9 E. 89th St.
New York, NY 10128

WHEELCHAIR ATHLETICS OF AMERICA
1475 West Gray
Houston, TX 77109

TRIATHLON

TRIATHLON FOR THE DISABLED
P.O. Box V-16
Palo Alto, CA 94304

WATER SPORTS

ACCESS TO SAILING
19744 Beach Blvd,
Huntington Beach, CA 92648

AMERICAN CANOE ASSOCIATION
7432 Alban Station Blvd.
Suite B–226
Springfield, VA 22150

AMERICAN WATER SKI ASSOCIATION
P.O. Box 21
Jackson Gap, AL 36861

HANDICAPPED SCUBA ASSOCIATION
1104 El Prado
San Clemente, CA 92672

NATIONAL OCEAN ACCESS PROJECT
P.O. Box 33141
Washington, DC 20033–0141

U.S. ROWING ASSOCIATION
11 Hall Pl.
Exeter, NH 03833

WEIGHTLIFTING

UNITED STATES
  WEIGHTLIFTING FEDERATION
39 Michael Pl.
Levittown, PA 19057

WHEELCHAIR RACING

CANADIAN WHEELCHAIR
  SPORTS ASSOCIATION
1600 James Naismith Dr.
Gloucester, Ontario,
Canada KI B 5N4

INTERNATIONAL WHEELCHAIR
  ROAD RACERS CLUB, INC.
30 Myano Lane
Stamford, CT 06902

MUSCLES (MICHIGAN UNITED SPORTS CHAIR
  LEAGUE ENDURANCE SERIES)
10030 Whitewood Rd.
Pinckey, MI 48169

NATIONAL WHEELCHAIR ATHLETIC ASSOCIATION
3595 East Fountain Blvd.
Colorado Springs, CO 80910

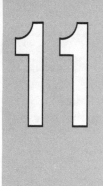

EIGHT MYTHS ABOUT MEN

S ay you're twenty-two years old. You find a few extra hairs on the shower drain and make the mistake of telling your mother about it. "Don't worry about it," she says reassuringly. "Your grandfather was bald by the time he was thirty-five, and nobody had a better life than he did." You freeze, remembering the biology teacher who said that if your mother's father was bald, it's a genetic inevitability that you will be, too. Was he right?

Myths, says the dictionary, are legendary stories whose truth is accepted uncritically. Which is not to say that they're not occasionally true. The following are nine commonly held beliefs about male health, sexuality and behavior. Some of them have a basis in fact. Some are wildly inaccurate. Some split the difference.

MYTH 1: PENIS SIZE DOESN'T MATTER

True in theory. False everywhere else.

"I've seen 17,000 men in my practice, and not one has said that a woman told him his penis is too small," says Cappy Rothman, M.D., a Los Angeles urologist and director of reproductive medicine at Century City Hospital in Los Angeles. "Sexually, penis size is not an issue."

Sure. Just like "It's not whether you win or lose, it's how you play the game." If winning isn't everything, you might ask, how come no one goes for the bronze? No matter what men—and women—claim to believe, penis size remains a very real issue for many.

"It probably doesn't matter," says Bernie Zilbergeld, Ph.D., an Oakland, California, therapist and author of *The New Male Sexuality: The Truth About Men, Sex and Pleasure*. "But the topic sure comes up a lot in therapy. One reason is the wider myth that for men, bigger is better. Bigger car, bigger income, bigger house—bigger man. Men are concerned about adequacy in many ways, and this is one of them." Zilbergeld says the idea starts early. "When a small boy sees his father's penis, it looks huge, and this becomes the child's basis for deciding what he needs himself," he says. "Once the man's grown, the child in him remembers this gargantuan penis."

In adulthood, the problem usually stems from a discrepancy between self-perception and reality. "I had a male patient, a virgin, who thought his penis was much too small—and that caused him to lose his erections," Zilbergeld says. "I sent him to a surrogate sex partner, and right after their session together she called to tell me that his was one of the biggest, longest penises she'd seen. And this from someone who's seen a few!"

This kind of discrepancy probably stems from the fact that there's no real way for a man to measure himself against others. "Most men compare themselves in the locker room, when they're soft," Zilbergeld says. But evidence shows that a smaller penis, measured when limp, grows more proportionally than a penis that starts off larger. By the time both are erect, there may not be much difference between them. "The only erections most men see, other than their own, may belong to a Long Dong Silver or some other actor in a porno movie," Zilbergeld adds, "and they're no one to match yourself against. These guys are hardly the penis next door." Will men ever stop worrying about size? Zilbergeld isn't holding his breath: "No matter how much knowledge men have, no matter how much publicity we give to the fact that penis size doesn't matter, men have an underlying feeling that it does," he says.

MYTH 2: WOMEN ARE FATTER THAN MEN

False. Men are just as fat. But they're not as likely to do anything about it.

"Women diet more than men," says Jerry C. Sutkamp, M.D., author of *How to Help Your Man Lose Weight* and a weight-loss specialist for more than twenty years. "But, except in the black population, just as many men are fat. Men simply have a harder time facing the facts about their weight." At any given time, Sutkamp says, 50 percent of American women are dieting, compared to only 25 percent of men.

Much of the misconception about weight has to do with how we are brought up. "Girls are expected to be thin and self-conscious about their weight," Sutkamp says, "while boys try to build up their weight to achieve a 'big guy' image. If a woman is ten pounds overweight, she'll become self-conscious; a man will just think, 'I'll buy a bigger suit.' It's really a different mindset about appearance and health."

In terms of body composition, women are actually allowed a greater percentage of body fat than men are: a maximum of 25 percent verses 18 percent, respectively. And the differences between the sexes vary according to race. Among white Americans, for example, 42 percent of both men and women are considered obese, meaning they're at least 20 percent above their ideal body weight. Among black Americans, though, 45 percent of women are obese, compared to only 22 percent of men. Why the discrepancy? "There's no medical explanation," Sutkamp says. "The difference is probably due to environmental factors."

MYTH 3: MUSCLE CAN TURN TO FAT

False. No one's muscle can turn to fat.

"Muscle is muscle and fat is fat," Sutkamp says. "You can convert fat to energy, then use that energy to convert the remaining fat to muscle, but you just can't take muscle and turn it to fat."

Why do so many men have this misconception? "What happens is that as you exercise less, your lean body tissue shrinks and you put on more fat," Sutkamp says. And athletes have a tendency to keep up the training diet after the training days are over. "Athletes who stop training but keep eating 6,000 calories or so per day will get fat. The muscle is still there, but they're adding fat. Interestingly, as you get fatter, your body adds more muscle just to haul around the extra body weight. A 300-pound man has more muscle than a 195-pound man—it's used to carry the fat."

A related common myth is that you can just "firm up the fat." But, as Sutkamp points out, if you don't make real changes in your eating habits, what usually happens is that you firm up the muscle underneath the fat, and the fat stays where it is. No way around it: You've got to eat less fat and tone up your muscles if you want to get back the body you used to have.

MYTH 4: MEN CAN'T HAVE SEX WITH ONE OR NO TESTICLES

False. Sex yes, children maybe.

"With no testicles, you can still get an erection, but there will be no ejaculate and therefore no sperm," urologist Cappy Rothman says. "The testicles produce testosterone, the hormone that triggers the release of seminal fluid which carries sperm from the prostate. So, if the testicles are lost because of cancer or some other reason, a man can no longer ejaculate."

What if a man loses only one testicle, as is often the case in cancer? That's different. "A man with one testicle can have a normal, happy and healthy sex and reproductive life," Rothman says. "Just as we can live with one kidney, a man can be sexually active and fertile with only one testicle. In cancer cases, there may be some interference with a man's fertility due to other aspects of treatment—chemotherapy, for example," Rothman adds. "But if a testicle is lost due to trauma, testicular torsion or infection, there should be no problem."

Just make sure you protect the one that's left.

MYTH 5: IF YOUR MOTHER'S FATHER WAS BALD, YOU'LL BE BALD, TOO

False. Even the medical community used to believe this one, but it's just not so.

"It can be true that baldness is passed down from the maternal grandfather," says Richard W. Fleming, MD, cochairman of the division of facial plastic surgery at the University of Southern California School of Medicine. "But it's also true that baldness can be inherited from anybody in your family—the genetic link is not limited to the maternal side."

Baldness is genetic, but there is no set pattern of how it's passed along. "It doesn't skip a generation, and it's inconsistent in how it's handed down," Fleming says. As an example, he points to the Gibb brothers, better known as the Bee Gees. "Look at those three brothers—one has a full head of hair, one is thinning and one is bald. They all have the same parents and grandparents, yet their hairlines are completely different."

Other baldness myths abound. For example: Washing your hair too often will make it fall out; wearing a hat can cause baldness; working out too much can lead to hair loss. "There's just nothing to these," Fleming says. What about the role of stress? "Stress can cause hair loss," he notes, "but the hairs that you lose were already genetically programmed to fall out. Stress just speeds up the process."

MYTH 6: MEN CAN'T DO AEROBICS

False. But a beat that's a piece of cake for a 5' 4" woman will make the most graceful guy look like a stumblebum.

"It's not true that men are naturally lousy at aerobics," says aerobicist-to-the-stars Karen Voight. Though Voight's Los Angeles classes are approximately 50 percent male, that's not typical of the national scene. "I've done exhibition classes on tour in the Midwest in which there have been 200 women and four men," she says.

"A lot of men (and some women) assume they're too big or not coordinated enough, but the real reason men have trouble with aerobics is that most classes aren't tailored to their particular needs," Voight says. So what do men need from aerobics classes? For one thing, slower music. "Most men have a hard time keeping up," she says. "When I have a class with a lot of guys, the first thing I do is slow the music down."

Another physiological hurdle that holds men back in the aerobics studio, says Voight, is their inexperience in isolating their legs from their hips when exercising. She isn't sure why that's so but says the habit can be broken. In beginners' classes, she concentrates on using rhythms that let men practice independent leg movements, and they're more than willing—and able—if given the chance.

"On the whole," Voight says, "men are less self-conscious than women when learning a new movement. And they're more interested in getting a really good workout; if you bore them, they won't come back. They want to leave in a sweat, and given a chance to show it, they've got a lot of rhythm."

MYTH 7: MEN ARE MORE VIOLENT THAN WOMEN

True. And it's not just because men's fists are bigger.

"The statistics behind this fact are pretty compelling," says Robert Nsick, Ph.D., author of *Awakening from the Deep Sleep: A Practical Guide for Men in Transition* and a consultant at the Ann Arbor [Michigan] Center for the Family. "Ninety-five percent of violent acts within the family are committed by men."

Pasick believes that much of the problem with men and violence is due to the way men were—and are—raised. "Look at the role models we provide to boys: the Terminator, Rambo. Television and movies have become much more violent, and the images are aimed more at men than women."

Pasick dismisses the notion that men are simply stronger physically than women and therefore more likely to be accused of violence. "Skeptics say, 'Well, women hit too, just not as hard.' But the fact is, women don't hit as often as men. If a woman wants to inflict damage, she can do it with a weapon if her fists aren't up to the task. But women just don't commit as many violent acts as men." Men also tend to deny that violence has occurred, says Pasick, either by excusing their own behavior ("I just hit her once . . . ") or by blaming the victim ("She provoked me."). "This extends to society at large," adds Pasick, "so that police often do not make arrests in cases of domestic violence, and statistics may be underreported as a result."

MYTH 8: FLAT FEET POSE A HEALTH RISK

False. And they won't keep you out of the army, either.

"The number-one cause for rejection from the armed services during World War II was flat feet," says Daniel M. McGann, a podiatrist in San Marino, California, and author of *The Doctor's Sore Foot Book*. "At the time, it was widely believed that men with flat feet couldn't move as fast as those with elevated arches and thus would be injured more easily. Indeed, the term 'flat-foot' today is still synonymous with clumsiness, and even now many people believe being flat-footed is an unhealthy condition."

There are three basic arch-related conditions: flat feet, weak feet and high arches, McGann says. "People who are born with flat feet tend not to have trouble with them," he says. "Their feet are flat both at rest and when bearing weight. If you have what we call 'weak feet,' they are arched at rest but weaken when weight is put on them. But it's the third category—high arches—that can really cause problems, because they are the least flexible."

In 1989, the U.S. Army conducted a study which disproved the flat-feet myth and revealed that high arches may in fact result in more injuries. "So what happened in World War II," McGann says, "is that the services rejected men with flat feet and took those with high arches. The guys with the flat feet might have done a lot better in the field."

INDEX

abdominal pain, 45
Abdul-Jabbar, Kareem, 115
Accutane, 151–52
acne, 142
    adult onset of, 149–53
    rosacea, 151
    steroid-induced, 150
    treatment of, 150–52
    vulgaris, 150
actinic keratosis, 62
acupuncture, 71–72, 227
acyclovir (Zovirax), 250
Adamski, Tom, 290, 291
ADD (attention deficit disor-
    der), 102–5, 120
addiction, 225–32
    to alcohol, 226, 227–30
    of batterers, 285
    to cigarettes, 230–32
    to exercise, 356–59
    healthy habits vs., 307
adultery, 286–89
Adultery (Lawson), 286
aerobic capacity, as biomarker,
    303–4
aerobic exercise, 19, 49–50,
    181
    anti-aging and, 306–7
    bone strength and, 306,
        307, 308
    cholesterol and, 49
    fartlek workouts in, 356
    heart and, 14–15, 48, 49,
        50
    heart rate and, 32, 352–53
    intervals in, 350–52,
        354–55
    program of, 353–56
    sex and, 244–45
aerobics, 371
affirmations, 122–23
aging, 46, 90, 156, 163

athletes and, 314–17
biomarkers of, 17, 301–6
body image and, 310–13
brain and, 13
death and, 328–30
DHEA for, 310
family history and, 300,
    322–27
libido and, 256, 310,
    317–20
life expectancy and, 8, 35,
    53, 80, 81, 90, 301, 307
male menopause and,
    320–22
melatonin in, 309–10
muscle mass in, 301, 302,
    303, 304, 306, 308
sex differences and, 25–26
sexuality and, 317–20
slowing process of, 300,
    302, 306–9
agoraphobia, 101
AIDS (acquired immune defi-
    ciency syndrome), 30,
    219, 252–55
    relationships and, 294–95
alcohol, 38, 43, 51, 52, 69, 98,
    259
Alcoholics Anonymous, 226
alcoholism, 226–30
    CAGE Index for, 230
"alcoholism gene," 226
Alda, Alan, 3
allergies, 224, 326
alternative medicine, 38,
    70–82
    mind fitness and, 359–63
    self-healing as, 38, 86,
        113–30
    stress-related disorders and,
        85–86
alveoli, 14

American Academy of Medical
    Acupuncture, 72
American Board of Medical
    Specialties, 34
American Botanical Council
    (ABC), 75
American Cancer Society
    (ACS), 60, 66, 67
American Chiropractic
    Association, 70
American Dietetic Association,
    202
American Foundation for
    Urological Disease, 66
American Hair Loss Council,
    160, 161
American Journal of Cardiology,
    93
American Journal of Psychiatry,
    17
American Yoga Association,
    118
amino acids, 156, 180, 181,
    182
Anatomy of an Illness (Cousins),
    113, 125
Anderson, David E., 323
androgenetic alopecia (male
    pattern baldness), 157
Anger: The Misunderstood
    Emotion (Tavris), 279
angina pectoris, 39–40, 72
anorexia, 171, 172, 174
    "reverse," 172
ANRED (Anorexia Nervosa
    and Related Eating
    Disorders Association),
    175
Antibiotic Paradox, The (Levy),
    218
antibiotics, 43, 54, 63, 69, 76,
    147, 151, 217–18, 249

antioxidants, 156, 201, 202, 227, 231
antrium, 21
anxiety, performance, 262–64
anxiety disorders, 99–102
Any Man Can (Fithian and Hartman), 240
appearance-consciousness, 131–34
see also grooming
arthritis, 20, 72, 326
Association for Voluntary Surgical Contraception, 247
Association of Applied Psychophysiology and Biofeedback, 121
asthma, 211, 326
atherosclerosis, 47–48, 227
see also heart attack, heart disease
attention deficit disorder (ADD), 102–5, 120
autogenics, 227
Awakening from the Deep Sleep (Pasick), 372
azoospermia, 247
AZT, 253
Azulfidine, 259

backaches, 15–16, 73, 176
risk-profile quiz for, 16
Bailey, Covert, 166
baldness, 140
attitude toward, 139, 162
heredity and, 370–71
remedies for, 157–60
testosterone and, 157–58
treatment costs for, 160–62
Baldwin, Bruce, 88
Ballentine, Rudolph, 121
Bannister, Roger, 115
Barbach, Lonnie, 236, 237–38
Barnett, Rosalind, 88
basal metabolic rate (BMR), 169–71
as biomarker, 303
Bassett, Arthur, 216
Batten, Mary, 271
batterers, 282–86, 372
behavior therapy, 101, 109

benign prostate hyperplasia (BPH), 64–65, 76
Benson, Herbert, 116–17, 126
beta-carotene, 156, 203–4, 231
bioenergetics, 72–73
biofeedback, 38, 86, 104, 119–21
biomarkers, 301, 306–7
aerobic capacity, 303–4
blood pressure, 301, 305
blood-sugar tolerance, 304
BMR, 303
body-fat, 303
bone density, 8, 17, 305–6
cholesterol, 304–5
internal temperature, 306
muscle mass, 301, 302, 303, 304, 306, 308
strength, 302, 306, 307, 308
Biomarkers (Evans, Rosenberg and Thompson), 301
biorhythms, 199
biotin, 156, 207
birth control, male, 246–48, 261–62, 322
contraceptive implants, 247
Bjorntorp, Per, 180
bladder control problems, 55
Blair, Steven, 165
bleeding, 43
Block, Gladys, 202, 204
blood cells, 13, 14–15, 17
blood pressure, 32, 51, 53, 180
as biomarker, 301, 305
high (hypertension), 42, 43, 46, 49, 51, 213
touch and, 274–75
see also heart attack, heart disease
blood-sugar tolerance, 304
Bloomfield, Harold H., 97, 98, 278
Bly, Robert, 4, 137
bodybuilding, *see* weight lifting
body fat, 167–71
as biomarker, 303

sex differences in, 369
test for, 166–67
body image, 131–77
aging and, 310–13
healthy, 136
"ideal," 139–40
obsession with, 134–36, 173
body types, 136, 138–39
body weight, 9, 15, 16, 20, 64, 139
self-image and, 162
bones, 9, 15, 16–17, 19
density of, as biomarker, 8, 17, 305–6
marrow of, 17
Bonhomme, Jean, 81
Bosley, L. Lee, 159
botanical medicines, *see* herbalism
Bowlus, Thomas, 93, 94
Braiker, Harriet B., 92, 93, 94
brain, 9–10, 19, 48
aging of, 13
cross-training of, 360–61
of men vs. women, 10–13
brain stem, 10
Branum, Donald, 174
breakfasts, one-minute, 193–94
Brigman, Keith, 363
bronchioles, 14, 211
bronchus, primary, 14
Brothers, Joyce, 131, 133, 134
bruises, 43–44
bulimia, 172, 173, 174
Burke, Ed, 351, 353, 356
Burnison, Chantal, 158
bursitis, 20
Byrd, Randolf, 127

Cado, Suzana, 245
caffeine, 38, 200, 210–16
bronchodilation and, 211
pain relief and, 211–12
calcium, 16, 17, 196, 202, 207
calcium channel blockers, 53
Callaway, Wayne, 164, 165
Campbell, Anne, 281

Campbell, Susan Rockwell, 263, 264
cancer, 29, 30, 149, 196, 198, 309
    coffee and, 213
    see also carcinomas; *specific cancers*
Capps, John T., III, 161
carbohydrates, 170, 199
    blood pressure and, 305
carcinomas:
    basal-cell, 149
    squamous-cell, 149
cardiopulmonary system, 13–15
cardiovascular:
    disease, *see* blood pressure; heart attack, heart disease
    exercise, *see* aerobic exercise
    system, aging of, 303, 306
cartilage, 16
Cash, Thomas, 161
CAT (coital alignment technique), 238, 239–40
Catalona, William, 67
catecholamine, 114
Catron, Sarah, 276
Center for Marital and Sexual Studies (CMSS), 241, 244
Center for Science in the Public Interest (CSPI), 179
Centers for Disease Control and Prevention (CDC), 219
centiums, 23
central nervous system, 10
cerebellum, 9–10
cerebrum, 9–10
Chalker, Rebecca, 22
chancres, 249
checkups, medical, *see* physical examination
chest pain, 38–42, 44
chiropractic, 73–74
chlamydia, 248, 249, 250
cholesterol, 15, 19, 32–33, 49, 50–51, 52, 196
    alcohol and, 227
    as biomarker, 304–5
    coffee and, 213

Chopra, Deepak, 114
Choudhury, Rajashree, 122
Chung, Fung-lung, 214
chyme, 21
cigarettes, *see* smoking
circulatory system, 14–15, 31, 47–48
Clanton, Gordon, 92
Clark, Nancy, 199–200, 210
cluster headaches, 37
coffee, 200, 210–13
cognition, sex differences in, 11
cognitive therapy, 109
coitus interruptus, 246
cold sores, 154
Cole, Louanne, 245
Coleman, Ellen, 211
collagen injections, 152
colon cancer, 326
Colvin, James, 298, 299
Comfort, Alex, 239
Coming Plague, The (Garrett), 217
commitment:
    analytical approach to, 272–74
    families and, 297
    instinct and, 271–72, 273
    quiz, 273–74
    weight training and, 340
condoms, 246, 250, 251
conflicts, 279–82
    domestic violence and, 282–83, 372
    rules of engagements in, 282
    sex differences and, 281–82
    zero-sum disputes and, 280–81
Conney, Allan, 214, 215
Connor, William E., 99
contaminants:
    cleaning, 222–23
    food-poisoning, 221–22
contraceptives, *see* birth control, male
copper, 156, 202, 208
Corbett, Tom, 223, 225
coronary-artery disease, 48, 227

    see also heart attack, heart disease; stroke
coronary heart disease, *see* heart attack, heart disease
corpus callosum, 11
cosmetic surgery, 131, 134
Coué, Emile, 123
coughing, 41, 44
Cousins, Norman, 113, 114, 125–26
cracked tooth syndrome (CTS), 24
creatinine, 33
cryotherapy, 251
cryptosporidium, 219
Csikszentmihalyi, Mihaly, 128–30
Cyoctol, 158
cysteine, 156
cytomegalovirus, 253

Dahlkoetter, JoAnn, 361
Dancing Healers (Hammerschlag), 127
Darwinian medicine, 47
Davidson, Joy, 137–38, 266–67
DBCP (dibromochloropropane), 260
DeLeo, Vincent, 141, 143
depression, 96–99
dermabrasion, 152
dermatitis, seborrheic, 153
dermis, 22
DeVillers, Linda, 319
Dexedrine (dextroamphetamine), 104
DHEA (dehydroepiandrosterone), 310
diabetes, 33, 326
    muscle mass and, 302
Diamond, Seymour, 37
diaphragm, 14, 350
diazoxide, 158
dibromochloropropane (DBCP), 260
diet and nutrition, 9, 15, 17
    anti-aging, 307
    cholesterol and, 50–51, 180
    fat intake and, *see* dietary fat intake

diet and nutrition (*cont.*)
hair and, 156
healthy lifestyle, 178–200
heart and, 50, 180
hypertension and, 32, 51,
53, 180
mineral ODAs, 204, 207,
208, 209–10
"pleasure revenge" in,
331–32
prostate and, 64, 65
protein in, 180–83, 199
salt-restricted, 51, 305
skin problems and,
154–56
supplements, 201–4
30-day menu for, 183–95
ulcers and, 69
vitamin ODAs, 204, 207,
208, 209
see also minerals; vitamins
dietary fat intake, 15, 50, 167,
169–70, 178–80
biomarkers and, 303, 305
low-fat foods and, 51, 165,
179
waist-to-hip ratio and,
180
Dieter's Dictionary, The (Vash),
169
dieting, 162–75
men and, 368–69
weight loss and, 162
yo-yo, 162–63
digestive system, 20–21, 42,
68–69
dihydrotestosterone (DHT),
157–58
disease, *see* illness; *specific diseases*
Doctor's Sore Foot Book, The
(McGann), 372
*Doctors' Vitamin and Mineral
Encyclopedia, The*
(Hendler), 201
domestic violence, 282–86,
372
dopamine, 112, 227
Dougherty, Carol, 290, 291
drinking, *see* alcohol
Druck, Ken, 293
Duesberg, Peter, 252

Eastwood, Clint, 138
eating disorders, 171–75
Ebola virus, 220
echinacea, 76
ectomorphs, 137, 138
best sports for, 138
eczema, 155
Eddy, Mary Baker, 125
Edelson, Todd, 299
Effexor, 98
Eichel, Edward, 239, 240
ejaculation, 241, 243
Ellison, Carol, 237
"embodiment," 136
embolism, pulmonary, 41–42
Emerging Viruses (Morse), 219
emotions, 3–5, 6
addictive behavior and,
225–32, 356–59
anger and, 12, 92, 93–94,
95–96, 114; *see also* conflicts
body and, 359–60
bone density and, 17
brain processing of, 11–12
food and, 198–200
grief, 328–30
toxic, 84, 91–96, 114
violence and, 282–86, 372
see also mental well-being;
*specific emotional prob-
lems*
endomorphs, 137, 139
best sports for, 139
endorphins, 71, 99, 200, 225,
227
environmental health, 216–25
ephedra, 74
epidermis, 21–22
epididymis, 24
erection problems, 45–46,
255–57
performance anxiety and,
263–64
eroticism, life-partner,
277–79
esophageal cancer, 215
Evans, William, 301–2, 304,
305, 306
excretory system, 21
exercise, 5, 17, 21, 99,
168–69

addiction and, 173,
356–59
aerobic, *see* aerobic exercise
aging athletes and, 314–17
anaerobic, 49–50, 354
anti-aging, 307; *see also*
aerobic exercise; weight
lifting
for back and abs, 176
body fat and, 168–69
cross training, 315
emotions and, 359–63
fitness craze and, 331–34
intensity of, 168
mental well-being and,
111–12, 360
metabolic rate and, 169–70
overtraining and, 43, 173,
359
physically challenged and,
362–66
risk factors and, 49–50
sperm count and, 258–59
strength-building, *see*
weight lifting
stretch and warm-ups,
334–37
visualization and, 360–62
weight-bearing, 17
weight lifting and, *see*
weight lifting

Fahrion, Steven, 120
Fair, William, 67
family:
health and, 53, 226,
270–71
medical history of, 300,
322–27
men's role in, 1–2, 3, 5
relationships in, 297–99
separate-spheres concept
of, 1–2, 3
social restructuring of, 1–3
family and marital therapy, 110
fantasies, sexual, 244–46,
279
Fariner, Dave, 355
Farrell, Warren, 133
fast foods, 194–95
fatherhood, changing role of,
1, 2, 3, 5

fatigue, 42
fats, *see* dietary fat intake
fatty acids, essential (EFA), 155, 156
feelings, *see* emotions
feet, flat, 372–73
Feirstein, Bruce, 133
female roles, *see* women
fenfluramine, 165
fertility, 261–62
    genetic counseling and, 260
finasteride, oral, 157–58
Fithian, Marilyn, 240, 244
fitness, *see* aerobic exercise; exercise; weight lifting
fitness craze, 331–34
Fit or Fat (Bailey), 168
Fleming, Michael, 323
Fleming, Richard W., 159, 370
Fletcher, Anne, 163
flow, 127–30
Flow (Csikszentmihalyi), 128
food:
    comfort, 200
    health benefits of, 155, 195–200, 204–10
    low-fat, 51, 165, 179
    -mood connection, 198–200
    see also diet and nutrition
Fox, Hannah, 257
"free PSA" test, 65
free radicals, 155–56, 196, 231
Freudian psychoanalysis, 110–11
Friedman, Meyer, 126–27
friendships:
    gay/straight, 295–97
    intimacy and, 289–91
    male bonding and, 291–94
Fry, William F., 113, 114
Fujiki, Hirota, 214
Full Catastrophe Living (Kabat-Zinn), 89
Fumento, Michael, 252
fundus, 21

Gainer, Sandra, 34
Garfield, Charles, 357, 358
garlic, 75, 76, 197–98

Garrett, Laurie, 217
gastrointestinal (G.I.) problems, 20–21, 42, 68–69
"Gay/Straight Friendships" (Feirstein), 295–97
gender roles, *see* men; women
generalized anxiety disorder, 100
genetic counseling, 260
George, Mark, 12
Gibbons, Larry, 51
Gilchrest, Barbara, 148
ginger, 76
ginkgo, 76
ginseng, 74, 76
Glasser, William, 357
Glickman, Adam, 246
Gohagan, John, 67, 68
Goldberg, Herb, 292
Goldberg, Kenneth, 263
Goldman, Ron G., 98, 99
Goldstein, David, 49
gonorrhea, 248, 249, 250
good looks, concept of, 136–40
Goodman, Joel, 113, 114
Goodwin, Frederick, 97–98
Gottman, John M., 280
Goulston, Mark S., 107–9, 328, 329, 330
Greeley, Andrew, 126
Green, Robert L., 134
grief, 328–30
Griffiths, Roland, 213
grooming, 22, 61, 140–45
    aging and, 310–13
guided imagery, 124–25

habits, *see* addiction; lifestyle, healthy
hair, 22, 23
    aging and, 312–13
    diet and, 156
    flap surgery, 159, 161
    grooming of, 143–44
    loss of, *see* baldness
    transplants, 159, 161
Halsted, Charles, 228
Hammerschlag, Carl, 127
Harman, S. Mitchell, 320
Hartman, William, 240–44
Hayward, Fred, 80–82

Hazards of Being Male, The (Goldberg), 292
headaches, 35–38, 326
    triggers of, 38
    see also lifestyle, healthy
health problems, *see* alternative medicine; illness; physical examination; malpractice, medical
heart, 14–15
    muscle, 18, 19
    palpitations, 39, 53
    rate, aging and, 304; *see also* heart rate, target
heart attack, heart disease, 5, 8, 9, 32, 33, 38–40, 42, 43, 48, 49, 53–54, 196, 233, 270
    atherosclerosis and, 47–48
    prevention of, 48–53, 326
    silent, 39, 43, 54
    "spiritual," 270
    symptoms mimicking, 39–42, 69
    walking and, 334
    warning signs of, 38–40, 43, 44
heartburn, 42
heart rate:
    maximum (MHR), 353
    resting (RHR), 32, 352–53
heart rate, target:
    program for, 353–56
    recovery and, 351–52
Heartscan, 32
Helicobacter pylori, 69
Helping Athletes with Eating Disorders (Thompson), 173–74
hematuria, 55
hemorrhoids, 43
Hendler, Sheldon Saul, 201, 202–3, 204
herbalism, 74–76
    uses of, 37, 75–76
heredity, 322–27
    see also illness
herpes, genital, 249–50, 251
herpes simplex 1 virus, 154
hernias, 56–57
    hiatal, 42
    inguinal, 57

Hilton Head Metabolism Diet,
   The (Miller), 170
Hine, Jean, 231
Hite, Shere, 275
HIV (human immunodefi-
   ciency virus), 29, 44,
   219, 253–55
hoarseness, 44
Hodgson, Michael, 224
holistic health, *see* alternative
   medicine
home, hazards of, 220–25
homeopathy, 76–78
homosexuals, 294–97
hormones, sex, *see* testosterone
Hot Monogamy (Love), 277
Hot Zone, The (Preston), 220
How to Heal Depression
   (Bloomfield), 97
How to Help Your Man Lose
   Weight (Sutkamp), 368
Hudson, Rock, 252
Huebner, Charlie, 363
human papilloma virus
   (HPV), 248
humor:
   sexiness and, 276
   therapy, 113–15
Hurlbert, David, 237
hypermasculine body shape,
   140
hypertension, 32, 42, 43, 46,
   49, 51, 213
   as biomarker, 301, 305
   see also heart attack, heart
   disease; stroke

ICSI (intracytoplasmic sperm
   injection), 261, 262
illness:
   body weight and, 9, 15, 16,
      20, 64
   detection of, *see* physical
      examination
   heredity and, 322–27
   infectious, 217–19
   lifestyle-related, 5, 9, 43
   mental, 10, 12, 17, 83–84,
      96–105; *see also* emo-
      tions
   prevention of, 48–53, 65

   risk factors and, 9, 28, 42,
      47–53, 149, 270,
      325–26
   of special concern to men,
      47–69, 80–82
   untreated symptoms of, 47
   warning signs of, 35–47,
      60, 61, 62–63, 149
   see also specific illnesses
impotence, 240, 255–57
   performance anxiety vs.,
      263
Inderal, 256
Indurain, Miguel, 32
infectious diseases, 217–19
insulin sensitivity, 304
intimacy, see relationships
in vitro fertilization, 261
iron, 54, 196, 202, 208
Iron John (Bly), 4

James, William, 113
Jantz, Gregory L., 172, 174
Johnson, Magic, 252
Johnson, Virginia, 264
Johnston, Richard B., 259
joints, 15, 19–20
Joseph, Bruce J., 265–66
Journal of Manipulative and
   Physiological Therapeutics,
   73
Journal of Marriage and the
   Family, 272
Joy of Sex, The (Comfort), 239,
   319–20
Jungian analysis, 109–10

Kabat-Zinn, Jon, 89, 116
Kaeser, Lisa, 248
Kaminer, Wendy, 332
Kaplan, Helen Singer, 256
Kaposi's sarcoma, 253
Keen, Sam, 256
Kegel, Arnold, 243
Kennedy, Gail, 293
Kennon, Tom, 357
keratoses, 148, 149
Kern, Marc F., 229, 230
Khalsa, Waheguru S., 215–16
kidney stones, 56
Kissinger, Henry, 137
Klein, Calvin, 133

Kleiner, Susan, 183
Klysa, Elise, 332
Kornhaber, Arthur, 127
Kosich, Daniel, 138
Kubo, Isao, 214, 215
Kuhlman, Kathryn, 125
Kurtz, Irma, 292

Lasch, Christopher, 4
Lawson, Annette, 286
Lebow, Fred, 173
Lerner, Joey, 103, 105
Lesser, Gershon M., 53
Levy, Stuart, 218
Lewis, Collins, 228, 229
libido, 256, 310, 317–20
Lieber, Charles, 228
Lieberman, Shari, 201, 202,
   204
life expectancy, 8, 35, 53, 80,
   81, 90, 301, 307
lifestyle, healthy, 178–234
   addictions and, 225–32
   eating and, 178–200; *see*
      also diet and nutrition
   sleep and, 232–34
ligaments, 19–20
limbic system, 12
lipoproteins, see cholesterol
Litt, Jerome, 153
liver disease, 227
Louganis, Greg, 115
Love, Patricia, 277–78
lovemaking, romance and,
   274–77
Love Secrets for a Lasting
   Relationship (Bloomfield),
   278
lumps, mysterious, 45
lungs, 13–14
   chest pain from, 40–42
Lyme disease, 219

McClure, R. Dale, 259
McEwen, Bruce, 10
McGann, Daniel M., 372–73
McNab, Diana, 360, 362
McPherson, Aimee Semple,
   125
Macrodantin (nitrofurantoin),
   259
McSweegan, Edward, 220

Madame Bovary (Flaubert), 286
Magic of Sex, The (Stoppard), 239
magnesium, 155, 209
Mahoney, Mike, 160, 161
Maier, Daniel, 322–23, 324
Malley, Kirk, 161–62
malpractice, medical, 27, 33–35
Mannino, David, 222
Man Talk (Kurtz), 292
March of Dimes, 260
Margolies, Eva, 256
Marks, Robin, 148
marriage:
   commitment vs., 272
   monogamy and, 274–79
Martin, John, 361
masculinity:
   archetype of, 3–4
   changing standard of, 1–2, 3–5
   new role model of, 3–4
   repressed emotions and, 3–5
massage therapy, 78–79
Masters, William, 263–64
Matarasso, Alan, 132, 138
Matarasso, Seth L., 150, 152, 153
Mathew, Ninan T., 36
matrix, 23
Mayer, Toby G., 159
meditation, 115–18
melanomas, 62–63, 147, 149
melatonin, 309–10
men:
   addictions and, 225–32
   aerobics and, 371
   aggression and, 13, 93
   anger and, 12, 92, 93–94, 95–96, 114; *see also* conflicts
   body image and, 131–77
   bonding and, 291–94
   conventional medicine and, 80–82
   domestic violence and, 282–86
   emotions and, 3–5, 6, 12, 83, 91–96, 135, 136, 137–38

grief of, 328–30
health-risk factors and, 9, 28, 42, 47–53
jealousy and, 92, 94
life expectancy of, 8, 35, 53, 80, 81, 90, 301, 307
love and, 53, 270, 276, 277; *see also* relationships
low-maintenance bodies of, 8, 25
media depiction of, 3–4
multiorgasmic, 240–44
myths and, 367–73
"new," vanity and, 6, 131–34
performance anxiety in, 262–64
and redefinition of manhood, 1–7
roles of, 1–2, 3, 4, 86–87
sense of identity and, 134–35
sex differences and, *see* sex differences
as sex objects, 139–40
sexuality of, 235, 239–69; *see also* sexuality
stages of, 13, 17, 25–26
touch and, 274–75
violence and, 282–86, 372
visual-spatial ability of, 11
Men, Women and Aggression (Campbell), 281
Men in Groups (Tiger), 293
menopause, male, 320–22
Men's Fitness, 153, 340
Men's Health Network, 20, 82
men's movement, 133, 137, 256
mental well-being, 83–130, 360
   food and, 198–200
   see also emotions
menu, 30-day high-performance, 183–94
   fast foods and, 194
   tailoring of, 195
Merchant, Kirk, 140–41
Mertz, Gregory, 250
mesomorphs, 136–37, 139
   best sports for, 139

metabolic rate, basal (BMR), 169–71
migraine headaches, 36–37, 326
Miller, Alexander, 150, 151
Miller, Mark, 283, 285
Miller, Peter M., 170
Mind as Healer, Mind as Slayer (Pelletier), 86
mind-body health, *see* alternative medicine
minerals:
   bone and, 305
   calcium, 16, 17
   chelation of, 203
   copper, 156, 202, 208
   food sources of, 155, 195–98, 207–10
   food vs. supplements of, 201–10
   iron, 54, 196, 202, 208
   magnesium, 155, 209
   ODA chart of, 207, 208–10
   zinc, 155, 156, 202, 210
   see also diet and nutrition; vitamins
minoxidil (Rogaine), 159–60, 161
Mitchell, Mark, 106
moisturizer, 22, 142, 153
monogamy, 274–79
Montgomery, Jim, 73
Mooney, W. Terrence, 89
Morison, Warwick, 146
Morse, Stephen, 219
Morton, Julia, 215
MRI (magnetic-resonance imaging), 13
muscle mass, 9, 50, 140, 181
   biomarker of, 301, 302, 303, 304, 306, 308
   weight lifting and, 302, 303, 304, 306, 307
muscles, muscular system, 15, 18–19, 20
   "emotional," 229
   fat vs., 369
   heart, 18, 19, 47
   involuntary, 18
   mass, *see* muscle mass
   PC, 243
   respiratory, 14

muscles, muscular system
  (*cont.*)
  skeletal, 18
  smooth, 18
  twitch fibers of, 302
  vaginal, 237
  voluntary, 18
  warming up of, 334–37
  weight lifting and,
    349–50; *see also* weight
    lifting
myocardial infarction, see
  heart attack, heart disease
Myth of Heterosexual AIDS,
  The (Fumento), 252

Nader, Ralph, 34
nails, 22, 23
  grooming of, 145
National Cancer Institute, 60,
  67, 68, 201
National Center for
  Homeopathy, 78
National Center for Patients'
  Rights, 34
National Headache
  Foundation, 38
National Institute for
  Occupational Safety and
  Health (NIOSH), 260
National Society of Genetic
  Counselors, 260
naturopathy, 79
Neiman, David, 111
nervous system, 9, 10, 73
neurotransmitters, 10, 36,
  104, 112
New Honest Herbal, The
  (Tyler), 75
New Male Sexuality, The
  (Zilbergeld), 367–68
New Our Bodies, Ourselves, The
  (Boston Women's Health
  Collective), 264
New York Road Runners Club
  Complete Book of Running
  (Lebow), 173, 315
nitrofurantoin (Macrodantin),
  259
Noble, Ernest P., 229
norepinephrine, 112

Novack, Brian H., 267–68
Novick, Nelson Lee, 146, 153
Now That I'm Married, Why
  Isn't Everything Perfect?
  (Page), 278
nutrition, *see* diet and nutri-
  tion

obesity gene, 164
obsessive-compulsive disorder (OCD), 100, 101–2
Ochs, Len, 120
ODA (optimal daily
  allowances), 201,
  204–10
1-RM (one resistance movement), 302
Oretic, 256
orgasms:
  aging and, 318–20
  men and, 240–44
  women and, 236–38
Orlistat, 165
Ornish, Dean, 50, 52, 116,
  179, 270
Ostroff, Stephen, 217
"Our Bodies, Ourselves?"
  (Hayward), 80–82
Outbreak (movie), 220
overtraining, 43, 173
  biomarkers and, 307
  warning signs of, 359
  weight training and, 341
overweight, *see* body weight;
  dieting

Page, Susan, 278
panic disorders, 100–1
parenting, *see* family; fatherhood, changing role of
Pasick, Robert, 372
Pauling, Linus, 201
Paulsen, Alvin, 247
PCIO 31, 158
PC muscle, 243
Pelletier, Kenneth, 86, 87, 90,
  127
penile cancer, 61
penile enlargement, 267–69
penis, 61, 235, 251
  size of, 140, 264–69,
    367–68

see also birth control, male;
    erection problems;
    orgasms
Perfect Fit, The (Eichel), 239
performance anxiety, 262–64
pericarditis, 40
peripheral nervous system, 10
Peters, Keith, 332
PET (positron-emission
    tomography) scan, 12
physical examination, 27–35
  checklist for, 29
  doctor-shopping for, 27,
    33–35
  heredity and, 326
  informed patient and, 30
  phases of, 28–31
  screening tests in, 29–31, 32
  test results of, 31–33
  see also illness
Pill, male contraceptive, 247
"pioneer spirit," 4
Pisetsky, David S., 326
pleurisy, 40–41, 43, 44
Pneumocystis carinii, 253
pneumonia, 40
pneumothorax, spontaneous,
    42
PNI (psychoneuroimmunolo-
    gy), 116
Podell, Ron, 265, 267
Pollock, Michael, 334
Pope, Harrison G., Jr., 172,
    173
Positive Addiction (Glasser),
    357
Posner, Joel, 90
post-traumatic stress disorder
    (PTSD), 100, 102
posture, 175–77
Poteet, John, 333, 334
prayer, 125–27
Preston, Richard, 220
Private Parts (Taguchi), 318
Proscar, 64
prostate, 63–65
prostate cancer, 63–68
  prevention of, 65, 326
  PSA controversy and,
    66–68
Prostate Cancer Support
    Groups Network, 66

prostate-specific antigen (PSA) test, 29, 65, 66–68
prostatitis, 63–64, 65
protein, 180–83, 199
sources of, 181, 183
Prozac, 98, 164, 174, 256
Pruett, Kyle, 4
pseudofolliculitis barbae (shaving bumps), 142
psyche, male, see emotions
Public Citizen, 34
Puig, Carlos, 159

quiz:
back-attack-risk-profile, 16
commitment, 273–74

Rapoport, Alan M., 326
razor, electric, 141, 143
RDA (recommended dietary allowance), 201–2
RDI (Reference Daily Intake), 17
Real Men Don't Bond (Feirstein), 133
Real Men Don't Eat Quiche (Feirstein), 133, 295
Real Vitamin and Mineral Book, The (Liebermann), 201
Reamy, Kenneth, 236
Reed, Harold M., 268
Reich, Wilhelm, 73
Relationship Events Scale (RES), 272–73
relationships, 270–99
barriers to intimacy in, 270
commitment and, 271–74
grief and, 329
health and, 270
relaxation response, 38, 52, 112, 118, 122, 126, 136
reproductive system, 24–25
resources, 78, 105, 175, 202, 212, 247
cancer and, 60, 66
malpractice and, 34
medical history, 324
pain and, 38, 72
relaxation and, 118, 121
of physically challenged, 364–66

sexuality and, 244, 260
respiratory system, 13–14
Retin-A, 151
rhythm method, 246
Richling, John, 348–50
Rigel, Darrell, 149
Rippe, James, 360, 362
risk factors, health, 9, 28, 42, 47–53, 149, 270
predisposition and, 325–26
Ritalin (methylphenidate), 104
Roberts, Oral, 125
Roehrs, Timothy, 234
Rogaine (minoxidil), 159–60, 161
romance, rekindled, 274–75
anticipation and, 275–76
boredom and, 274, 275
difficult times and, 277
nongoal-oriented, 275–76
spousal dating and, 276–77
touching and, 274–75
rosacea, 154
Rosen, Don, 87
Rosenberg, Irwin, 301, 302, 304, 305, 306
Rosenbloom, Chris, 181
Rosenfeld, Isadore, 39
Ross, Jon, 363
Rothman, Cappy, 246–47, 258, 259, 260–61, 367, 370
"rugged individualism," 4
Ryan, Edward J., 70

SAD (seasonal affective disorder), 43, 97
Samitier, Ricardo, 268
Santorelli, Saki, 91
Savin-Williams, Ritch, 292, 293–94
saw palmetto, 76
Schardt, David, 179
Scheman, Andrew, 153
Schneider, Max A., 228
Schrader, Steven, 260
Schwarzenegger, Arnold, 137, 138, 139, 172, 316
seborrheic dermatitis, 153
Second to None (Garfield), 357
Secrets Men Keep, The (Druck), 293

"Secrets of Making Love to the Same Person Forever," 266
Seinfeld, Jerry, 122, 258, 290
self-healing, 36, 86, 113–30, 226
self-tests:
back attack risk-profile, 16
hostility, 95–96
testicular cancer, 60
sensuality, 274–77
serotonin, 36, 112, 115, 199, 227
selective reuptake inhibitors (SSRI) of, 98
sex differences, 8–9, 14, 35, 49
aging and, 25–26
body fat and, 369
brain and, 10–13
emotions and, 11–12
foreplay and, 22
handling conflicts and, 281–82
health care and, 80–82
joint disease and, 20
life expectancy and, 8, 35, 53, 80, 81, 90, 301, 307
"male-ideal" and, 139–40
menopause as, 320–22
sexuality and, see sexuality
sex hormone, male, see testosterone
sexual desire, hypoactive, 256
Sexual Desire Disorders (Kaplan), 256
sexuality:
adultery and, 286–89
aging and, 317–20
AIDS and, 30, 219, 252–55
birth control and, 246–48, 261–62, 322
CAT and, 239–40
cerebral sex and, 244–46
fantasies and, 244–46, 279
fertility and, 261–62
gay men and, 294–97
impotence and, 255–58
libido, 256, 310, 317–20
multiple orgasms and, 240–44

sexuality (*cont.*)
  penile enlargement and,
    267–69
  penis size and, 140, 264–67
  performance anxiety and,
    262–64
  romance and, 274–77
  sperm and, 258–61
  STD and, 248–55
  testicles and, 370
  women and, 235–39
Sexual Selection (Batten), 271
shaving, 140–43
  bumps (pseudofolliculitis
    barbae), 142
  skin type and, 142
  thick beard and, 142
Sheehy, Gail, 320
Sheppard, Risa, 177
Sherman, Richard, 119, 120
Shope, Robert E., 220
Sibutramine, 164
sigmoidoscope, 29
Sime, Wes, 119
sinus headaches, 37–38
skeletal system, 15–17
skin, 21–22, 61–63, 131, 147
  aging and, 312–13
  common problems of,
    149–54
  dry, 142, 153
  shaving and, 142
  touch and, 274–75
skin cancer, 62, 147–49
  melanomas, 62–63
  risk factors for, 149, 326
  sun exposure and, 145–49
Skinner, Elia C., 67–68
Skopp, Martin, 333
sleep disorders, 232–34
  melatonin and, 310
Smart Exercise (Bailey), 166,
    168
Smith, Dan, 89–90
smoking, 38, 43, 48, 50, 69,
    155–56, 226, 230–32,
    259
social phobia, 100, 101
Solzhenitsyn, Alexander, 130
Somers, Virend, 233
Sound Mind, Sound Body
    (Pelletier), 86, 90

sperm, 258–61
  pesticide and, 260
  production of, 247
spinal cord, 10
spontaneous pneumothorax,
    42
Stand By Me, 294
Starrett, Barbara, 255
STD (sexually transmitted dis-
    eases), 248–55
Stern, Robert, 151
stimulants, 200, 210, 216
Stoney, Catherine, 180
stool, bloody, 43
Stoppard, Miriam, 239
strength, biomarker of, 302,
    306, 307, 308
strength-building exercises,
    see weight lifting
stress, 24, 36, 38, 42, 49, 50,
    52, 64, 69, 83, 227
  de-, 88, 91, 112
  exercise and, 359–60
  friendships and, 270
  post-traumatic (PTSD),
    100, 102
  reaction-response of,
    84–86
  -related disorders, 85–86
  self-healing of, 113–30
  sources of, 86–91
  sperm count and, 258
stretching, 334–37
stroke, 32, 33, 48, 71, 227
  movement and, 18
Strollo, Patrick, 234
sugar, 199–200
sunscreen, 146–48
supplements:
  DHEA (dehydroepiandros-
    terone), 310
  melatonin, 309–10
  mineral, *see* minerals
  vitamin, *see* vitamins
Sutkamp, Jerry C., 169–70,
    368, 369
SUZI (subzonal
    Insemination), 261–62
Swann, William B., Jr.,
    98–99
sweating, heavy, 44
Symptoms (Rosenfeld), 39

synaptic cleft, 10
synovial fluid, 19
syphilis, 248, 249, 250
Szpindor-Watson, Anne, 223,
    224–25

Taguchi, Yosh, 318
Tamura, Scott, 145
Tannen, Deborah, 281–82
Tavris, Carol, 279
tea, 200, 210, 214–16
teeth, 23–24
  grooming of, 144–45
temperature, body, as bio-
    marker, 306
tendinitis, 20
Tenover, Joyce, 321–22
tension headaches, 36
Terminator, 3
testicles, 370
testicular cancer, 25, 30,
    59–60
  self-exam for, 60
testosterone, 10, 13, 85, 229,
    258, 309, 318, 320–22
  baldness and, 157–58
  -enanthate (TE) injections,
    247
  impotence and, 257
Thau, Rosemarie, 247
therapy, 98, 104, 105–11
  action, short-term, 105–11
  alternative-medicine, 38,
    70–80
  self-healing, 86, 113–30,
    226
Thin for Life (Fletcher),
    163–64
Tiger, Lionel, 293
30-day high performance
    menu, 183–95
Thomas, Paul, 201
Thompson, Catherine, 328,
    329
Thompson, Jacqueline, 301
Thompson, Ron A., 173–74
thrombocytopenic purpura, 44
Tricomin, 158
touching, 274–75
  erotic, 275
Trusting Heart, The
    (Williams), 95–96

Tollefson, Mark, 137
20-minute workout, for
    weight lifting, 348–50
Tyler, Varro E., 75, 213
Type-A behavior, 54, 69, 83,
    126, 213

ulcers, 69
Ullman, Dana, 77
ultra fast CT (computerized
    tomography) scanner, 32
Undressing the American Male
    (Margolies), 256
Updike, John, 8, 131, 235,
    300
ureters, 25
urethra, 24, 54
urinary tract, 24–25
    problems of, 46, 55–56
U.S. News & World Report, 8

valerian, 76
vanity, 6, 131–34
    see also grooming
Vanity Fair, 320
varicoceles, 57–59
vas deferens, 24–25, 247
vasectomy, 246–47
Vash, Peter, 169, 170, 171
vegetables, health and, 155,
    195–98, 204–10
venereal disease, 248
villi, 21
visualization, 124–25, 227
    exercise and, 360–62
vitamins, 195–98
    A, 155, 179, 203–4
    B, 44, 154, 155, 156, 205
    beta-carotene, 156, 203–4,
        231
    biotin, 156, 207
    C, 44, 155, 202, 203, 206,
        231
    D, 17, 179, 202, 206
    E, 65, 155–56, 179, 203,
        206, 231

fat-soluble, 179
folic acid, 44, 155, 203,
    208
food sources of, 155,
    195–98, 204–7, 208,
    209
food vs. supplements of,
    201–10
K, 206
ODA chart of, 204–7, 208,
    209
skin problems and defi-
    ciency of, 154–56
see also diet and nutrition;
    minerals
Voight, Karen, 371
volunteerism, 52–53

Wacker, Frans, 49
Walden (Thoreau), 84
Walker, Philip, 167
walking, 334
Wallace, Margaret, 323
warning signs and symptoms
    of disease, 35–47, 60,
    61, 62–63, 149
warts, genital, 248, 249,
    250–51
Wear, Pamela, 324
Weary, Peyton, 147
weight, body, *see* body
    weight
weight lifting, 17, 19, 21, 50,
    182
    aging and, 316–17
    anti-aging and, 302, 303,
        304, 306–7
    basics of, 340–42
    cracked tooth syndrome
        and, 24
    gym equipment and,
        344–47
    routine of, 342–48
    strength-building and, 302,
        303, 304, 306–7
    terminology of, 337–40

20-minute workout and,
    348–50
weight loss, sudden, 45
Wellbutrin, 98
Wetcher, Kenneth, 12, 93,
    94, 95
*What to Do When He Has a
    Headache* (Wolfe), 256
When Harry Met Sally, 290,
    291
White, Arthur H., 175–76
Whitehead, E. Douglas, 268,
    269
Whitman, Walt, 19
*Why Men Are the Way They
    Are* (Farrell), 133
Williams, Redford, 95–96
Wilmore, Jack, 168
Wirth, James B., 171–72
Wolf, Steve, 120–21
Wolfe, Janet L., 256
women, 8–9, 22, 25
    cognition and, 11
    emotions and, 11–12
    "male-ideal" and, 139–40
    orgasm and, 236–38
    relationships and, 270
    roles of, 1–2, 3
    sexual anatomy of, 238–39
    sexuality and, 235–38
    touch and, 274–75
    see also sex differences
wrinkles, 22, 131, 147,
    155–56

Yanovski, Susan Z., 163, 164
yoga, 117–18, 121–22
yohimbe, 76
You Just Don't Understand
    (Tannen), 281

Ziccardi, Donald, 133
Zilbergeld, Bernie, 237, 367
zinc, 155, 156, 202, 210
Zoloft, 256
Zovirax (acyclovir), 250

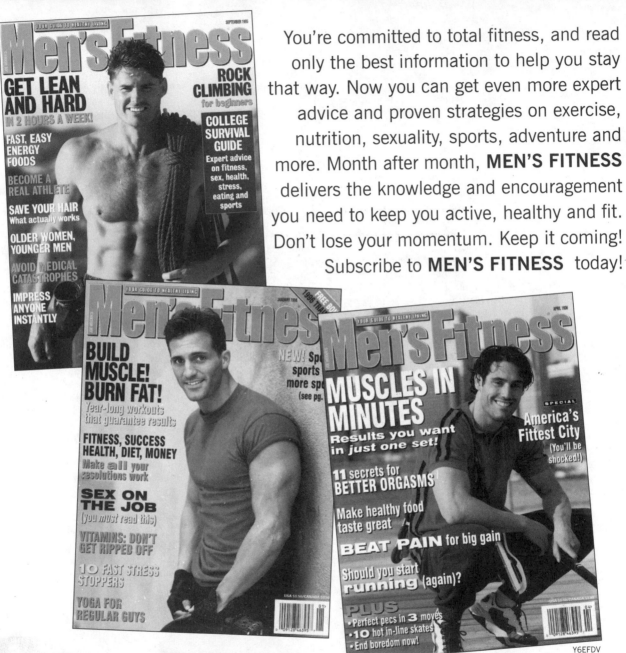